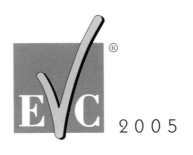

EVC® 2005

UNEXPECTED CHALLENGES IN VASCULAR SURGERY

© 2005 by Blackwell Publishing
Blackwell Futura is an imprint of Blackwell Publishing

Blackwell Publishing, Inc., 350 Main Street, Malden, Massachusetts 02148-5020, USA
Blackwell Publishing Ltd, 9600 Garsington Road, Oxford OX4 2DQ, UK
Blackwell Science Asia Pty Ltd, 550 Swanston Street, Carlton, Victoria 3053, Australia

First published 2005

ISBN-13: 978-1-4051-34705
ISBN-10: 1-4051-3470-4

Unexpected challenges in vascular surgery / edited by Alain Branchereau, Michael Jacobs.
      p. ; cm.
  ISBN 1-4051-3470-4
  1. Blood-vessels--Surgery. 2. Blood-vessels--Surgery--Complications.
  [DNLM: 1. Vascular Surgical Procedures--adverse effects. 2. Perioperative Care. 3. Postoperative Complications--prevention & control.] I. Branchereau, Alain. II. Jacobs, Michael, MD.

  RD598.5.U59 2005
  617.4'1301--dc22

                        2005000402

A catalogue record for this title is available from the British Library

Acquisitions: Gina Almond
Production: Julie Elliott
Set in France by Odim

For further information on Blackwell Publishing, visit our website:
www.blackwellcardiology.com

The publisher's policy is to use permanent paper from mills that operate a sustainable forestry policy, and which has been manufactured from pulp processed using acid-free and elementary chlorine-free practices. Furthermore, the publisher ensures that the text paper and cover board used have met acceptable environmental accreditation standards.

Notice: The indications and dosages of all drugs in this book have been recommended in the medical literature and conform to the practices of the general community. The medications described do not necessarily have specific approval by the Food and Drug Administration for use in the diseases and dosages for which they are recommended. The package insert for each drug should be consulted for use and dosage as approved by the FDA. Because standards for usage change, it is advisable to keep abreast of revised recommendations, particularly those concerning new drugs.

UNEXPECTED CHALLENGES IN VASCULAR SURGERY

Edited by

ALAIN BRANCHEREAU, MD
University Hospital, Marseille, France

&

MICHAEL JACOBS, MD
University Hospital, Maastricht, The Netherlands

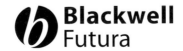

LIST OF CONTRIBUTORS

Jérôme ALBERTIN
Service de Chirurgie Vasculaire et Thoracique
Hôpital Arnaud de Villeneuve
371, avenue du Doyen Gaston Giraud
34295 Montpellier Cedex 5, France

Eric ALLAIRE
Départment de Chirurgie Vasculaire
Hôpital Henri Mondor, Université Paris XII
94000 Créteil, France

Jens-Rainer ALLENBERG
Abteilung für Gefässchirurgie
Ruprecht-Karls-Universität Heidelberg
Kirschnerstrasse 1
69120 Heidelberg, Germany

Pierre ALRIC
Service de Chirurgie Vasculaire et Thoracique
Hôpital Arnaud de Villeneuve
371, avenue du Doyen Gaston Giraud
34295 Montpellier Cedex 5, France

Bernadette AULIVOLA
Chirurgia Vascolare, Università di Bologna
Policlinico S. Orsola, Via Massarenti 9
40138 Bologna, Italy

Ali BADRA
Service de Chirurgie Vasculaire
Hôpital de la Cavale Blanche
Centre Hospitalier Universitaire de Brest
Boulevard Tanguy-Prigent
29609 BREST Cedex, France

Jean-Pierre BECQUEMIN
Départment de Chirurgie Vasculaire
Hôpital Henri Mondor, Université Paris XII
94000 Créteil, France

Jean-Philippe BERTHET
Service de Chirurgie Vasculaire et Thoracique
Hôpital Arnaud de Villeneuve
371, avenue du Doyen Gaston Giraud
34295 Montpellier Cedex 5, France

Luca BERTOGLIO
Divisione di Chirurgia Vascolare
Università "Vita-Salute"
Scientific Institute H. San Raffaele
20132 Milan, Italy

Dittmar BOECKLER
Abteilung für Gefässchirurgie
Ruprecht-Karls-Universität Heidelberg
Kirschnerstrasse 1
69120 Heidelberg, Germany

Pierre BONNET
Service d'Anatomie Humaine, Université de Liège
Service d'Urologie, Centre Hospitalier Universitaire
B 35, Sart Tilman
4000 Liège, Belgium

Alain BRANCHEREAU
Faculté de Médecine de Marseille
Université de la Méditerranée
Assistance Publique Hôpitaux de Marseille
Hôpital La Timone, Service de Chirurgie Vasculaire
13385 Marseille Cedex 05, France

Pascal BRANCHEREAU
Service de Chirurgie Vasculaire et Thoracique
Hôpital Arnaud de Villeneuve
371, avenue du Doyen Gaston Giraud
34295 Montpellier Cedex 5, France

Chiara BRIOSCHI
Divisione di Chirurgia Vascolare
Università "Vita-Salute"
Scientific Institute H. San Raffaele
20132 Milan, Italy

Marcus BROOKS
St Mary's Hospital
Hammersmith 66, Harley Street
London W1N 1AE, United Kingdom

Jaap BUTH
Department of Vascular Surgery
Catharina Hospital, PO Box 1350
5602 ZA Eindhoven, The Netherlands

Fabio Massimo CALLIARI
Divisione di Chirurgia Vascolare
Università "Vita-Salute"
Scientific Institute H. San Raffaele
20132 Milan, Italy

Piergiorgio CAO
S.C. di Chirurgia Vascolare
Azienda Ospedaliera di Perugia, Via Brunamonti
06122 Perugia, Italy

Roberto CHIESA
Divisione di Chirurgia Vascolare
Università "Vita-Salute"
Scientific Institute H. San Raffaele
20132 Milan, Italy

Efrem CIVILINI
Divisione di Chirurgia Vascolare
Università "Vita-Salute"
Scientific Institute H. San Raffaele
20132 Milan, Italy

Albert CLARÁ
Servício de Cirugía Vascular
Hospital del Mar, Paseo Maritimo 25-29
08003 Barcelona, Spain

Marc COGGIA
Service de Chirurgie Vasculaire
Hôpital Universitaire Ambroise Paré et
Faculté de Médecine Paris-Ile de France Ouest
92100 Boulogne-Billancourt, France

Valérie COPPIN
Department of Vascular Surgery
University Hospital of Gasthuisberg, Heerenstraat 49
3000 Leuven, Belgium

Kim DAENENS
Department of Vascular Surgery
University Hospital of Gasthuisberg, Heerenstraat 49
3000 Leuven, Belgium

Michiel DE HAAN
Department of Radiology
University Hospital Maastricht, PO Box 5800
6202 AZ Maastricht, The Netherlands

Paola DE RANGO
S.C. di Chirurgia Vascolare
Azienda Ospedaliera di Perugia, Via Brunamonti
06122 Perugia, Italy

Luca DEL GUERCIO
Divisione di Chirurgia Vascolare
Università "Vita-Salute"
Scientific Institute H. San Raffaele
20132 Milan, Italy

Pascal DESGRANGES
Départment de Chirurgie Vasculaire
Hôpital Henri Mondor, Université Paris XII
94000 Créteil, France

Isabelle DI CENTA
Service de Chirurgie Vasculaire
Hôpital Universitaire Ambroise Paré et
Faculté de Médecine Paris-Ile de France Ouest
92100 Boulogne-Billancourt, France

Gabriele DUBINI
LaBS - Laboratory of Biological Structure Mechanics
Department of Structural Engineering
Politecnico di Milano
20132 Milan, Italy

Markus ENZLER
Klinik Hirslanden
Witellikerstrasse 40
8029 Zurich, Switzerland

Jean-Noël FABIANI
Département de Chirurgie Cardio-Vasculaire
Hôpital Européen Georges Pompidou
20, rue Leblanc
75015 Paris, France

Gian Luca FAGGIOLI
Chirurgia Vascolare, Università di Bologna
Policlinico S. Orsola, Via Massarenti 9
40138 Bologna, Italy

Inge FOURNEAU
Department of Vascular Surgery
University Hospital of Gasthuisberg, Heerenstraat 49
3000 Leuven, Belgium

Andreu GARCÍA-LEÓN
Servício de Cirugía Vascular
Hospital del Mar, Paseo Maritimo 25-29
08003 Barcelona, Spain

Mauro GARGIULO
Chirurgia Vascolare, Università di Bologna
Policlinico S. Orsola, Via Massarenti 9
40138 Bologna, Italy

Olivier GOËAU-BRISSONNIÈRE
Service de Chirurgie Vasculaire
Hôpital Universitaire Ambroise Paré et
Faculté de Médecine Paris-Ile de France Ouest
92100 Boulogne-Billancourt, France

Pierre GOUNY
Service de Chirurgie Vasculaire
Hôpital de la Cavale Blanche
Centre Hospitalier Universitaire de Brest
Boulevard Tanguy-Prigent
29609 BREST Cedex, France

Roy GREENBERG
Departments of Vascular Surgery
and Biomedical Engineering
Desk S-40, 9500 Euclid Ave
Cleveland, Ohio 44195, USA

Gildas GUERET
Département d'Anesthésie-Réanimation
Hôpital de la Cavale Blanche
Centre Hospitalier Universitaire de Brest
Boulevard Tanguy-Prigent
29609 BREST Cedex, France

George HAMILTON
University Department of Surgery
Royal Free Hampstead NHS Trust
Pond Street, Hampstead
London NW3 2QG, United Kingdom

Krassi IVANCEV
Endovascular Center
Malmö University Hospital
SE 205 02 Malmö, Sweden

Michael JACOBS
Department of Vascular Surgery
University Hospital Maastricht, PO Box 5800
6202 AZ Maastricht, The Netherlands

Isabelle JAVERLIAT
Service de Chirurgie Vasculaire
Hôpital Universitaire Ambroise Paré et
Faculté de Médecine Paris-Ile de France Ouest
92100 Boulogne-Billancourt, France

Pierre JULIA
Département de Chirurgie Cardio-Vasculaire
Hôpital Européen Georges Pompidou
20, rue Leblanc
75015 Paris, France

Jur KIEVIT
Department of Vascular Surgery
Catharina Hospital, PO Box 1350
5602 ZA Eindhoven, The Netherlands

Hisham KOBEITER
Départment de Chirurgie Vasculaire
Hôpital Henri Mondor, Université Paris XII
94000 Créteil, France

Riitta LASSILA
Department of Hematology
Division of Coagulation Disorders
Helsinki University Central Hospital
PO Box 340 - Haartmaninkatu 4
00029 Hus, Finland

Christian LATRÉMOUILLE
Département de Chirurgie Cardio-Vasculaire
Hôpital Européen Georges Pompidou
20, rue Leblanc
75015 Paris, France

Mauri LEPÄNTALO
Department of Vascular Surgery
Helsinki University Central Hospital
PO Box 340 - Haartmaninkatu 4
00029 Hus, Finland

Lina LEURS
Department of Vascular Surgery
Catharina Hospital, PO Box 1350
5602 ZA Eindhoven, The Netherlands

Christopher D LEVILLE
Departments of Vascular Surgery
and Biomedical Engineering
Desk S-40, 9500 Euclid Ave
Cleveland, Ohio 44195, USA

Raymond LIMET
Service de Chirurgie Cardio-Vasculaire et
Thoracique, Centre Hospitalier Universitaire
B35, Sart Tilman
4000 Liège, Belgium

Martin MALINA
Department of Vascular Surgery
Malmö University Hospital
SE 205 02 Malmö, Sweden

Enrico MARIA MARONE
Divisione di Chirurgia Vascolare
Università "Vita-Salute"
Scientific Institute H. San Raffaele
20132 Milan, Italy

Charles MARTY-ANE
Service de Chirurgie Vasculaire et Thoracique
Hôpital Arnaud de Villeneuve
371, avenue du Doyen Gaston Giraud
34295 Montpellier Cedex 5, France

Agostino MASELLI
Istituto di Radiologia, Sezione Angiografia
Azienda Ospedaliera di Perugia, Via Brunamonti
06122 Perugia, Italy

Germano MELISSANO
Divisione di Chirurgia Vascolare
Università "Vita-Salute"
Scientific Institute H. San Raffaele
20132 Milan, Italy

Volker MICKLEY
Abteilung für Gefässchirurgie
Stadtklinik Baden-Baden, Balger Strasse 50
D-76532 Baden-Baden, Germany

Xavier MONTAÑÁ
Instituto Cardiovascular, Hospital Clínic
Universidad de Barcelona, Villarroel 170
08036 Barcelona, Spain

André NEVELSTEEN
Department of Vascular Surgery
University Hospital of Gasthuisberg, Heerenstraat 49
3000 Leuven, Belgium

Michel NONENT
Service de Radiologie
Hôpital de la Cavale Blanche
Centre Hospitalier Universitaire de Brest
Boulevard Tanguy-Prigent
29609 BREST Cedex, France

Lucia NORGIOLINI
S.C. di Chirurgia Vascolare
Azienda Ospedaliera di Perugia, Via Brunamonti
06122 Perugia, Italy

Soundrie PADAYACHEE
Department of Ultrasonic Angiology
Guy's & St. Thomas' Hospital, Lambeth Palace Road
London SE1 9RT, United Kingdom

Clarismundo PONTES
Instituto Cardiovascular, Hospital Clínic
Universidad de Barcelona, Villarroel 170
08036 Barcelona, Spain

Jan A RAUWERDA
VU University Medical Center
Department of Surgery
De Boelelaan 1117, P.O. Box 7057
1007 MB Amsterdam, The Netherlands

Vincent RIAMBAU
Instituto Cardiovascular, Hospital Clínic
Universidad de Barcelona, Villarroel 170
08036 Barcelona, Spain

Begoña ROMÁN
Faculdad de Filosofía
Universitat Ramon Llull, Calle Claravall 1-3
08022 Barcelona, Spain

Lydia ROMANO
S.C. di Chirurgia Vascolare
Azienda Ospedaliera di Perugia, Via Brunamonti
06122 Perugia, Italy

Gabrielle SARLON
Faculté de Médecine de Marseille
Université de la Méditerranée
Assistance Publique Hôpitaux de Marseille
Hôpital La Timone, Service de Chirurgie Vasculaire
13385 Marseille Cedex 05, France

Hardy SCHUMACHER
Abteilung für Gefässchirurgie
Ruprecht-Karls-Universität Heidelberg
Kirschnerstrasse 1
69120 Heidelberg, Germany

Geert Willem SCHURINK
Department of Vascular Surgery
University Hospital Maastricht, PO Box 5800
6202 AZ Maastricht, The Netherlands

Francesco SETACCI
Divisione di Chirurgia Vascolare
Università "Vita-Salute"
Scientific Institute H. San Raffaele
20132 Milan, Italy

Björn SONESSON
Department of Vascular Surgery
Malmö University Hospital
SE 205 02 Malmö, Sweden

Andrea STELLA
Chirurgia Vascolare, Università di Bologna
Policlinico S. Orsola, Via Massarenti 9
40138 Bologna, Italy

Guido STULTIËNS
Department of Vascular Surgery
Catharina Hospital, PO Box 1350
5602 ZA Eindhoven, The Netherlands

Jesper SWEDENBORG
Department of Vascular Surgery
Karolinska University Hospital
17176 Stockholm, Sweden

Peter TAYLOR
Department of Vascular Surgery
Guy's & St. Thomas' Hospital, Lambeth Palace Road
London SE1 9RT, United Kingdom

Yamume TSHOMBA
Divisione di Chirurgia Vascolare
Università "Vita-Salute"
Scientific Institute H. San Raffaele
20132 Milan, Italy

Nicolas VALERIO
Faculté de Médecine de Marseille
Université de la Méditerranée
Assistance Publique Hôpitaux de Marseille
Hôpital La Timone, Service de Chirurgie Vasculaire
13385 Marseille Cedex 05, France

Reuben VEERAPEN
Service de Chirurgie Vasculaire et Thoracique
Hôpital Arnaud de Villeneuve
371, avenue du Doyen Gaston Giraud
34295 Montpellier Cedex 5, France

Antoine VERHAEGHE
Service de Radiologie
Hôpital de la Cavale Blanche
Centre Hospitalier Universitaire de Brest
Boulevard Tanguy-Prigent
29609 BREST Cedex, France

Fabio VERZINI
S.C. di Chirurgia Vascolare
Azienda Ospedaliera di Perugia, Via Brunamonti
06122 Perugia, Italy

Francesc VIDAL-BARRAQUER
Servício de Cirugía Vascular
Hospital del Mar, Paseo Maritimo 25-29
08003 Barcelona, Spain

Sailaritta VUORISALO
Department of Vascular Surgery
Helsinki University Central Hospital
PO Box 340 - Haartmaninkatu 4
00029 Hus, Finland

Willem WISSELINK
VU University Medical Center
Department of Surgery
De Boelelaan 1117, P.O. Box 7057
1007 MB Amsterdam, The Netherlands

John WOLFE
St Mary's Hospital
Hammersmith 66, Harley Street
London W1N 1AE, United Kingdom

August YSA
Servício de Cirugía Vascular
Hospital de Cruces, Plaza de Cruces s/n
48903 Baracaldo (Vizcaya), Spain

PREFACE

In ancient medicine, men of all cultures and civilizations faced the problems of hemorrhage and the first attempts to control a bleeding vessel actually represent the beginning of vascular surgery. During the last decades, vascular surgery has evolved to a mature specialization and, despite impressive innovation and technical developments, the modern vascular surgeon still meets challenges during and after vascular and endovascular procedures. These challenges are often unforeseen and unexpected and the spectrum ranges from small problems to catastrophes. It is the duty and the responsibility of the vascular and endovascular surgeon to recognize and subsequently to solve these complications in an adequate and efficient manner.

The subject of this year's European Vascular Course is "Unexpected challenges in vascular surgery" and twenty-six chapters describe the wide range of problems arising in daily vascular and endovascular practice. Displacement and migration of stents and endografts, dissection and rupture, unintentional occlusion of visceral arteries and aortic neck problems are all potential complications encountered in endovascular repair. In open surgery, unexpected anatomy, difficult clamping, perforation, calcified arteries, ureteral lesions and mycotic aneurysms can cause serious dilemmas which require prompt solutions. In addition to this, endovascular and surgical treatment of carotid and peripheral arterial disease comprises significant hurdles which necessitate immediate diagnosis and treatment.

We greatly appreciate the contribution of all authors and the editorial assistance of Nicolas Valerio and Dirk Ubbink, as well as the Blackwell Publishing team including Vicki Donald and Gina Almond. We are indebted to our course manager Iris Papawasiliou and our secretaries Annie Barral and Claire Meertens. Marie-France Damia and the ODIM team are highly acknowledged for their superb work and printing of this textbook.

The support of the medical and biomedical industry is crucial for the accomplishment of this book and we are grateful to our major sponsors for their continued contribution.

XI

Marseille - Maastricht, 2005

Alain Branchereau   -   Michael Jacobs

CONTENTS

XIV

1

LUCK, COMMON SENSE OR A SYSTEMATIC APPROACH: WHAT IS BEHIND THE SUCCESSFUL MANAGEMENT OF UNEXPECTED CHALLENGES IN VASCULAR SURGERY?

ALBERT CLARÁ, AUGUST YSA, ANDREU GARCIA-LEÓN
BEGOÑA ROMÁN, FRANCESC VIDAL-BARRAQUER

Professions are social constructs that survive insofar as they bring value to the communities they serve: otherwise they tend to disappear. Beyond the human sphere of our profession, it is certainly the need to decide about health and disease under conditions of uncertainty and the subsequent assumption of responsibility in our actions that pragmatically make our profession socially necessary. In the extreme edge of this proposition, unexpected surgical challenges (USCs) appear as one of those scenarios where this social need becomes more evident.

The best of our wisdom and skill is always expected every time USCs appear. Surprisingly, however, little attention has been paid to these problems over the last several years in scientific meetings, surgical journals and specialized books. Surgeons' strategy to prevent and manage USCs does not seem to be an issue openly discussed within the profession. Some of the most successful managed challenges may become widely reported. However, this is not often the case for many other scenarios. In particular, the knowledge from errors and failed approaches may be little-known beyond a small group of surgeons or may fade into oblivion.

In this chapter, the authors will provide a second-order approach, more reasonable than rational, to the problem of USCs in vascular surgery. It will begin by framing the concept of USC and disclosing its intriguing nature. Next, the decision-making process of 150 vascular surgeons surveyed facing 8 USCs will be analyzed. To conclude, the strengths and limitations of their background approach will be discussed from the perspective of the strategy of other non-medical organizations which have to deal frequently with the unexpected (aircraft carriers, nuclear power stations, etc.).

The nature of unexpected surgical challenges

Our common second-order knowledge about USCs can be easily summarized in two simple ideas. First, USCs are usually infrequent but also unsuspected intraoperative problems in which the surgeon is involved in a challenging decision and/or action. Second, the expertise of the surgeon is usually a determining feature of their successful prevention and management.

Beyond this brief description, little more can be said in general to define USCs. They are currently one of the least reported and openly discussed issues within scientific meetings, surgical journals and specialized books. Some determining factors may lie behind such obscurity and their careful appraisal may help to better understand the nature of USCs.

THE INCIDENCE OF USCs

The great knowledge acquired over the last decades in standard vascular surgery has probably resulted in a lower incidence of USCs during procedures and, consequently, in professionals' decreasing interest in the remaining very occasional problems (for which practical consequences are often difficult to ascertain). However, in this apparent loss of interest, the dynamic nature of USCs does not appear to have been taken in consideration. Currently, a leaking anastomosis is not usually seen as challenging, even for residents. However, this may not be the case, even for experienced surgeons, if the deployment device of an endograft cannot be removed from the patient. New available technologies (such as endovascular and minimally invasive surgery) result inevitably in new USCs. As these procedures evolve and become widely used, surgeons will have to deal with new USCs. Furthermore, as many procedures become partly replaced, an increasing group of surgeons, especially the younger generation, will become more vulnerable to those USCs associated with older

viable techniques which are performed infrequently. Thus, there appears to be no justification for diminishing the interest in USCs on the basis of their incidence.

SUBJECTIVITY OF THE TERMS "UNEXPECTED" AND "CHALLENGING"

Aortic rupture during cross-clamping is both unexpected and challenging for (almost) every vascular surgeon and represents a good example of an USC. However, the interpretation of what is an unexpected appearance or challenging management is partly determined by the characteristics of the surgeon. The factors which influence a surgeon in the appraisal of a surgical problem as an USC are not unexpected and include: age, number and complexity of surgical procedures performed, skill, mindfulness, and decision-making ability. Often all these characteristics are gathered together under the term *expertise* (defined as skillfulness by virtue of possessing special knowledge). However, this term is sometimes inexact and does not allow for an evaluation of the relative significance of each of its components. For example, operating on a patient with an embolic acute limb ischemia without embolectomy catheters may be both unexpected and challenging for any surgeon younger than 60 years old. However, this may not be the case for our most senior colleagues who, regardless of their professional experience, skill and mindfulness, may remember scenarios like this from their early years in practice. However, although the appraisal of a surgical problem as an USC may depend partly in the characteristics of the surgeon, there would be easy to find a common and tacit opinion about what surgical scenarios can be considered as USCs for the majority of surgeons with average experience.

SOME USCs MAY APPEAR BY ACTION OR OMISSION OF THE SURGEON

In hindsight, many USCs could have been foreseen. This is common knowledge for surgeons. However, little is done to disclose this wisdom within the community of surgeons. Without doubt, ethical and legal responsibilities and, especially, the current *success* culture in which we operate prevent many opportunities to improve our wisdom and skill for managing such problems. Very few surgeons can afford the presentation of bad results or surgical complications directly related to their work without raising doubts about their reputation. The current scenario in which a great number of USCs reported in meetings or surgical journals consist of heroical managed problems whose origin lies more on the patient than on the surgeon is not only of little instructive value but is also far removed from the reality of most USCs.

USCs May not be Evaluated Properly by our Current Methodological Tools

The mathematical models in which the most frequently used statistical tests are based cannot explain adequately situations which are: very occasional in appearance; complex in nature; or qualitatively flawed. It is not just a question of time and the accumulation of data. It is true that certain parts of reality can be explained by regression models, but many other phenomena show graphical displays with obstinately bad behavior: for example, with regions where multiple correlations between x- and y-values can be obtained [1]. Planets may travel according to Newtonian predictions but, winds may result in hurricanes, a properly placed clamp may rupture the artery, and our opinion about a patient can change depending on the day. Discontinuity is both the norm and the exception in the real world. It is unclear to where our present methodology will evolve, but it is clear that our current statistical tools provide only rough approximations in answer to simple questions.

Knowledge about USCs is Essentially Tacit

Without doubt, every vascular surgeon knows about USCs more than they will reveal. The importance of this tacit knowledge was established by the scientist and philosopher Michael Polanyi. Central to Polanyi's thinking was the belief that creative acts are charged with strong personal feelings and commitments. Arguing against the then dominant position that science was value-free, Polanyi sought to bring into being a creative tension between reasoned and critical interrogation with other more tacit forms of knowledge [2]. Tacit knowledge is the knowledge that we have without realizing it. An

example of tacit knowledge is knowing how to do something without being able to explain it adequately. Tacit knowledge is difficult to make explicit because it depends largely on deliberations, subjective insight, intuition and action-based skills that surgeons acquire by virtue of their experience, reasoning ability, and mindfulness. Capturing tacit knowledge may be undertaken only by reasonable rather than rational approaches. With this purpose, among others, in mind, the *Vascupractice* study was designed.

The Vascupractise study

The *Vascupractice* study is a questionnaire survey on vascular surgeons from Spanish vascular departments designed to evaluate what is behind their therapeutic choices in the resolution of USCs.

Participants and Methods

Development of the Vascupractice questionnaire. A structured questionnaire with open answers, entitled *Vascupractice*, was designed specifically for this study. It was developed and revised on the basis of several discussions among four vascular surgeons and two general surgeons. The final survey consisted of eight USCs (see cases in Results Section) and ten items covering personal and professional variables.

All USCs were adapted from real cases to place the participating surgeons before a problem which could occur in practice. They varied in degree with respect to the following factors:

1 - unexpected appearance,
2 - advisable time to decide and act,
3 - number of therapeutic options,
4 - conventional nature of therapeutic options,
5 - technical demands of the procedure,
6 - surgeon's involvement in their origin,
7 - opportunity to adopt a conservative attitude,
8 - immediate risk for the patient,
9 - use of new technologies,
10 - appearance at inconvenient hours.

Special care was taken to ensure that all cases had to be considered and managed by the attending surgeon and that more than one therapeutic choice existed.

The therapeutic choice for each USC was an open answer question. Immediately after each answer, participating surgeons were asked to evaluate what had been behind their attitude by choosing, from five options, the one or two preceding factors (from five) most involved in each decision. Proposed preceding factors were:

1 - *previous experience* as a surgeon or assistant in an exact or similar case,

2 - *referred experience* by another surgeon in a person-to-person approach or by attending a meeting,

3 - *published experience* read in a surgical journal or book,

4 - *previous layout* of this potential problem as a mental exercise,

5 - *common sense* of the surgeon (which included intuition, the application of basic principles of surgery, tacit knowledge and all such wisdom not included in the previous preceding factors). Participating surgeons were then asked to rate the chosen one or two preceding factors to add a total of 5 points.

The remaining items of the questionnaire inquired about the professional profile of the interviewed surgeon (for example: years of practice, on-call service, career status, job in a teaching hospital, hospital of their residency program, status as endovascular surgeon), whereas others inquired about their personal profile (for example: age, sex). Their status as endovascular surgeons was recorded as follows:

1 - usually not involved in such procedures,

2 - occasional participation in endovascular techniques,

3 - regular participation in the majority of endovascular cases performed at their department. This classification was left somewhat imprecise to avoid any attempt to identify the surgeon.

Sample and procedures. A convenience sample of 150 licensed vascular surgeons, aged between 29 and 60 years, from 52 Spanish public hospitals, was selected to participate in the study. Participating surgeons were surveyed by telephone without prior warning. Questionnaires were carried out by a vascular surgeon. Participation was voluntary and confidential. The main topic and scope of the questionnaire was only revealed if the surgeon agreed to participate at the time. Otherwise, an appointment was scheduled.

Immediately after some brief instructions, participating surgeons were asked to reveal quickly their therapeutic choice for the 8 USCs. Preceding factors were chosen and rated after each case, except for answers such as "I do not know what I would do" or

"It would never happen to me". The majority of interviews were completed in 15 minutes. Some minor modifications to clarify the cases were done once 10 surgeons were surveyed. No changes in the questionnaire were done thereafter. No comprehensive difficulties were observed and no additional information was provided beyond what was already known for each USC. Whenever additional information was requested, the surveyed surgeon was advised to include their considerations in their answer.

Statistical analysis. The results of the questionnaires were entered into a database. All open format answers were codified in numeric variables and grouped thereafter. Case and surgeon characteristics were described using measures of central tendency for continuous variables and frequency distributions for categorical variables.

Associations among categorical variables were assessed by chi square tests, whereas associations between continuous variables and a categorical variable were examined through non-parametric tests (Mann Whitney U, Kruskal Wallis H). To evaluate changes in the surgeon attitudes related to seniority, bivariate associations of number of years in practice (in sixtiles) with the mean value of each preceding factor for each case and for the combined 8 cases were carried out.

RESULTS

Characteristics of participating surgeons. One hundred and fifty licensed vascular surgeons from 52 vascular departments of Spanish public hospitals participated in the survey. Two surgeons directly declined the participation in the study and were replaced. Of the 150 surgeons surveyed, 118 (78.7%) were men. Median age was 40 years, with a range of 29 to 60 years. Ninety-four (62.7%) worked in hospitals with a vascular residency program. One hundred and thirty-four (89.3%) performed vascular on-call services at their hospitals. One hundred and twenty-three (82%) were registrars and 27 (18%) unit or department heads. Median of years in practice (including residency) was 14.5, with a range of 5 to 37 (5-7 years in 17.3%, 8-10 years in 18%, 11-14 years in 14.7%, 15-18 years in 17.3%, 19-24 years in 18% and 25-37 years in 14.7%). Older and experienced surgeons were characterized by male sex ($p = 0.002$, $p = 0.004$); belonging to institutions with residency program ($p < 0.001$, $p < 0.001$); not doing on-call services ($p < 0.001$, $p < 0.001$); and having a head position ($p < 0.001$, $p < 0.001$).

Forty-one surgeons (27.3%) did not perform or participate in endovascular procedures, 83 (55.3%) did perform or participate in such techniques sometimes and 26 (17.3%) did perform or participated regularly in all or the majority of endovascular procedures performed at their department. There was a significant relationship between involvement in endovascular procedures and male sex (p = 0.005), head position (p = 0.011), age (p = 0.003) and years of practice (p = 0.001).

Therapeutic choices and background attitudes for the eight unexpected surgical challenges. In the present section, the general therapeutic approach and the mean score given to each preceding factor for each USC will be presented.

Case 1. *Aortobifemoral graft implantation by a left retroperitoneal approach. During the blind tunneling from the aorta to the right groin, the right external iliac vein is injured at some point and bleeding only ceases by finger pressure within the tunnel. What would you do?*

One hundred and forty-eight surgeons provided a therapeutic attitude based on a mix of previous experience (mean 39.2%), referred experience (5.4%), published experience (2%), previous layout (3%) and common sense (50.4%). The remaining two surgeons declared that such a problem would never happen to them.

Even though it was stated that "bleeding only ceased by finger pressure in the tunnel", 27 surgeons (18.2%) kept as their first choice a conservative measure: gauze packs to stop the bleeding by tamponade. These surgeons based their attitude more in previous experience than the remaining 121 (tending to an active solution), whose attitude was more based in referred experience and common sense (p < 0.001).

One-hundred and thirty surgeons proposed three different approaches for an active solution as a first or second choice: inguinal approach opening the inguinal ligament if needed in 24 (18.5%); right retroperitoneal approach in 69 (53%); and conversion of the left retroperitoneal into a transperitoneal approach in 37 (28.5%). Mean age and years of experience associated with these approaches were respectively 44, 42 and 38 years (p = 0.01) and 19, 16 and 12 years (p = 0.003). The background attitude favoring an inguinal approach was more based in previous experience than that of the remaining two approaches, more based in common sense (p < 0.001).

Case 2. *Reversed saphenous vein bypass from the common femoral to the upper anterior tibial artery. During the preparation of the harvested vein, the graft is unexpectedly sucked by the canula and goes directly to the aspirator-reservoir. What would you do?*

One hundred and forty-seven surgeons provided a therapeutic attitude based in a mix of previous experience (mean 15%), referred experience (11.3%), published experience (8%), previous layout (6.7%) and common sense (59%). The remaining three surgeons declared that such problem would never happen to them.

The main question in this case was whether the vein should be retrieved from the aspirator reservoir in order to use it after an "adequate cleaning". This therapeutic option was favored by 26 (17.7%) surgeons whose attitude was more based in referred experience than that of surgeons tending toward using an alternative graft (alternative vein 74.4%, other grafts 25.6%) whose attitude was more based in published experience, previous layout of the problem and common sense (p < 0.001).

Case 3. *Open surgical repair of a 5.5 centimeter abdominal aortic aneurysm (AAA) in a 69-year-old man. Immediately after doing the mid-line laparotomy, the surgeon discovers four 1-cm subcapsular hepatic nodules whose intraoperative pathologic analysis reveals to be metastases of an adenocarcinoma. In the abdominal exploration, no other nodules or primary tumors are found. What would you do with the AAA?*

One hundred and forty-seven surgeons provided a therapeutic attitude based in a mix of previous experience (mean 15%), referred experience (7.6%), published experience (12.5%), previous layout (8.3%) and common sense (56.6%). The remaining three surgeons declared that such problem would never happen to them.

The main question in this case was whether the aneurysm should be repaired once the abdomen was open. Ninety-one surgeons (61.9%) favored this option, 47 (31.9%) would have closed the abdomen, 8 were hesitant and would have decided according to the opinion of a general surgeon or an oncologist, and the remaining surgeon would have performed a palliative technique on the aneurysm (banding and/or aneurysmorraphy). No significant differences in the magnitude of the preceding factors or in the characteristics of the surgeon were found between the two main choices.

Case 4. *Acute limb ischemia secondary to a bifurcated graft limb thrombosis. Preoperative angiography* reveals patent profunda femoral and popliteal arteries. During the groin graft revision, the surgeon finds a suspiciously purulent collection around the graft, which seems to be limited to the groin. How would you revascularize the acute ischemic limb?

One hundred and forty-seven surgeons provided a therapeutic attitude based in a mix of previous experience (mean 38.6%), referred experience (6.7%), published experience (20.3%), previous layout (7.6%) and common sense (26.8%). The remaining three surgeons declared that they would not do anything else to the patient and were considered as missing answers.

This case raised many interesting questions. Surgeons provided up to almost 40 different therapeutic choices considering several anatomic approaches, graft materials and the value of an intraoperative gram stain of the suspiciously purulent collection. Remarkably, 27 (18.4%) surgeons favored directly a standard approach to the limb graft thrombosis delaying the eventual treatment of the graft infection until the patient had recovered from the acute ischemia and the possible infection had been studied adequately. These surgeons were characterized by a higher proportion of chiefs (p = 0.026) and their attitude was more based in common sense than that of the remaining 120 surgeons, more prone to other techniques and whose attitude was more based in referred experience.

Within those 120 surgeons not favoring a standard treatment of the limb graft thrombosis, 27 (22.5%) would have done a standard or an alternative technique according to the result of an intraoperative gram stain of the suspiciously purulent collection. The remaining 93 surgeons (77.5%) would have revascularized the patient's limb directly by alternative techniques. These two types of surgeon did not differ significantly in their background attitudes or professional characteristics.

Case 5. *Typical common femoral embolic acute ischemia (three days evolution) with healthy arteries. The surgeon opens the common femoral artery and takes away the embolus. The profunda femoral artery has back bleeding. The surgeon asks for an embolectomy catheter to remove the secondary thrombus at least from the superficial femoral artery and the nurse states that no catheters are available at that moment. What would you do?*

One hundred and thirty-eight surgeons provided a therapeutic attitude based in a mix of previous experience (mean 12.3%), referred experience (7%), published experience (4.3%), previous layout (1.4%) and common sense (75%). The remaining twelve surgeons declared not knowing what to do (6 cases) or that such problem would never happen to them (6 cases).

Forty-nine surgeons (29.7%) would not have improvised an alternative technique to remove the clot from the superficial femoral artery. Essentially, they would have performed an intraoperative angiogram before closing the wound and asked for embolectomy catheters from another institution. Once the catheters had arrived several hours later, the patient would be reconsidered for surgery. Alternatively, 97 (70.3%) surgeons favored up to 15 alternative techniques (alone or in combination) to the catheter embolectomy, including retrograde flushing from the popliteal artery, limb expression, fibrinolisis, alternative catheters with some sort of balloon at their edge, aspiration cannulas, bypass and so forth. The attitude of these surgeons was more based in referred and published experience than that of more conservative ones (p = 0.001). No other personal or professional characteristics differed significantly between both groups.

Case 6. *A 76-year-old man with a ruptured AAA is on the operating table. The patient is stable with a systolic blood pressure of 100 mmHg but is oligo-anuric. The surgeon is going to initiate an open surgical repair but the anesthesiologist says that blood derivatives will take one hour to arrive to the OR because of cross-matching problems. What would you do?*

One hundred and forty-nine surgeons provided a therapeutic attitude based in a mix of previous experience (mean 21%), referred experience (4%), published experience (6%), previous layout (6%) and common sense (63%). The remaining surgeon declared that such problem would never happen to them.

Ninety-six surgeons (64.4%) favored an immediate surgical repair without blood-matched derivatives and considering cell saver, isogroup blood or nothing else. Forty-eight surgeons (32.2%) would have delayed the laparotomy one hour, provided that the patient remained hemodynamically stable. Curiously, these surgeons were older (p = 0.012), more experienced (p = 0.002) and had a more senior position (p < 0.001). There were almost no significant differences between the background attitude of these two groups of surgeons.

The remaining 5 surgeons would have favored an occlusion balloon (3 cases), and endograft (1 case) or a variable attitude depending on whether the patient had been intubated or not.

Case 7. *Endovascular repair of a 6-centimeter AAA (2-centimeter neck length) in a 78-year-old man with creatinine levels within normal range. In the postdeployment angiogram, the surgeon notices that one renal artery has been completely covered by the endograft (the other renal artery is patent). What would you do?*

One hundred and thirty-three surgeons provided a therapeutic attitude based in a mix of previous experience (mean 20.1%), referred experience (12.2%), published experience (11.3%), previous layout (5.3%) and common sense (51.1%). The remaining 13 surgeons declared to have no experience or not enough knowledge to answer the case properly.

Ninety-three surgeons (69.9%) favored a wait-and-see conservative attitude whereas the remaining 40 surgeons (30.1%) would have tried to provide an active solution by open or endovascular procedures. The attitude of surgeons favoring a conservative approach was more based in previous and referred experience and in previous layout than that of active surgeons whose attitude was more based in common sense (p < 0.001). None of the professional characteristics, even their status as endovascular surgeons, differed significantly between these two groups. However, among surgeons prone to an active solution, those most experienced in endovascular surgery would have favored an endovascular solution rather than an open surgical repair (p = 0.005).

Case 8. *Simple percutaneous transluminal angioplasty of a common iliac artery in the operating room. During completion angiography, a contrast-media extravasation is seen and the patient initiates signs of hemodynamic instability. What would you do?*

One hundred and forty-nine surgeons provided a therapeutic attitude based in a mix of previous experience (mean 29.1%), referred experience (8.8%), published experience (22.8%), previous layout (6.8%) and common sense (32.5%). The remaining surgeon declared to have no experience or not enough knowledge to answer properly.

Thirty surgeons (20.1%) would have immediately reinflated the balloon, regardless of whether their subsequent action was to be open surgical or endovascular. The remaining 119 surgeons (79.9%) made no mention of this maneuver and exposed their direct solution to the ruptured iliac artery. These latter surgeons had declared a lesser involvement in endovascular procedures than the first ones (p < 0.001).

Fifty-two surgeons (36.1%) would have performed an open surgical repair of the iliac artery whereas 92 (63.9%) would have approached the case through an endovascular solution. Remarkably, the attitude of surgeons favoring a direct surgical approach was more based in previous experience and common sense, while surgeons prone to an endovascular approach were more sensitive to published experience (p < 0.001). Surgeons frequently involved in endovascular procedures showed a higher but non-significant (p = 0.1) preference for the endovascular solution.

Considering both cases 7 and 8, there were no significant differences between the therapeutic choices favored by surgeons with no experience in endovascular procedures and those with occasional experience. The statistically significant differences observed in the cross-tabulations of cases 7 and 8 were exclusively determined by the therapeutic choices of those surgeons most regularly involved in such procedures.

Changes in the background attitudes towards unexpected surgical challenges with increasing years of surgical practice. The scores given by each surgeon to the preceding factors of each case were gathered together in a single score for each preceding factor per surgeon. The mean relative value of this single score for each preceding factor was then evaluated according to the number of years of surgical practice (in sixtiles) (Fig. 1). Common sense was the highest rated preceding factor (Fig. 2). Its relative importance ranged from 26.8% to 75% depending on the case. Even though common sense in 30-year-olds may not be the same as that in 60-year-olds, there were no significant differences in the mean value given to common sense with increasing years of practice.

Previous experience was the next highest rated preceding factor (Fig. 3). Its relative importance ranged from 12.3% to 39.2% depending on the case. As expected, surgeons based their therapeutic choices increasingly on previous experience as seniority increased (p = 0.002).

Remarkably, referred experience, published experience and previous layout (Figs 4,5,6, respectively) were much less rated by participating surgeons (4-12.8%, 2-22.8%, 1.4-8.3%, respectively). Their relative

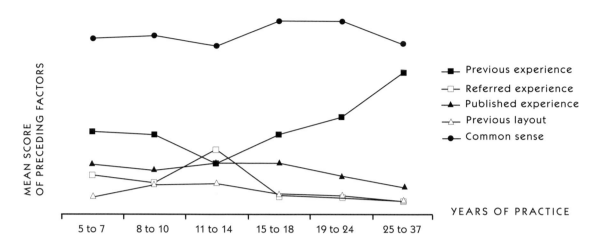

FIG. 1 Changes in the mean score of the 5 preceding factors rated by the surgeons in their therapeutic attitude towards 8 unexpected surgical challenges (combined) according to the number of years of surgical practice (in sixtiles).

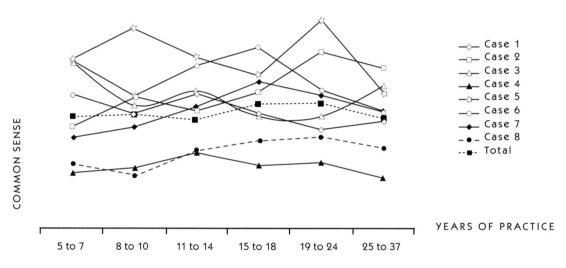

FIG. 2 Surgeons' therapeutic attitude towards 8 unexpected surgical challenges: changes in the mean score given to *common sense* according to the number of years of surgical practice (in sixtiles).

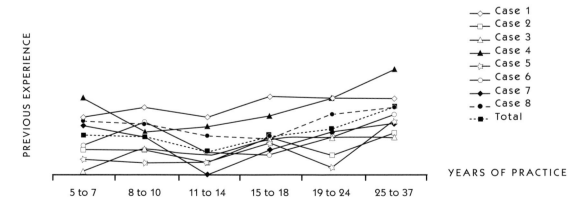

FIG. 3 Surgeons' therapeutic attitude towards 8 unexpected surgical challenges: changes in the mean score given to *previous experience* according to the number of years of surgical practice (in sixtiles).

1
8

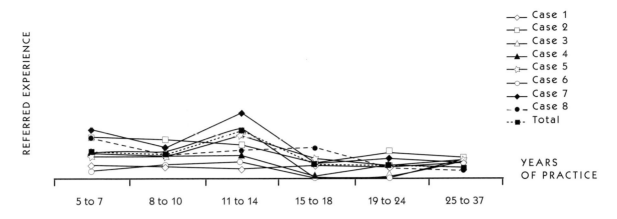

FIG. 4 Surgeons' therapeutic attitude towards 8 unexpected surgical challenges: changes in the mean score given to *referred experience* according to the number of years of surgical practice (in sixtiles).

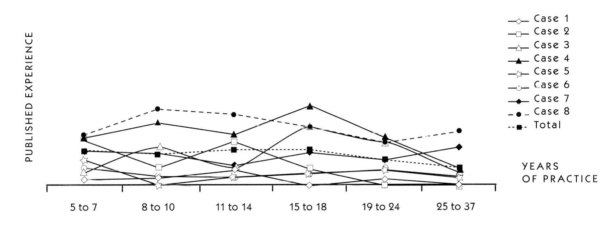

FIG. 5 Surgeons' therapeutic attitude towards 8 unexpected surgical challenges: changes in the mean score given to *published experience* according to the number of years of surgical practice (in sixtiles).

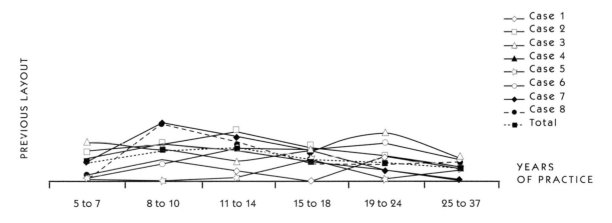

FIG. 6 Surgeons' therapeutic attitude towards 8 unexpected surgical challenges: changes in the mean score given to *previous layout* according to the number of years of surgical practice (in sixtiles).

importance decreased as seniority increased, although this tendency was only significant for referred experience (p = 0.001).

Figure 7 illustrates the relative importance of previous experience compared to the alternatives combined in a single group (referred experience added to published experience and previous layout) according to the number of years of practice. Surgeons tended to give more value to their own experience than to other sources of knowledge (referred, published or previous layout) from their 15-18 years of surgical practice (residency included).

Discussion

THE VASCUPRACTICE STUDY

Previous experience was not the highest rated but the most valued preceding factor among surveyed surgeons. Whenever a surgeon had previous experience in an exact or similar case, this knowledge was a determining factor on how they would have managed the patient. This conclusion cannot be supported by the numerical results of the study but based on tacit data appraised from the 150 interviews done. The weight given to previous experience was higher as seniority increased, although there was a slight decrease of its importance at mid-

age, in which surgeons were more sensitive to referred experience. If this finding is true, it could be explained by the residual effect of residency training. Surgeons use to be conscrvative about their therapeutic attitudes. During their initial years practicing as licensed professionals, surgeons may feel more comfortable following the rules of practice that they have learnt during their residency. Several years later, surgeons conscious of the limitations of their learned approach may become more sensitive to the experience of others until they accumulate enough personal experience.

The mean score given to referred and published experience was never important, but was still less so as professional seniority increased. It may be easy to understand why published experience was not important in the choices of surgeons (because of reporting bias), but it is more difficult to explain why referred experience was not valued by surgeons. Perhaps it may be also related to some disclosure bias. Oral reporting of USCs may be determined by certain features (such as positive outcome, heroical management), except in the most intimate professional relationships. This is common knowledge for surgeons. Therefore, a certain scepticism may underlie the consideration of the listener surgeon where these surgical problems are frequently complex and the context is subjective. Curi-

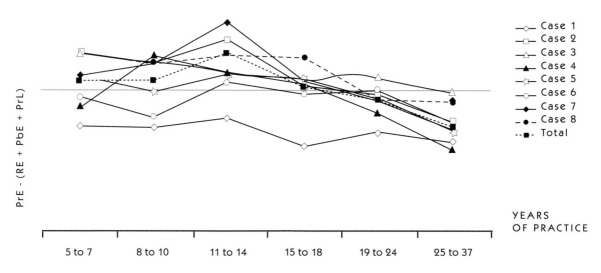

FIG. 7 Surgeons' therapeutic attitude towards 8 unexpected surgical challenges: comparison between the mean score given to previous experience and that resulting from the sum of referred experience, published experience and previous layout according to the number of years of surgical practice (in sixtiles). Note that only after 15 to 18 years of practice (residency included), previous experience becomes more important in surgeons' decisions than the sum of other alternative sources of knowledge (common sense excluded).

ously, previous layout of potential USCs did not appear to be a frequent practice within surgeons of all ages. Perhaps in other sectors this practice may be more common.

The value given to common sense remained stable over the years of surgical practice. This does not mean that common sense remains the same at different ages. Common sense may involve tacit knowledge, the application of general principles of surgery and intuition in different proportions and these may change over time. Both tacit knowledge and intuition may improve with experience. Junior surgeons may be able to follow the general principles of surgery but their tacit knowledge is limited and their intuition may end sometimes in improvisation. Common sense may reflect the best and the worse of ourselves. We all should be concerned in reducing the relative score given by surgeons in their thirties to common sense.

Pilots are trained to manage unexpected challenges in flight simulators. Open surgery, laparoscopic and endovascular simulators will be very welcome in teaching hospitals in the foreseeable future. In the meantime, a simple way to improve the performance of surgeons in USCs may be simply to talk about them. Finding a place for such practical issues during courses or scientific meetings or creating an anonymous and world-wide accessible database of USCs may improve the score given to referred experience (directly) and previous layout (indirectly). The resulting scenario, adapted from Figure 1, is shown in Figure 8.

WHAT SURGEONS CAN LEARN FROM HIGH RELIABILITY ORGANIZATIONS

Good management of the unexpected is mindful management of the unexpected. That conclusion comes from careful study of organizations that operate under very trying conditions. These organizations, collectively referred to as High Reliability Organizations (HROs), include nuclear power generating plants, aircraft carriers, firefighting crews, power grid dispatching centers, air traffic control systems, emergency departments and hostage negotiation teams [3].

The following is how one navy veteran describes life on a carrier [4]:

Imagine that it's a busy day, and you shrink San Francisco airport to only one short runway and one ramp and one gate. Make planes take off and land at the same time, at half the present time interval, rock the runaway from side to side, and require that everyone who leaves in the morning returns the same day. Make sure that the equipment is so close to the envelope that it's fragile. Then turn off the radar to avoid detection, impose strict controls on the radios, fuel the aircraft in place with their engines running, put an enemy in the air, and scatter live bombs and rockets around. Now wet the whole thing down with seawater and oil, and man it with twenty-year-olds, half of whom have never seen an airplane close-up. Oh, and by the way, try not to kill anyone.

HROs have developed ways of acting and styles of leading that enable them to manage the unexpected better than most other kinds of organizations. HROs manage the unexpected through five processes:

1

11

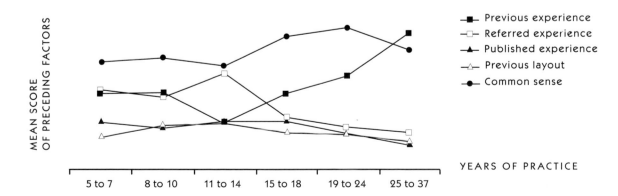

FIG. 8 Hypothetical scenario (adapted from Fig. 1) of surgeons' attitudes towards unexpected surgical challenges resulting from an open and frequent discussion of these problems within the professional community.

1 - preoccupation with failures rather than successes,
2 - reluctance to simplify interpretations,
3 - sensitivity to operations,
4 - commitment to resilience,
5 - deference to expertise [3].

The first three processes are preventive measures and may be of interest for surgeons. The key difference between HROs and other organizations in managing the unexpected often occurs at early stages, when the unexpected may give off only weak signals of potential trouble. The overwhelming tendency is to respond to weak signals with weak responses. Mindfulness preserves the capability to see the significant meaning of weak signals and to give strong responses to them.

PREOCCUPATION WITH FAILURE

HROs are preoccupied with their failures, both the large and the mostly small instances. They view any failure, no matter how small, as a window on the system as a whole [3]. Small failures (such as an inadequate sterile dressing of the patient, a deficient bladder catheterization or the infusion of prophylactic antibiotics once the procedure has been started) should be treated as signs of potential larger problems within the system, such as: poor communication among professionals in the operating room; blurred hierarchies; or inadequate training protocols. People assuming that success demonstrates competence are more likely to drift into complacency, inattention and predictable routines. Complacency increases the likelihood that unexpected events go undetected and accumulate into bigger problems.

HROs also show preoccupation with failure by promoting error disclosure. HRO encourage reporting of errors and questioning. For example, they elaborate on experiences of a near-miss for what can be learned and they are wary of the potential liabilities of success [3]. In order for this to occur, people need to feel safe to report incidents, or they will ignore them or cover them up. The key of the question is that HROs treat any failure as a symptom that something is wrong with the system. The best HROs encourage and reward error reporting, even going so far as to reward those who have committed them. A seaman on the nuclear carrier Carl Vinson reported the loss of a tool on the deck. All aircrafts already airborne were redirected to land bases until the tool was found and the seaman was commended for his action the next day at a formal ceremony

[5]. A climate of openness makes people more willing to: report and discuss errors; work toward correcting them; and learn more about complex systems. Technology can always surprise the surgeon.

RELUCTANCE TO SIMPLIFY

Another way HROs manage for the unexpected is by being reluctant to accept simplifications. Once an end-point is established, people tend to simplify and overlook small warning signals of potential problems. A simple example from the operating room illustrates this tendency to simplification. An endovascular aortic repair has lasted much longer than expected. It is time to close the femoral arteries. These vessels were already diseased and now are a little bit worse. The surgeon is somewhat exhausted but proud to have been able to fix a complex aneurysm. The femoral repair that would have been done if this femoral surgery had been the single case of the day would be probably more precise (and lasting) than what actually is going to be done. Surgeons should be reluctant to accept simplifications like this. Small moments of inattention and misperception can escalate into serious postoperative complications.

An additional way to fight against simplification is the interaction of people who have diverse expectations. Coming back to the previous example, suppose that the vascular surgeon on call is requested to finish the procedure. His expectations, beyond the interest of the patient, are clear: no redo procedures should be done to this patient in the next 24 hours. It is not just interaction by itself that decreases simplification and increases mindfulness. It is the fact that the interaction is among people who have diverse expectations. This diversity enables people to see different things when they "view" the same event [3]. The efficacy of preoperative clinical sessions, where patients are presented and discussed among several surgeons, may depend largely on this fact.

SENSITIVITY TO OPERATIONS

Unexpected events usually originate in what psychologist James Reason calls *latent failures* [3]. Latent failures are "loopholes in the system's defenses, barriers and safeguards whose potential existed for some time prior to the onset of the accident sequence, though usually without any obvious bad effect". Many of these latent failures are discovered only after the fact of an unexpected event. Two clear examples of latent failures within a surgical department are surgeons half-trained in new technologies and those with partial inattention to minor cases as a consequence of workload, dedication to curricular activities or simply convenience.

Surgeons who occasionally undertake or assist in endovascular procedures may be considered as a loophole in the system if they are expected to act as endovascular surgeons in an unexpected challenge. They are supposed to know endovascular skills but their practical behavior (see *Vascupractice* results) is closer to that of surgeons with no experience in endovascular surgery than to those regularly involved in these procedures.

Sensitivity to operations means treating all daily activities as important ones. Unnoticed findings in a chest X-ray are probably more common in patients with minor surgical problems, such as a toe amputation, than in patients with a complex vascular disease. When activities are treated as equally important, most initial stages of anything unexpected are noticed and seldom progress.

Sensitivity to operations is facilitated by real-time information. Normal operations may reveal deficiencies (deficient knowledge of how the portable X-Ray device works or how to perform a thoracotomy) that are "free lessons" that signal the potential for unexpected events. But these lessons are visible only if there is frequent assessment of the overall safety of the organization. Surgeons, from the head of the organization downwards, should be in continuous communication during daily activities and exchange information about the status of patients and activities. For obvious reasons, the early morning meeting has been considered one of the most important daily activities. People in HROs are aware of the close tie between sensitivity to operations and sensitivity to relationships. For this reason, HROs appraise frequently the extent to which managers maintain continuous contact with the front line and the extent to which they are accessible when important situations develop [3].

Conclusion

Surgeons should not aspire to become experts in USCs. If that is the case, the surgeon is probably on the wrong track. USCs are infrequent and diverse events and significant experience may only be gained if the surgeon has a special predisposition to "provoke" them. The key to the management of USCs is clearly their prevention. High reliability organizations provide useful strategies for a mindful prevention of the unexpected. When the unexpected appears, however, the surgeon should not trust themselves completely to luck. Common sense, explicit experiences (own, referred or published) and previous layout can be very useful tools for managing the unexpected. However, while common sense and personal experience may improve only with seniority, a systematic approach based in a previous layout of the problem enlightened by the experience of others, may be learned and applied from the beginning. Training simulators with consensus solutions for unexpected problems are probably the future. In the meantime, the best we can do for our colleagues is to disclose, without taboos or complexes, our most hidden but instructive experiences. Obviously, a proper and confidential space and some change in surgeons' attitudes (culture of failure) may be needed. However, in the end this challenge will be to the benefit of our patients.

1

13

REFERENCES

1 Woodcock AER, Davis M. *Catastrophe Theory*. New York: EP Dutton, 1978; pp 11-23.
2 Polanyi M. Personal Knowledge Towards a Post Critical Philosophy. *The University of Chicago Press*, Chicago; pp 3-407.
3 Weick KE, Sutcliffe KM. Managing the unexpected. *Assuring high performance in an age of complexity*. San Francisco: Jossey-Bass (University of Michigan Business Scholl Management Series) 2001; pp 1-83.

4 Weick KE, Roberts KH. Collective mind in organizations: heedful interrelating on flight decks. *Administrative Science Quarterly* 1993; 38: 357-381.
5 Landau M, Crisholm D. The arrogance of optimism: notes on failure avoidance management. *Journal of Contingencies and Crisis Management* 1995; 3: 67-80.

2

CHALLENGES IN ENDOVASCULAR THORACIC ANEURYSM REPAIR

CHRISTOPHER LEVILLE, ROY GREENBERG

Endovascular treatment of thoracic aortic disease continues to be an area of significant investigation at many centers across the world. Since the advent of endovascular grafts, many patients with a variety of diseases of the aorta undergo less invasive treatment options. Open surgical repair for thoracic aortic disease is now reserved for patients with adequate pulmonary function and relatively moderate risk factors. The morbidity associated with conventional treatments has been linked to patient risk factors [1] and thus endovascular grafting has had a significant impact as a primary treatment for many patients. However, thoracic aortic disease is a broad term that includes patients with aneurysm, dissection, ulceration, fistula, or combinations of these. Although early trials with thoracic grafts treated many types of complex pathologies, most of the larger multicenter studies have been limited to favorable anatomic situations. Nonetheless, all studies have confirmed the added complexity of the thoracic bed in contrast to infrarenal aneurysms [2]. Improved devices and refined techniques have pushed thoracic grafting into more difficult regions of the aorta including severe tortuosity, complex aortic dissections, and aneurysms involving branch vessels.

Aortic pathology and imaging

In parallel with endovascular graft development, strides in cross-sectional imaging techniques have been invaluable for the assessment of patients and planning treatment [3]. It is important to remember that the entire aorta must be studied when thoracic aortic pathology is suspected as delivery planning must include an assessment of the pelvic vasculature (Fig. 1). Thus, contrast bolus timing and rapid image acquisition during a single breath hold remain critical. Studies must include non-contrast

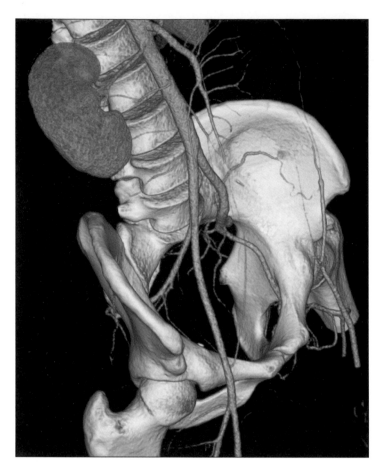

FIG. 1 This reconstruction of a pelvic CT in a patient with bilaterally palpable femoral pulses was performed on a patient with a thoracic aneurysm as part of a planning study. Clearly the absence of an external iliac artery will partake in the delivery planning.

and arterial phases preoperatively, while delayed imaging is more useful postimplantation or to assist with the identification of coincident end-organ pathology (such as liver or renal lesions). Image assessment using three-dimensional techniques is mandatory for planning and sizing of endovascular devices reside within the thoracic aorta. Reconstruction of images perpendicular to a calculated centerline of flow can allow for accurate diameter measurements within tortuous regions. This technique alleviates problems relating to inaccurate diameter measurements resulting from short or long axis lengths within non-circular aortic segments.

The aortic arch is the most difficult area to assess radiographically as a result of the naturally complex three-dimensional structure. In addition to a significant incidence of variable anatomy, the high flow dynamics make this region particularly susceptible to device planning and deployment-related errors. Thus, after the ascending aorta is assessed for length and its tortuosity, a thorough understanding of the arch anatomy is crucial with respect to sealing and fixation zone determinations. It is the inherent tortuosity within the transverse arch which most significantly influences the stent-graft options. Device flexibility and deliverability are limited and, therefore, must correspond to the inherent anatomy. Additional consideration must be given to the relevance of any coronary circulation based off the internal mammary arteries, as well as the collateral vertebral flow.

Current investigational (USA and Asia) and commercial (Europe and Australia) grafts

An ideal thoracic stent-graft would be able to accommodate a tortuous arch, provide adequate proximal and distal sealing areas, and be deployed easily and secured in both straight and tortuous segments. The stent-graft should also have an acceptable long-term durability which means that it is free from migration, associated with a minimal endoleak rate, and encourages aneurysm sac shrinkage. The current thoracic stent-grafts have various capabilities, usually differing in flexibility and mode of fixation. Therefore, when reviewing available stent-grafts it is important to note that modifications to the designs are continuously being made in response to perceived problems. Specific anatomy or pathology will likely lend one to choose one design over another. For example, an acute type B dissection may not require secure fixation given the absence of an aneurysm, but the fragile nature of an acutely dissected aorta mandates the need for a flexible graft. Conversely, a fusiform aneurysm of the descending aorta would be best treated by a graft with secure fixation and fabric that is conducive to aneurysm resorption. Currently, within the USA, there are no FDA approved devices. A number of devices are commercially available in Europe, Australia and other countries.

GORE TAG EXCLUDER® GRAFT

The TAG Excluder® *(W.L. Gore, Flagstaff, AZ, USA)* is constructed with nitinol stents and lined with expanded polytetrafluorethylene (ePTFE). Initial studies in the thoracic aorta included stabilizing nitinol bars along the length of the stent, which were prone to fracture [4]. Current grafts do not have this feature and also have a modified ePTFE lining to decrease the incidence of type IV endoleak or seroma formation. The Excluder® is currently the most flexible stent-graft and is delivered through a 20-24 French system. It does not have fixation barbs and has a *pull-cord* mechanism for release. The graft deploys from the middle out to prevent any *wind-socking*, minimizing deployment inaccuracies. However, the graft deploys rapidly rather than allowing for a slow, controlled release.

MEDTRONIC TALENT® GRAFT

The Talent® device *(Medtronic/AVE, Fort Lauderdale, FL, USA)* is similar to its sister abdominal graft in that it incorporates a proximal uncovered non-barbed stent intended to assist with fixation. It has an outer nitinol skeleton with an inner lining of polyester fabric. Its delivery system differs from the Gore system by having its own sheath delivery which is introduced over a stiff wire. The stent is then unsheathed using a sheath pullback method, which is usually done in the setting of induced hypotension or temporary asystole. The delivery system is 22-25 French and is somewhat stiff. Debate exists with respect to the need or benefit of a proximal uncovered stent and the company has considered introducing a non-bare stent design.

COOK TX1/TX2® GRAFTS

The TX1® is a single body graft constructed from stainless steel Gianturco-Z stents and standard thickness polyester. There is no uncovered proximal stent, but the proximal sealing stent does include barbs that protrude through the fabric which are designed to engage the aorta within the sealing region. The distal aspect of the device has the option of an uncovered stent, which may help to prevent retrograde migration of the stent into an aneurysm sac. The two piece system (TX2®) is similar, with the exception that the proximal and distal fixation components are separated. The first component includes the proximal sealing stent fixation system, while the distal component docks inside the first (with a prescribed overlap) and contains the distal fixation system. This type of construction avoids the need for a single device to cover extensive distances and simplifies planning. The Z-stents within the graft body are shorter than the abdominal counterpart, making the graft more flexible than the Talent®, but not as flexible as the TAG® device.

Universal problems

PROXIMAL NECK MODIFICATIONS

The proximal landing zone for thoracic aortic repair really requires a minimum of 15 millimeters to establish adequate proximal sealing. Parallel, straight segments are ideal but uncommon given the tortuosity of the proximal descending thoracic aorta. Sizing the stent-graft 10%-15% greater than the outer wall-outer wall diameter of the aorta improves sealing and fixation [5]. In the treatment of aortic dissection, the upsizing of the graft is less important, and is between 0%-10% depending on the pathology. Coverage of the left subclavian artery can be performed with little morbidity, but if poor collateral flow is present or if a left internal mammary artery (LIMA) cardiac bypass graft is present, then subclavian bypass is warranted. Carotid to left subclavian bypass is usually done prior to stent-graft placement, to preserve the required flow (if necessary) and allow brachial access to the carotid system. This operation is performed through a supraclavicular neck incision with placement of an interposition graft [6]. In the absence of a subclavian aneurysm, ligation of the subclavian artery proximal to the vertebral artery is performed at this time to prevent backflow to the aorta and possible type II endoleak. If the proximal subclavian artery cannot be safely dissected at this time, later endovascular occlusion is possible. A drain is usually placed perioperatively to monitor for lymph leak. If more proximal coverage of the aortic arch is required for a proximal seal zone for the stent-graft, coverage of the left common carotid artery may be required, albeit rarely, and a subsequent carotid-carotid-subclavian bypass can be performed in preparation for placement of this proximal thoracic stent-graft [7]. This is used uncommonly in our institution and reserved for resolution of proximal leak issues in the setting of acute presentations rather than for primary operations. Alternatively, elephant trunks are combined with a second stage endovascular approach in these cases. The required median sternotomy is surprisingly well tolerated in contrast to a left lateral thoracotomy. The elephant trunk can be implanted immediately distal to the left subclavian artery (Fig. 2) or, alternatively, between the left common carotid and left subclavian. The endovascular device is then placed through a femoral introduction point to bridge the short proximal graft to the distal healthy aorta.

DISTAL NECK MODIFICATIONS

Mesenteric bypass techniques have been described, allowing thoracoabdominal graft coverage through the visceral segment [8,9]. These techniques either derive visceral flow from the infrarenal aorta or one of the iliac vessels (Fig. 3). It can be accomplished through using a medial visceral rotation or through a left retroperitoneal incision. We prefer to use the latter technique. If the right renal artery must be included also, a transperitoneal exposure through the retroperitoneal incision can be accomplished. Following this, a series of thoracic grafts can be inserted (usually the maximum length is about 20 centimeters to limit the deployment friction), overlapped appropriately, and then combined with a bifurcated abdominal device if necessary. Although paraplegia (0 out of 13 patients at our institution) and serious neurologic deficit (1 out of 13 patients with left leg weakness) is relatively uncommon despite the degree of aortic coverage, the numbers of treated patients are small. Given

the requirement for essentially an aortic repair, this option can hardly be considered minimally invasive and will likely be replaced with branched and fenestrated techniques, as described later.

DEVICE INTRODUCTION

When accurate deployment of the proximal stents appears to be difficult because of tortuosity, two methods of assistance have been described. The use of exceptionally stiff wires can be helpful to a certain point, but ultimately, if the tortuosity is severe, these will kink or cause the device to kink. In this situation, the use of a less stiff wire in conjunction with right brachial access is helpful and described as a "through and through" technique. Tension placed along the wire (which must be protected from contact with the brachiocephalic vessels with a catheter or sheath) creates a rail allowing the stent-graft to be tracked, thus negotiating complex

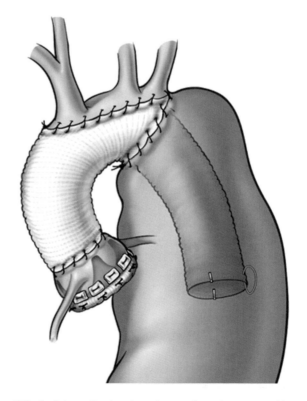

FIG. 2 Schematic drawing of an arch replacement with a distal elephant trunk demonstrates the creation of a proximal sealing and fixation zone. This is then treated with an endovascular graft to complete the descending thoracic aneurysm repair. As evident from this drawing, proximal aortic and cardiac pathology is repaired at the time of the elephant trunk creation.

angles into the transverse arch. However, once the delivery system resides within the arch, either the device must be introduced into the innominate artery, or a loop of wire into the ascending aorta must be created by advancing wire pinned between the stent-graft and sheath inserted from the arm. It is critical to realize that tortuosity within the arch is inherent and difficult to deal with. Thus, if compounding issues, such as tight or calcific iliac arter-

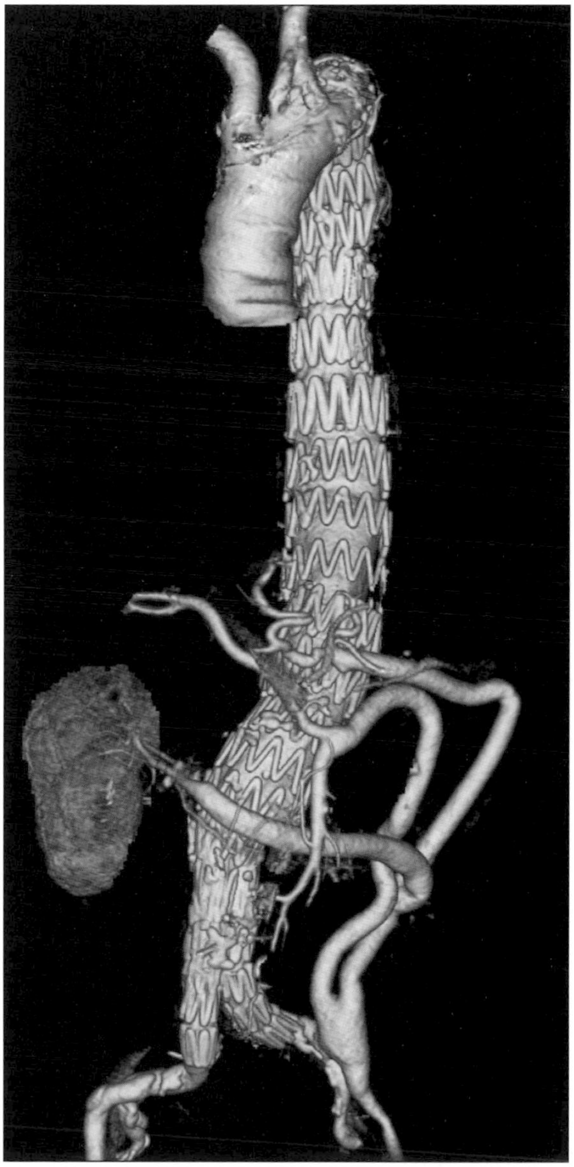

FIG. 3 This depicts a mesenteric revascularization procedure that was based off the left iliac artery, followed by thoracic stent grafting, and distally, with a bifurcated abdominal device.

ies, also exist, these should be dealt with prior to device insertion with the use of conduits.

ENDOLEAKS AND SAC BEHAVIOR

Following stent-graft deployment, ballooning is variably used. If needed, the graft orientation to the proximal vasculature can be adjusted slightly with balloon inflation, but if avoidable, simple graft deployment is preferred. Proximal endoleaks are extremely disappointing and much more difficult to treat than proximal leaks within the abdominal aorta. Most frequently, such an event is treated with an extension cuff if adequate room exists between critical brachiocephalic vessels. In the absence of enough room, consideration must be given to subclavian coverage, extra-anatomic bypass, and conversion to open repair or the use of fenestrated/ branch vessel grafts.

Type II endoleaks are less common in the thoracic aorta than in the abdominal aorta. They can arise from a non-ligated left subclavian artery that is covered by the prosthesis or may result from intercostal vessels. Again, the latter are more difficult to treat than patent IMA or lumbar vessels, given the paucity of sizable collateral access vessels. Type III endoleaks most frequently result from modular joint mis-alignments, particularly when overlap sections are seated with an angulated aortic region. In these cases, additional overlap, proximally or distally, with additional radial force is necessary. The use of Palmaz stents is uncommon within the thoracic aorta as a result of the larger inherent diameter, significant tortuosity, and higher flow rates, all of which complicate deployment. Furthermore, deployment of Palmaz stents within very tortuous aortic segments is considered potentially dangerous.

The aneurysm sac within the thoracic aorta interacts differently with surrounding structures than is seen in abdominal aneurysms. The thoracic aorta, as it curves through the aortic arch, creates an enclosed region for the pulmonary vasculature. The proximity of the aorta to the bronchial tree and esophagus also create concerns. Finally, there is a limited amount of space within the chest for pulmonary reserve and, therefore, the sac behavior after device implantation is critical. Any patient with a growing thoracic aneurysm is likely to be at a greater risk for compromise of the lung, esophagus or pulmonary vasculature. Thus, it is imperative that any patient exhibiting aneurysmal growth is carefully evaluated for the presence of an endoleak and receives treatment.

MIGRATION

Distal fixation of the thoracic stent-graft appears to be as critical as the proximal segment with respect to long-term device durability. Through the development of the first generation thoracic stent-grafts, it was noted that a significant number of grafts suffered from proximal migration of the distal stent, as well as distal migration of proximal stents, as the stent-grafts were driven into the aneurysm by persistent hemodynamic forces. However, migration is extremely hard to detect within the thoracic aorta, unless three-dimensional imaging techniques are used to calculate the distance between the fixation sites of the implanted graft and the neighboring branches at each follow-up. Ideally, a minimum length of two centimeters for distal fixation would be present, but again, this is simply not the case. Many factors delineate the risk of migration and include: the presence of active fixation systems of the device, the aortic diameter, tortuosity, and the patient's hemodynamic status. As the aortic diameter increases in size, the application of adequate radial force becomes more difficult. Furthermore, tortuous segments are best handled by landing either proximal or distal to that acute angulation rather than within it. The latter circumstance can result in the endograft resting on a pivot, which is not ideal for fixation or sealing. Ultimately, the decision has to be made as to the health of the aorta in the implantation regions. Ideally, devices would extend from normal aorta to normal aorta. In the abdominal situation, this means from the renal arteries to the internal iliac arteries, as we cannot tell where a proximal or distal neck ends. To accomplish the same goal within the thoracic aorta requires extensive coverage of intercostals vessels and the incorporation of tortuous segments that may be best left out of the repaired region. Thus, a balance must be struck between the desired length of coverage, optimal fixation, and the risk of complications.

Extensive aortic replacement has been associated with increased risks of neurologic deficits and should be viewed in context of collateral spinal cord perfusion through the lumbars, hypogastric arteries and vertebral circulation. The presence of concurrent aneurysms (abdominal or iliac in nature) and the timing or need for treatment for these merits discussion. Clearly, the type of stent-graft utilized may influence the ability to clamp an aorta or combine the devices within the visceral or iliac segment for a staged approach. Simultaneous treatment has

been avoided by most, following Dake's report of a higher incidence of paraplegia in these circumstances [10].

Branched and fenestrated thoracic aortic grafts

The development of branched vessel and fenestrated techniques to treat patients with complex aortic anatomy has been encouraging. Such techniques have allowed stent-graft coverage in areas involving major aortic branch vessels which drastically increase the number of patients amenable to minimally invasive repair. Such extensive aneurysms which typically involve the visceral or arch vessels are associated with significant morbidity and mortality following conventional surgery, and thus may well be associated with the greatest benefit from an endovascular approach. When considering a device that involves a fenestration or branch, substantial planning is required. Not only must the exact size and orientation of the incorporated vessels be determined, but how the device will be situated within that aortic segment is critical.

Fenestrated devices have been described most frequently for treatment of juxtarenal aneurysms [11]. Branched grafts have also been described with application to preserve hypogastric pelvic blood flow. The aortic arch is also a potential area where fenestrated and branch vessel devices may become increasingly applicable [12]. However, it is important to realize that fenestrated grafting for thoracic lesions is less intuitive than that for abdominal aneurysms. The complicating factors again relate to the inherent tortuosity of the proximal sealing zone and the extensiveness of required coverage. The simplest form of fenestration is a scallop, or hemi-oval, cut within the proximal or distal graft component to accommodate a branching vessel. These designs have been successfully used to extend repairs deep into the arch or stretch into the visceral segment. Typically, the scallop is placed within an extension (and, therefore, is relatively short) which is coupled with a more conventional thoracic graft. This technique improves the rotational ability, and decreases deployment friction, thus assisting with deployment accuracy. Orientation markers placed onto the constrained device, along with markers denoting the fenestration, assist with rotational orientation. However, rotational ability is imperative following partial deployment, as exact alignment prior to complete graft expansion is impossible. This is accomplished to a certain extent with the use of restraining wires (Fig. 4), whereby the graft is free of the withdrawn delivery sheath but remains attached to the delivery system proximally and distally. It is also constrained to a lesser diameter using a tethering technique which is released only after proper orientation is achieved. This technique works beautifully in non-tortuous segments, such as the distal thoracic aorta in the region of the visceral vessels. Unfortunately, it does not help within the arch. Even the most straightforward arch anatomy is not amenable to conventional fenestration techniques because rotational orientation is lost once current devices traverse the requisite angulation. Therefore, the technique has been altered. Preloaded wires and catheters within proximally fenestrated thoracic grafts are used to cannulate the desired branch vessels selectively. The wire, which resides within the constrained implant, transcends through the fenestration and is advanced into the proximal aorta prior to sheath withdrawal and graft deployment. Snares inserted from the brachial vasculature are used to capture the wire(s) and assist with orientation. Constraining wires then allow for partial graft deployment and balloons are placed over the snared wires bridging the branch vessel and fenestration. As the graft-constraining wire is removed, the device is forced to deploy over the balloons which accommodate the brachiocephalic architecture. Stents are then placed within the branch extending into the aorta to ensure patency of the incorporated vessel.

Fenestrations are simpler distally. Distal extensions with small, large or scalloped fenestrations can be designed. Following insertion through a femoral vessel, the graft material (still tethered) is deployed and access into the device from above is obtained using a brachial puncture. The fenestration(s) is (are) cannulated and access into the desired branch is established. Balloons or guides can be placed into the branches that are then stented, if so desired.

The substitution of stent-grafts for the stents that bridge into the branched vessels, alters the device from a fenestrated graft into a branched graft. However, this requires that a seal be established between the aortic device and bridging stent-graft, as well as distally within the branch vessel. This is more complex than simple fenestrations, requires larger sheaths for deployment of stent-grafts as opposed to stents, and cannot transcend long segments of open spaces (very large non-thrombus filled sacs). However, it is extremely useful for thoracic aneurysms that extend proximally or distally to involve only one component of the arch or visceral segments. Although this technology is appealing and promising, there are several potential problems. With the increase used of branched vessel devices, there can be an increased incidence of component separation. Current designs usually place the fenestrations within extensions and, therefore, it is imperative that adequate overlap exist or, if not present, it is supplemented with additional components. Kinking and occlusion of branch vessels resulting in branch vessel loss is also possible. This is obviously an issue as vessel loss may result in death or serious cerebrovascular compromise. The planning of these advanced grafts is increasingly difficult and precision is mandatory or else both acute and chronic vessel loss will be the rule rather than the exception.

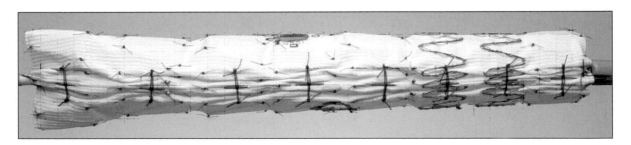

FIG. 4 Fenestrated and branch grafting requires rotational movement following partial graft deployment allowing for appropriate rotational orientation. Thethering wires *(shown below)* allow the graft to remain partially constrained following sheath withdrawal, preserving some rotational ability.

Conclusion

Thoracic stent grafting continues to have great potential for treating a variety of patients with thoracic aortic pathology. Patients with thoracic aortic disease frequently have significant co-morbidities and an endovascular treatment option has the prospect of improved patient outcome. More recent studies of thoracic stent-grafts are showing this to be true. Caution must be exercised with respect to choosing a device with attributes that will provide for the best long-term solution for the patient. This is frequently specific to the disease (aneurysm or dissection) and anatomy. Failures relating to fixation systems, endoleaks and acute technical difficulties are well described and, therefore, it is incumbent upon treating physicians to exercise judgment in choosing both devices and patients. Although extra-anatomic bypass techniques can potentially extend the application of this technology into more proximal or distal aortic segments, fenestrated and branched grafting will ultimately allow for minimally invasive treatment of the entire aorta.

REFERENCES

1 Svensson, L, Crawford E, Hess KR et al. Variables predictive of outcome in 832 patients undergoing repairs of the descending thoracic aorta. *Chest* 1993; 104: 1248-1253.

2 Semba CP, Mitchell RS, Miller DC et al. Thoracic aortic aneurysm repair with endovascular stent-grafts. *Vasc Med* 1997; 2: 98-103.

3 Greenberg RK. Secor JL Painter T. Computed tomography assessment of thoracic aortic pathology. *Semin Vasc Surg* 2004; 17: 166-172.

4 Ellozy SH, Carroccio A, Minor M et al. Challenges of endovascular tube graft repair of thoracic aortic aneurysm: midterm follow-up and lessons learned. *J Vasc Surg* 2003; 38: 676-683.

5 Greenberg R, Risher W. Clinical decision making and operative approaches to thoracic aortic aneurysms. *Surg Clin North Am* 1998; 78: 805-826.

6 Criado FJ, Clark NS, Barnatan MF. Stent-graft repair in the aortic arch and descending thoracic aorta: a 4-year experience. *J Vasc Surg* 2002; 36: 1121-1128.

7 Svensson LG, Kim KH, Blackstone EH et al. Elephant trunk procedure: newer indications and uses. *Ann Thorac Surg* 2004; 78: 109-116.

8 Greenberg R, Resch T, Nyman U et al. Endovascular repair of descending thoracic aortic aneurysms: an early experience with intermediate-term follow-up. *J Vasc Surg* 2000; 31: 147-156.

9 Flye MW. Choi ET. Sanchez LA et al. Retrograde visceral vessel revascularization followed by endovascular aneurysm exclusion as an alternative to open surgical repair of thoracoabdominal aortic aneurysm. *J Vasc Surg* 2004; 39: 454-458.

10 Dake MD, Miller DC, Semba CP et al. Transluminal placement of endovascular stent-grafts for the treatment of descending thoracic aortic aneurysms. *N Engl J Med* 1994; 331: 1729-1734.

11 Greenberg RK, Haulon S, Lyden SP et al. Endovascular management of juxtarenal aneurysms with fenestrated endovascular grafting. *J Vasc Surg* 2004; 39: 279-287.

12 Chuter TA, Buck DG, Schneider DB et al. Development of a branched stent-graft for endovascular repair of aortic arch aneurysms. *J Endovasc Ther* 2003; 10: 940-945.

3

LATE AORTIC WALL PERFORATION AFTER SUCCESSFUL THORACIC ENDOAORTIC RECONSTRUCTION

JENS-RAINER ALLENBERG
HARDY SCHUMACHER, DITTMAR BOECKLE

3
23

Since the general availability of commercially manufactured devices in the 1990s, current technological innovations in thoracic endografting enable surgeons to treat high-risk patients with different thoracic pathologies, who would not be candidates for conventional open surgery. Although potentially less invasive with lower in-hospital complications, the mid-term effectiveness and long-term durability of the devices are unproven and have to be evaluated. This new technology has mainly evolved by learning from failures. *Completely new hazards and unexpected severe adverse events (difficult deployment, graft migration, endoleak, material fatigue) may occur after endo-aortic surgery but these are not associated with classical open surgery. Secondary interventions have been used to improve later outcomes of many devices. The potential for breakdown of the mechanical parts (textile and/or stent) of the endograft is challenging. The purpose of this paper is to analyze a large single-center experience over the last 8 years with thoracic endografting in 110 patients in order to identify the incidence of device failure and modes and causes of later material fatigue, focusing on aortic wall perforation after primarily successful endovascular reconstruction of the thoracic aorta.*

The challenge of thoracic endoprosthesis design and durability for complex morphology

The treatment goal of thoracic endografting is to eliminate the rupture risk by excluding the diseased aortic wall from the systemic arterial pressure. Incomplete seal, called endoleak, has to be considered as a failure mode of this technique. By classifying endoleaks as graft-related and non-graft-related, the overall importance of device stability in the clinical results of this technique could be clearly demonstrated. Manufacturers and engineers have developed several devices with different technical options, such as passive fixation by only the radial force of the stent or active fixation by attachment systems including barbs and hooks. However, because most devices are simply derivatives of known abdominal aortic aneurysm (AAA) endoprosthesis, they are not specifically designed for the unique features of the aortic arch (complex tortuosity and displacing hemodynamic forces). Their performance is suboptimal and should be further improved. Although several mechanical and technical stent graft problems have been mastered and improved, device fatigue remains one of the most challenging causes for procedure failure (Table I). Manufacturers try to improve device durability by design modifications based on analysis of clinical long-term behavior.

Unique clinical properties of different pathologies require specific thoracic endografts

In thoracic aortic endovascular treatment, the following specific issues indicate the need for tailor-made approaches.
- The majority of thoracic pathologies are in close proximity to the left subclavian artery at the distal arch (Table II). Therefore, the essential proximal landing zone of at least two centimeters in length involves this very tortuous segment.
- Several severe curvatures along the thoracoabdominal aorta and at the distal arch (serpentine profile) make it considerably difficult to advance the sheath without force and subsequently release the endograft smoothly and precisely without damage (Fig. 1).

- The pulsatile displacement jetstream forces on endovascular grafts are higher than those dealing with by infrarenal endografting. Distal migration of the proximal portion of the graft and proximal migration of the distal part of the endograft can be the result of these forces.
- The larger stent dimensions challenge technicians to match radial forces with desired flexibilities. To obtain sufficient radial force, the large diameter stents are very long. However, long stent configuration shows an inadequate alignment with the arch.
- The intended columnar strength by a longitudinal bare was thought to be necessary. This spine wire is very vulnerable to material fatigue in a bent position [2].
- The tortuosity, especially at the aortic arch and thoracoabdominal segment, makes accurate total endograft length calculations in the centerline very difficult and requires the surgeon to trombone

| Table I | POSSIBLE CAUSES AND MODES OF LATE ENDOGRAFT FAILURES * |

1 Deployment problems

 a) Delivery system torque causing endoprosthesis misalignment

 b) Endograft damage from insertion forces

 c) Misplacement of proximal or distal attachment/anchoring zone

 d) Failure to appose arterial wall (proximal and/or distally)

2 Migration

 a) Patient attachment zone enlargement

 b) Device structural failure

 c) Inadequate friction with increased displacement forces

3 Device structural failure

 a) Separation of tromboned components (design limitations, inadequate overlap, morphology induced traction)

 b) Prosthesis fabric failure (fabric disruption, angle stent impact trauma)

* Modified from J. Beebe [1]

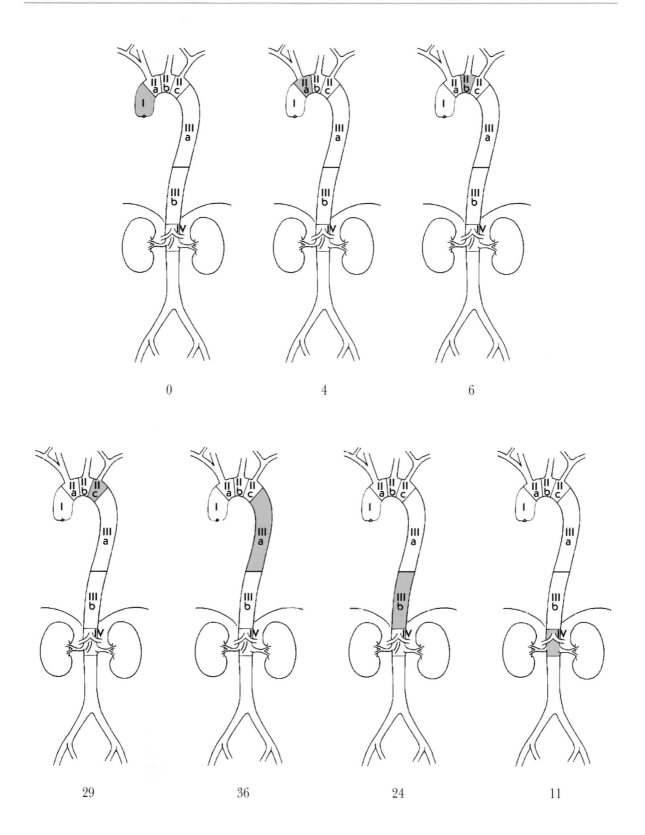

Table II: classification and distribution of the thoracic lesions in 110 patients treated between March 1997 and November 2004 in Heidelberg.

several endografts to cover the diseased aortic segment sufficiently.

- Endografting aortas in young patients with traumatic transection is very challenging. The aortic compliance, the sharp angulated distal arch and the small aortic diameter (range of 16 to 20 millimeters) make sizing very problematic, resulting in inadequate aortic arch alignment and large oversize by up to 20%.

- Endoluminal caliber mismatching can occur in aortic dissection, with a large diameter in the proximal landing zone and a small collapsed true lumen (Fig. 2).

- There are different degrees of wall vulnerability in distinct thoracic lesions with a fragile dissection membrane in acute aortic dissection.

- Traumatic proximal bare stent anchoring at the distal arch can occur, with cases of late aortic perforation [3,4].

- There can be heavy pulsatile movements of the endograft caused by poor compliance with proximal and distal migration.

- Endograft collapse due to excessive oversizing (more than 20%) can occur, resulting in heavy graft crimping with subsequent lumen obstruction and fatal outcome.

- Manipulation inside the curved arch is associated with cerebral infarction, arch perforation or intimal injury with retrograde type A dissection.

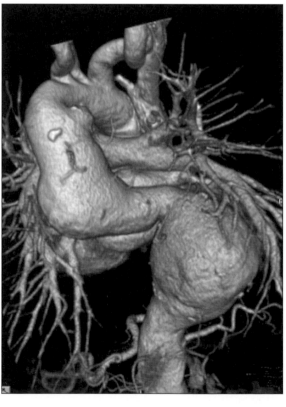

FIG. 1 Serpentine curvature in the thoracoabdominal segment of the aorta.

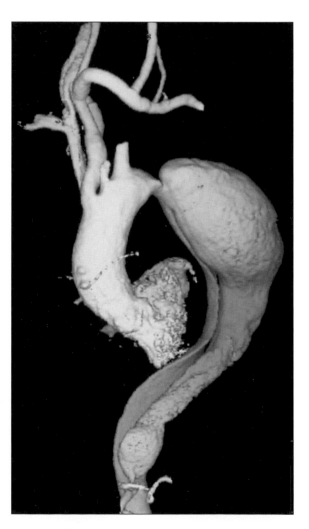

FIG. 2 Chronic expanding aortic dissection Stanford type B. Problematic endograft selection: the ideal tapered straight device is not available yet.

Characterization of the graft textile and stent frames of current thoracic endoprostheses

Almost all endoluminal stent-graft systems are designed to be placed endovascularly in the straight portion of the descending thoracic aorta and most of them are specifically designed for the endovascular treatment of aneurysms. However, some endograft systems are even contraindicated in patients treated for thoracic aneurysms where it is required to place the proximal edge of the covered stent-graft material beyond the top of the aortic arch. In our series, this was inevitable and necessary in two thirds of our patients. Creases and kinks occur when a straight tubular graft is curved and this will result in a mismatch between the graft and the aortic arch *(armadillo effect)* (Fig. 3).

The *Talent®* stent-graft (Fig. 4) is a self-expanding straight endoprosthesis composed of a polyester graft fabric and a stent scaffold made from nitinol wire. The stent is composed of a series of serpentine springs stacked in a tubular configuration. The springs are connected by full-length connecting bars, producing a flexible yet fully supported stent frame. Each stent-graft end is available with a bare uncovered spring (FreeFlo®), a graft-covered spring design (ClosedWeb®) or an alternating spring graft-covered design (OpenWeb®).

The *Talent®* system is contraindicated in patients with thoracic pathologies that require placement of the proximal edge of the covered stent-graft material beyond the top of the aortic arch. The *Talent®* endograft's Achilles heel is the proximal bare uncovered spring stent and the longitudinal con-

necting bar for supporting the stent frame. When being forced into a curved position, it is only a matter of time before these will break as a result of material fatigue. This also happened with the first generation *Excluder TAG®* which lead to a voluntary withdrawl and the relaunch of a modified device without this longitudinal backbone wire.

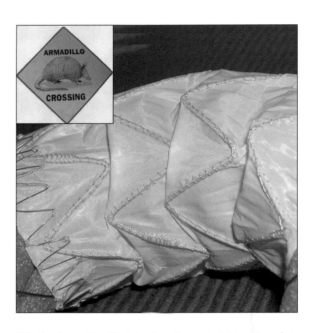

FIG. 3 *Armadillo* effect, i.e. bending a straight endograft in a curved position: the large size stents show an accordion effect with heavy crimping of the graft itself. Endografts deployed in a kinked aortic arch often show a poor opposition and alignment of the stent-graft to the wall (inner curvature) of the arch, resulting in proximal type I endoleak or late rupture at the outer curvature.

3
27

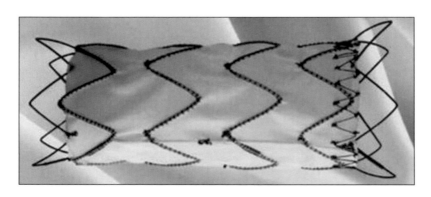

FIG. 4 The *Talent®* system (FreeFlo®).

The *Zenith*® TAA endovascular graft (Fig. 5) is a woven polyester graft supported on a skeleton of self-expandable large-size Gianturco Z-stents. At the distal and proximal graft margins, the Z-stents are attached to the inner surface, and elsewhere the stents are sutured on the external surface to reduce guidewire entanglement. A ring of proximal and distal barbs promotes active fixation. The proximal barbs protrude through the graft material, the distal barbs ring is located on an open Z-stent.

The *Zenith*® TAA endovascular graft is supplied pre-loaded in an introducer sheath with a working length of 75 centimeters. The *Zenith*® system is not recommended for heavy angulation at smaller than 45 degrees and a radius of the distal arch of smaller than 35 millimeters. The *Zenith*® endograft is preloaded in a teflon introducer sheath and secured by two locking trigger-wires (top and bottom).

The *Excluder TAG*® endograft (Fig. 6) is made of expanded polytetrafluoroethylene (ePTFE) graft material and is supported by a nitinol wire along its external surface. An ePTFE sleeve is used to constrain the endoprosthesis on the leading end of the delivery catheter. Deployment of the graft starts in the middle of the device and extends towards both ends of the graft simultaneously.

The longitudinal wire in the first generation device was used to support the columnar strength and to stabilize the graft during deployment. In 2001, W.L. Gore decided to suspend worldwide distribution after detection of wire fractures of TAG devices during follow-up of patients enrolled in the US clinical trials. These fractures were identified on X-ray films ranging from 3 to 39 months after implantation. The fracture rate within the US feasibility Study was approximately 33%.

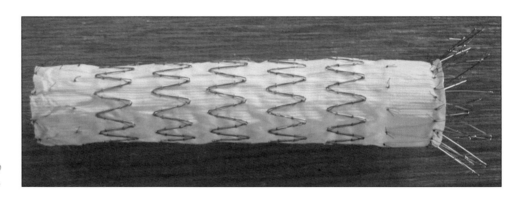

FIG. 5 The *Zenith*® TAA system.

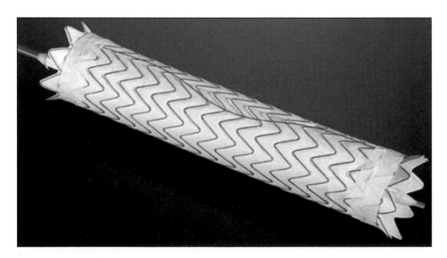

FIG. 6 The *Excluder TAG*® system.

Personal experience

Over an 8-year period in our department (Table II, III), 110 patients underwent endovascular thoracic aortic aneurysm repair. A total of 3 patients out of this subset (2.7%) had late aortic wall perforation as identified with radiographic studies or the analysis of the explanted endograft devices. The median follow-up period was 30 months, with a range from 1 to 74 months.

CASE HISTORIES OF THE THREE PATIENTS WITH LATE AORTIC WALL PERFORATION DURING FOLLOW-UP

Case 1. Mediastinal perforation with suspected chronic infection due to spine wire fracture three years after successful thoracic EVAR for post-traumatic aneurysm

A 43-year-old man (with a history of hypertension, diabetes mellitus, smoking, asymptomatic high-grade carotid artery stenosis and myocardial infarction with subsequent threefold coronary stenting)

underwent urgent thoracic stent-graft repair for a symptomatic 7-centimeter post-traumatic saccular thoracic aneurysm. He suffered from a car accident fourteen years before with subsequent undiagnosed traumatic transection. Angiography (Fig. 7) confirmed a contained ruptured aneurysm. The 3D aortic morphometry demonstrated a proximal landing zone of 34 millimeter length distal to the left subclavian with 32 millimeters in diameter suitable for endoluminal treatment. There was no documentation of growth and expansion rates available as no imaging had been performed previously. Indication for urgent treatment was based on severe chest pain lasting two weeks and the increasing size with a significant rupture risk. An *Excluder TAG®* endoprosthesis (40-200 millimeters) was deployed in general anesthesia under adenosine induced cardiac arrest via transfemoral approach. Completion angiography showed successful exclusion of the aneurysm, no endoleak and a patent left subclavian artery. Follow-up surveillance with plain chest X-ray and CT scan was performed before discharge, at 3, 6 and 12 months and then annually. The patient had

Table III	ETIOLOGY AND INDICATION FOR THORACIC ENDOGRAFTING IN 110 PATIENTS OVER AN 8-YEAR PERIOD *		
Etiology	*Elective procedure N = 48*	*Emergency procedure N = 62*
Thoracic aortic aneurysm	20	15
Anastomotic aneurysm	1	
Thoracic-abdominal aneurysm	8	3
Type A dissection		4
Type B dissection	13	17
Plaque rupture	6	
Mycotic plaque rupture		2
Traumatic rupture		9
Patch rupture		3
Aortobronchial fistula		9

* At the Department of Vascular and Endovascular Surgery, Euprecht-Karls-University, Heidelberg

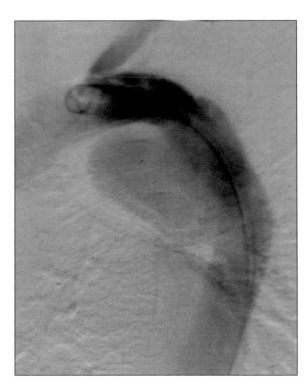

FIG. 7 Post-traumatic false saccular aneurysm in the proximal descending aorta.

an uneventful postoperative course without stent-graft migration until the 43rd postoperative month. At that time, plain X-ray and CT-reconstruction demonstrated a spine wire fracture (Fig. 8). Another 3 months later (46 months after stent-graft placement) the patient presented with back pain, elevated white blood cell count (WBC: 21000 cells/mm^3), elevated CRP (23 mg/dl), and fever (38.7°C). Blood cultures were negative. CT-images revealed an inflammatory aneurysm wall with air in the aneurysm sac (Fig. 9), suggesting chronic infection. The proximal fractured segment of the spine wire was also present in this location. An aortoesophageal fistula tract could not be proven by means of contrast enhanced crossectional imaging and endoscopic esophageal investigations. Given the fact that the patient's symptoms resolved with conservative treatment within a few days (normal WBC, CRP, no pain, no fever), that he was at high risk due to comorbidities, and that he also refused open stent-graft extraction at this time, restaging was to be redetermined after a 3-month period while the patient was put on oral antibiotics. A nuclear scan (white cell) was also discussed but not considered to be helpful at this stage. At 50 months, a CT scan (which acquired 16 simultaneous slices with a collimation of one millimeter with post processing on a Vitrea 2 workstation) confirmed persistent air around the stent-graft and spine wire fracture. The indication for surgical removal of the stent-graft was based on strong suspicion of chronic stent-graft infection in a potentially contaminated area. Staged carotid endarterectomy for a high-grade stenosis was performed before conversion.

Intraoperative findings were remarkable because of the observed chronic inflammation of a thickened aneurysm wall and a shrunk aneurysm sac. No purulent exsudate was observed around a well-incorporated graft. After proximal and distal clamping, the aorta was opened and the graft circumferentially dissected and removed carefully intact. The end of the proximal spine wire fragment extruded through the aorta (Fig. 10). Reconstruction was performed by a tube interposition with a silver coated polyester prosthesis. The stent-graft and aortic tissue cultures were sterile, despite the clinical and radiological findings. The patient was discharged home after an uncomplicated postoperative recovery. Today, he is alive and doing well after 12 months with no further adverse events.

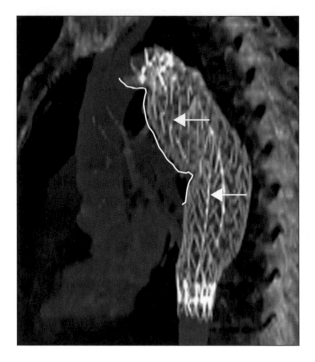

FIG. 8 CT reconstruction demonstrates *bulging/hernia* of the endograft into the former aneurysm sac (the device was severely oversized for the reasons discussed) and shows the broken spine wire *(arrows)*.

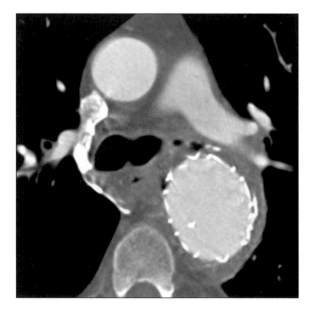

FIG. 9 CT images demonstrate an inflammatory wall reaction and air around the stent-graft as a radiological sign of chronic infection.

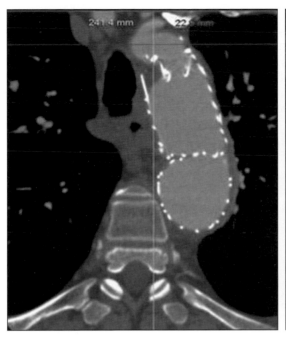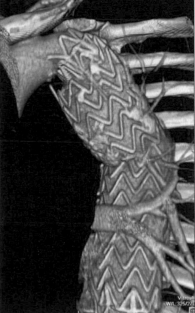

FIG. 10 Spine wire fracture with perforation of the broken wire into the mediastinum with suspected communication with the left main bronchus (air within the aneuysm sack) despite negative bronchoscopy.

Case 2. Contained ruptured type III endoleak due to infectious PTFE-material disruption three months after emergency thoracic EVAR for traumatic aortic transection

A 30-year-old male patient suffered from a violent high-speed frontal deceleration crash while driving a motor vehicle. The aortic injury was secondary to blunt chest trauma with severe lung contusion and head injury. Aortic injury was obscured by the presence of other serious injuries (polytrauma with injury severity score of 25): head trauma with open skull base fracture (orbita fracture, frontal sinus fracture with liquorrhea, complex middle face fractures); and bilateral open lower extremity fractures (open femur fracture and contralateral hip fracture). The initial chest X-ray revealed a widened mediastinum, irregularity of the aortic knob contour and presence of a left apical cap sign. The total body spiral computed tomography with three-dimensional reconstructions demonstrated a complete circumferential transection with separation of the aortic stumps. The typical rupture location was at the site of insertion of the ligamentum arteriosum. All the craniofacial, thoracic and potential abdominal injuries could be

evaluated at the same time. Immediate endovascular aortic repair followed in the hemodynamically stable patient before surgical approaches of the extremities and the craniofacial injuries. The endovascular procedure was uneventful with a complete sealing of the transection using a single *Excluder TAG®* (34-150 millimeters). In the following two weeks, eight distinct operations were performed to treat the multiple fractures. The postoperative control computed tomography scan at day 4 showed complete exclusion of the pseudoaneurysm. The left subclavian artery was intentionally covered without transposition. After complete restoration and rehabilitation, the 3-month follow-up CT scan surprisingly showed a midgraft type III endoleak (Fig. 11). At both endograft ends, a satisfactory seal could be achieved with no type I endoleak. The aortic wall was not completely healed and restored. There were also new hematoma in the mediastinum and in the pleural space. Plain X-ray studies from several angles could not detect any fracture or damage of the stent-graft. The patient had recovered without any clinical problems and was in perfect condition and he had no left arm ischemia or neurological deficits.

The indication for secondary urgent conversion was made. The intraoperative findings were astonishing and unexpected. There was a 2 x 2 centimeter abscess formation with direct contact to the endograft. In this area, the transected aortic wall was not yet healed, indicating that the endograft was directly exposed to the mediastinum. The cause for the type III endoleak detected in the CT scan was a bacterial degradation of the PTFE fabric. Analyzing the root cause for this abscess, the most likely explanation is a hematogenous infection of the residual mediastinal hematoma during the sequence of eight different craniofacial operations at the base scull with a high risk for infection. The intraoperative cultures were sterile. The endograft was explanted and the descending aorta was reconstructed using a silver-coated dacron tubegraft. The postoperative course was uneventful and two years later the patient is alive and well, without any signs of infection on the latest CT scan in July 2004.

Case 3. Contained ruptured type I proximal endoleak four years after urgent thoracic EVAR for symptomatic thoracoabdominal aneurysm

A 78-year-old woman with a prohibitive high-risk for conventional surgery (ASA III) was initially treated for a symptomatic thoracoabdominal aortic aneurysm Crawford type I with a maximal aortic diameter of 6.5 centimeters and severe back pain. In September 2001, we performed an urgent endovascular aortic reconstruction using three overlapping devices in reversed trombone technique (3 *Excluder TAG*® first generation: 40-200, 37-200 and 40-200 millimeters) with a total covered aortic length of 42 centimeters. At the 12-month follow-up CT scan, a proximal endoleak type I due to attachment zone enlargement of the proximal landing zone at the distal arch (progress of the aneurysmal disease) with endograft downstream migration was detected. To provide an adequate proximal sealing zone in the midarch segment, a partial transposition of the supra-aortic vessels was necessary. In November 2002, we planned a staged procedure: first, the supra-aortic vessel transposition (*debranching* technique to allow the placement of the endograft in the midarch position) and, in a second operation, endovascular repair with proximal extension. Via a carotid-carotid-subclavian crossover bypass (extrathoracic supraclavicular exposure), both the left subclavian and left carotid artery were transposed. Unfortunately, the general health condition deteriorated and both the patient and her general practitioner refused the planned second stage endorepair. This unusual course now provided the unique observation of the natural history of an untreated type I endoleak. In April 2004, the patient was admitted with a pulsatile tumor protruding through

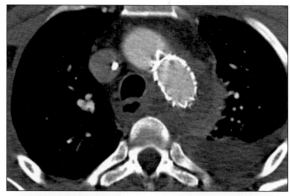
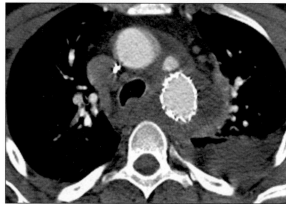
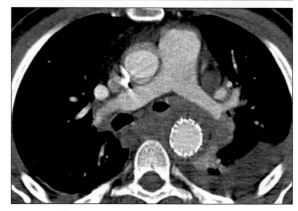

FIG. 11   3-month follow-up CT scan (A-C) showing type III endoleak with mediastinal and pleural hematoma. Perfect sealing at the proximal and distal attachment zone (no type I endoleak).

the ribs (Fig. 12). The CT scan revealed a contained aortic wall perforation about 25 centimeters distal to the proximal type I endoleak with a huge false aneurysm eroding the ribs. Despite the reduced physical condition in this 81-year-old woman, the endorepair was performed. We gained access to the heavily calcified and narrowed aortoiliac axis using a retroperitoneal approach with an aortic dacron conduit. The in-situ proximal endograft was pro-ximally extended up to the origin of the innominate artery (Fig. 12 D). However, the patient died four weeks later due to severe pneumonia.

General considerations

Endovascular repair of different thoracic pathologies [5-7] has been shown to be an attractive

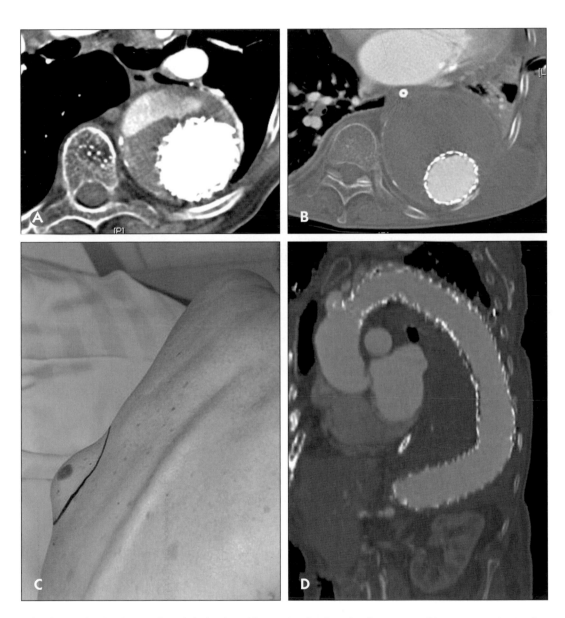

FIG. 12 A - Proximal type I endoleak after 12 months. B - Contained rupture with aneurysm protruding through the intercostal space. C - Pulsatile tumor on the back of the patient. D - Proximal endorepair showing extension to midarch after partial supra-aortic transposition.

alternative to open surgery with low periprocedural morbidity, mortality, and acceptable short-term results. However, very little is known about long-term (after 5 years) durability of both the device and the treated pathology. The Achilles'heel of endografts in the aortic position is definitely the durability of the devices. Well-described complications do exist and material fatigue requires long-term follow-up in order to assess the durability of stent-grafts and select potential patients for elective secondary conversion. Melissano et al. [8] reported on their experience with the *Endofit®* stent-graft system *(Endomed, Phoenix, AZ)* in 11 patients with subsequent conversion in 1 case due to collapse of graft-based stent fractures. In contrast to AAA endorepair, limited data on surgical conversion after thoracic endografting are available. Out of 110 patients being treated with thoracic stent-graft implantations for a variety of thoracic pathologies in our department since 1997, 6 patients needed conversion (2 primary, 4 secondary). Conversion, to some extent, can be a technically demanding procedure, especially when endografts are well incorporated and fixed in the distal arch covering the left subclavian artery. Based on our limited experience, elective planning of open stent-graft repair minimizes procedure-related complications. The presented cases further emphasize the need for consequent lifelong surveillance using standardized imaging protocols. Reports of infection involving aortic endografts are rare [9]. Multiple causes of late endograft infection are proposed: local contamination of the graft at implantation (which is not a realistic explanation of graft infection in our patient who never experienced postoperative fever or leucocytosis), and secondary infection by hematogenous spread.

There were no other infection signs over the years in our patient, who had no other wounds, ulcers or chronic bronchial infections. The search for the source of infection raised the question whether the fractured spine wire could cause an aortoesophageal and aortobronchial fistula (AEF, ABF). It is well-known that imaging studies hardly visualize AEF or ABF-tracts. It was not surprising that esophageal endoscopy and contrast enhanced fluoroscopy results were negative in our patient. The decision not to operate on the patient, when the CT scan at 47 months revealed little trapped air as indirect evidence of graft infection, was based on the fact that no clinical signs of infection were present and all cultures were negative. An aortobronchial fistula was excluded by bronchoscopy. Very little evidence for chronic stent-graft infection remains. In contrast, an inflammatory response to transmural extension of parts of the stent-graft is an alternative hypothesis and explanation for this entire process. The impact of wire form fractures in this particular case, but also in general, still remains unclear among endovascular specialists and industrial partners.

The phase II trial *(W.L. Gore, TAG)* in the USA reports an incidence of 18 wire fractures, the majority of which involve the longitudinal spine. Only one of these 18 patients required a stent-graft explant for an endoleak. Rapid response to the problem has been seen with completion of the phase III Gore study in June 2004 and the following removal of the longitudinal spine. The new Gore TAG® Thoracic Endoprosthesis *(W.L. Gore & Associates)* was released to the European market with a modified design: stronger ePTFE/FEP graft, sandwiched between existing layers, in order to provide the combination of longitudinal stiffness and device conformability and to replace the spine. The new design will offer more flexibility and sufficient radial force in kinked aneurysms and for fixation in the distal arch.

Potential causes for spine wire fracture are bending forces arising in the arch or in kinked aneurysms. Theoretically, excessive oversizing of the stent-graft may also be responsible for added stress leading to longitudinal spine fracture. Other issues which need to be considered are the sharp *herniation* of parts of the endograft into the pseudoaneurysm sac *(bulging)* and the high aortic compliance. In 1999, stent-graft oversizing was generally accepted with a margin up to 20%-25%, especially for the *Excluder TAG®* which was without active fixation and relied only on radial forces. The oversized diameter was chosen to overcome the aortic compliance, which is high in healthy walls, but not in transected or dissected aortic walls. Additionally, we had no other stent-graft size in stock in order to treat our urgent case. The patient showed no signs of rupture or drop of hemoglobin but he was considered to be symptomatic, due to ongoing severe untreatable chest pain. Even in a retrospective self-critical view, there was sufficient urgency to treat the patient and to use this oversized device.

Indication for conversion was material fatigue, partial transmural extension and risk of complete penetration of the entire endograft. The patient was young and without any risk for conversion (ASA II). Nevertheless, we retrospectively discussed the decision to convert the patient after four years. It obviously remains debatable whether a 43-year-old *(young)* patient should be treated endoluminally at all, bearing in mind that no long-term results of endovascular therapy of thoracic lesions are available. We believe, however, that the initial endovascular treatment in this patient was nevertheless justifiable because of high-risk comorbidities and an ideal aneurysm morphology. An uneventful 4-year postoperative course affirms retrospectively that decision. Thoracic endografting offers a minimally invasive alternative to patients with multiple comorbidities or traumatic injuries, especially in emergency surgery of the thoracic aorta. Long-term sequelae include endoleak, late rupture, migration, delayed retrograde aortic dissection and chronic endograft infection. The latter is of major concern, especially in patients with aortoesophageal and aortobronchial fistulas. Endografting in these patients can be considered at least as a bridging therapy.

Finally, the suspected endograft infection in this case remains uncertain. The more likely assumption is that stent-graft fatigue and an inflammatory response to longitudinal spine wire fracture and transmural extension of parts of the stent-graft caused the entire process.

Conclusion

The impact of stent-graft fatigue on long-term device stability needs to be investigated. Recognition or strong suspicion of endograft infection requires conversion with removal. Long-term follow-up after endografting is required to assess the durability of stent-grafts. Oversizing of stent-grafts in traumatic aortic rupture should not be more than 10%-15%. Better clinical results can be expected in the future given the rapid technological developments occurring in this field.

REFERENCES

1 Beebe HG. Late failures of devices used for endovascular treatment of abdominal aortic aneurysm. In: Gloviczki P (ed); *Perspectives in vascular and endovascular therapy* Vol 14, No.1. Thieme, New York 2001.

2 Bortone AS, De Cillis E, D'Agostino D, de Luca Tupputi Schinosa L. Endovascular treatment of thoracic aortic disease: four years of experience. *Circulation* 2004; 110: 262-267.

3 Breek JC, Hamming JF, Lohle PN et al. Spontaneous perforation of an aortic endoprosthesis. *Eur J Vasc Endovasc Surg* 1999; 18: 174-175.

4 Chen FH, Shim WH, Chang BC et al. False aneurysms at both ends of a descending thoracic aortic stent-graft: complication after endovascular repair of a penetrating atherosclerotic ulcer. *J Endovasc Ther* 2003; 10: 249-253.

5 Eggebrecht H, Baumgart D, Radecke K et al. Aortoesophageal fistula secondary to stent-graft repair of the thoracic aorta. *J Endovasc Ther* 2004; 11: 161-167.

6 Von Fricken K, Karamanoukian HL, Ricci M et al. Aortobronchial fistula after endovascular stent-graft repair of the thoracic aorta. *Ann Thorac Surg* 2000; 70: 1407-1409.

7 Malina M, Brunkwall J, Ivancev K et al. Late aortic arch perforation by graft-anchoring stent: complication of endovascular thoracic aneurysm exclusion. *J Endovasc Surg* 1998; 5: 274-277.

8 Melissano G, Tshomba Y, Civilini E, Chiesa R. Disappointing results with a new commercially available thoracic endograft. *J Vasc Surg* 39: 124-130.

9 Parra JR, Lee C, Hodgson KJ, Perler B. Endograft infection leading to rupture of aortic aneurysm. *J Vasc Surg* 2004; 39: 676-678.

3

35

4

PERIOPERATIVE STROKE AND PARAPLEGIA IN DESCENDING THORACIC AORTIC STENT GRAFTING

GEERT WILLEM SCHURINK, MICHIEL DE HAAN, MICHAEL JACOBS

Paraplegia and stroke are both devastating complications in the treatment of thoracic aortic pathologies. Due to several improvements in approach and technique, paraplegia and stroke rates following open thoracic and thoracoabdominal aortic repair have declined.

In open descending thoracic aortic aneurysm (TAA) and thoracoabdominal aortic aneurysm (TAAA) repair, it is recognized that the manifestation of paraplegia or paraparesis relates not only to aortic cross-clamp time, but also to multiple factors such as aortic dissection, previous aortic surgery, advanced age, preoperative renal insufficiency, diabetes, rupture, and, most significantly, aneurysm extent [1,2]. Incidence of stroke in open thoracic and thoracoabdominal surgery is about 2.5% [3]. Risk factors for stroke in open descending thoracic and thoracoabdominal aortic surgery were identified as aortic arch pathology, preexisting chronic renal failure and femoral arterial cannulation. Stroke is accompanied by a significant decrease in 3-year survival rates (43% in stroke patients vs. 85% in other patients). Stroke occurring in thoracic aortic surgery is an important risk factor for early and late mortality, particularly in patients of 70 years of age and older [4].

Endovascular repair of the thoracic aorta offers numerous advantages over open repair. Avoiding extensive surgical trauma, aortic cross-clamping and distal aortic perfusion will reduce episodes of hypotension and spinal cord reperfusion. However, despite these theoretical advantages, complications like paraplegia and stroke remain a realistic problem. By patient selection, preoperative diagnostics and implementing techniques derived from open repair, paraplegia and stroke rates after endovascular repair can probably be reduced.

Patient selection and preoperative workup

The first step in avoiding complications like stroke and paraplegia is to identify conditions and circumstances associated with a higher chance of developing these complications.

STROKE

A review of the literature identified severe aortic arch atheroma as an important risk factor for stroke. The odds ratio for stroke in patients with severe aortic arch atheroma is greater than four, and for mobile atheroma it is even greater than twelve [5]. Atheromas may also cause emboli during catheterization, balloon pump placement, and cardiopulmonary bypass. In thoracic stent grafting, the use of extra stiff guide wires and device manipulation in the aortic arch can easily dislodge atheroma, leading to cerebral and/or peripheral embolization. Imaging the aortic arch before stent-graft implantation is important in order to estimate the risk for atheroma dislodgement. Computed tomography angiography [6], magnetic resonance angiography [7], transesophageal echocardiography [8] and transcutaneus B-mode ultrasonography [9] are all validated techniques for identifying atheroma in the aortic arch.

In stent grafting of the proximal descending aorta for aneurysmal disease and dissections, the left subclavian artery is frequently covered in order to create a longer proximal sealing zone. Very little complications induced by this maneuver are reported [10,11]. It is important to identify patients in whom intentional occlusion without previous revascularization of the left subclavian artery is unwise. It is obvious that patients with patent left internal mammary - coronary bypass and left arm arteriovenous access shunts for hemodialysis will need carotid-subclavian bypass or subclavian transposition prior to stent placement. The possibility of neurological complications due to sealing off direct inflow into the left vertebral artery by covering the left subclavian artery can be elevated in cases of anatomical variations. Variations in normal anatomy in the extracranial vertebral artery are relatively frequent, ranging from asymmetry of both vertebral arteries to significant hypoplasia of one vertebral artery. The left vertebral artery diameter is often larger than the right and flow volume is significantly higher at the left side as compared to the right. Vertebral artery hypoplasia (defined as a diameter smaller than 0.22 centimeter or a flow volume of less than 30 mL/min) is not infrequent, with 7.8% at the right side and 3.8% at the left side in healthy individuals [12]. Beside these variations in normal anatomy, atherosclerotic occlusive disease of the innominate artery, proximal right subclavian artery or right vertebral artery can also be a reason for left vertebral artery dominancy.

A chronic subclavian steal syndrome due to subclavian stenosis or occlusion is usually well tolerated by the brain and arms. However, acute interruption of flow to the left subclavian artery can produce significant shunting from the carotid circulation across the posterior communicating arteries and the left vertebral artery to the left arm. This has been demonstrated in a canine model in which the subclavian artery was temporarily occluded [13]. After the occlusion, the subsequent reversal of blood flow through the left vertebral artery approximated the magnitude of normal forward flow through that vessel. Despite a compensatory increase in flow through the right vertebral and carotid arteries, the overall effect of this single manipulation was a 41% reduction in total cerebral blood flow. In the clinical situation, acute traumata of the subclavian artery leading to acute vertebrobasilar insufficiency has been reported as the cause for infarction of the occipital lobes and left internal capsule, resulting in cortical blindness with confabulation and neglect of visual deficit [14]. Both identification and quantification of vertebral artery diameter, velocities and flow volumes can be done accurately by duplex ultrasonography [15].

Left vertebral artery dominancy should be an indication for revascularization of the left subclavian artery before stent-graft deployment.

PARAPLEGIA

Paraplegia in thoracic stent grafting is induced by circulatory problems in the perfusion area of the anterior spinal artery of the spinal cord. The main causes are either embolic or as a result of direct occlusion of important inflow in the anterior spinal artery. The anterior spinal artery can receive blood supply from approximately 25 pairs of segmental arteries that arise from the aorta. In healthy individuals, in the cervical and upper thoracic region, the anterior spinal artery is supplied by multiple branches of both vertebral arteries and several radicular arteries. Usually one radicular artery provides the midthoracic spinal cord and three to five radicular arteries supply the anterior spinal artery in the lower thoracic and lumbar area. The arteria radicularis magna is the major radical spinal cord feeding artery in the thoracolumbar spinal cord (artery of Adamkiewicz) and usually arises between T8-12 (75%) and between L1-2 in only 10%. Nevertheless, this artery can originate from all segments between T5 and L5.

During the advancement of chronic aortic disease, a number of collateral pathways can develop when segmental ostia become occluded. First, segmental arteries can develop connections in the muscles along the vertebral column. Secondly, anastomoses between the anterior and posterior spinal arteries can account for some additional collateral circulation. The third collateral system is formed via the branches of the internal iliac arteries.

Considering these anatomical and pathophysiological considerations, a theoretical risk exists in occluding the left subclavian artery and subsequently blocking the most proximal inflow in the anterior spinal artery through the left vertebral artery. No cases of paraplegia due to left subclavian overstenting have been published.

One of the disadvantages of thoracic stent grafting is the inability to reattach intercostal arteries into the aortic graft. Thus, coverage of the lower intercostal arteries (T8-12) is a potential risk for disturbing spinal cord blood supply with subsequent paraplegia. However, several publications report on uncomplicated coverage of the T8-12 aortic segment [16,17] although covering an extensive part of the thoracic aorta is mentioned as a risk factor for paraplegia [18-20]. Conversion to open repair is also an event associated with increased paraplegia rate [19-21].

As previously mentioned, spinal cord blood supply frequent depends on collateral circulation in patients with a diseased aorta. For this reason, occlusion of proximal intercostal arteries, lumbar arteries and hypogastric arteries can lead to paraplegia.

The pathology of the infrarenal aorta has been recognized as a potential risk for paraplegia after endovascular treatment of the thoracic aorta. Both coexisting abdominal aortic aneurysm (AAA) and earlier repair of an AAA are associated with increased incidence of paraplegia after endovascular treatment of the thoracic aorta [21-23]. Furthermore, paraplegia is reported in several cases with concomitant endovascular repair of a thoracic aortic aneurysm and open repair of an AAA [21-24]. The Stanford University series reports endovascular treatment in 103 patients with descending TAAs [23]. Within this group, 19 patients underwent simultaneous open repair of their abdominal aortic aneurysm. Two of the 19 patients (11%) suffered from early paraplegia in contrast to one case of paraplegia in the remaining 84 patients (1%). This last patient had undergone aortic aneurysm repair in the past.

The first step in the prevention of paraplegia is the selection of patients at risk. The threshold for treating the thoracic aortic disease should be higher for this subgroup than for the low-risk group. Open repair with reattachment of intercostal arteries should be considered for patients with aneurysm morphology suitable for endovascular treatment but fit for surgery. Adjunctive protective measures can be taken for patients who undergo endovascular treatment.

Intraoperative risk management

STROKE

During the stent-graft procedure the risk of stroke can be limited by minimizing guide wire and device manipulations in the aortic arch. Pushing a partially deployed stent-graft forward or backward can dislodge atheroma and thrombus in the aorta with embolization in the cerebrovascular circulation.

Many manufacturers of stent-grafts recommend lowering the systemic blood pressure before deployment of the stent-graft in the distal aortic arch or proximal descending thoracic aorta. Even temporary asystole by infusion of adenosine has been advocated to prevent distal migration during stent-graft deployment [25,26] The influence of induced arterial hypotension during stent-graft deployment has been studied by von Knobelsdorff et al. [27]. In their study, the mean arterial pressure during deployment was decreased below 50 mmHg. Diastolic cerebral blood flow velocity during induced arterial hypotension decreased by 59%. Although neurological complications were not seen, this study shows that induced arterial hypotension has significant impact on cerebral circulation. By using stent-grafts which deploy very fast (e.g. TAG®, *W.L. Gore and Associates, Inc., Flagstaff, AZ, USA*) or devices with proximal and distal fixation to the central rod during deployment (e.g. Zenith® TX-1/TX-2, *William Cook Inc, Bloomington, IN, USA*), distal migration during deployment is minimized, indicating that hypotension is unnecessary.

For minimizing the risk of vertebral artery insufficiency, one should consider partial overstenting the subclavian artery when total overstenting is not needed for creating sufficient neck length. In our own experience, partly covered subclavian arteries at the end of the procedure will not thrombose during follow-up.

PARAPLEGIA

Cerebrospinal fluid (CSF) drainage is widely used in open thoracoabdominal aortic aneurysm repair and has proven to reduce paraplegia rate [28]. However, in endovascular treatment, CSF drainage is mainly used after paraplegia has occurred. CSF drainage has also been advised during procedures covering an extensive length of the thoracic aorta [18] and for concomitant endovascular thoracic and open abdominal aortic repair [21]. In our protocol for endovascular treatment of thoracic aortic pathology, CSF drainage is performed in patients treated for thoracic aortic aneurysms below T8 and in all patients with abdominal aortic aneurysm repair in their medical history.

Spinal cord function monitoring is a technique which is used to reduce paraplegia rate in open thoracoabdominal aortic repair [29]. Also, during thoracic endovascular procedures spinal cord function tests such as measuring motor-evoked potentials (MEP) can be performed. The problem arises when MEP-registration indicates significant spinal cord ischemia, potentially leading to paraplegia. Like in open repair, the first step is to elevate systemic blood pressure with the intention to raise the spinal cord perfusion pressure. In two of our own cases where MEPs dropped to 30% and 50% of their initial values, respectively, after deployment of thoracic stent-grafts, blood pressure elevation lead to significant improvement of the spinal cord function without postoperative paraplegia. This elevated blood pressure level is the minimal pressure to be maintained during the first postoperative days. If blood pressure management does not restore MEP-amplitudes, management of spinal cord ischemia becomes more complex. Although tried in home-made devices [30,32], no commercially available devices are available.

If blood pressure regulation does not have the desired effect, conversion to open repair, removal of the stent-graft and intercostal artery reattachment is the only chance to restore spinal cord function

[32]. However, the time necessary for conversion and reattachment of segmental arteries can be too long to prevent permanent neurological damage.

MEP-registration during temporary proximal and distal balloon exclusion of the thoracic aneurysm with axillofemoral bypass as a means of distal aortic perfusion could be a way to predict the spinal cord function outcome in these patients [33,34]. Using this technique, stent-graft placement can be abandoned in case of non-correctable spinal cord ischemia. We treated a 60-year-old man with an 8-centimeter thoracoabdominal aneurysm between a previously implanted thoracic stent-graft and an infrarenal tube graft. The stent-graft was placed two years earlier for a ruptured thoracic aneurysm (Figure, A). The tube graft was performed shortly after the rupture for a 10 centimeter infrarenal aneurysm. He could not undergo open repair because of extremely poor cardiac function. We performed an external axillofemoral bypass first to establish distal aortic perfusion during balloon occlusion at the level of the thoracic stent-graft and the infrarenal tube graft (Figure, B and C). No changes in MEP were noted during ten minutes of balloon occlusion, indicating that endovascular exclusion of the thoracoabdominal aneurysm was possible without paraplegia. Before deployment, the mesenteric and renal arteries were revascularized with grafts anastomosed to the abdominal tube graft. Postoperatively, the patient could move both legs normally.

Other methods generally used in open TAAA repair, such as administration of steroids, could also reduce the risk of paraplegia during and after endovascular repair of descending thoracic aneurysms. Our protocol for distal descending TAAs (T8-12) is almost similar to open TAAA-protocol, including CSF-drainage and administration of steroids. Also, assessment of spinal cord function by means of the MEP monitoring is carried out.

Postoperative management of neurological complications

STROKE

The incidence of postoperative stroke after endovascular treatment of thoracic aortic aneurysms and dissections varies considerably. In the largest series reported, Buffolo et al. [35] do not describe a single case of stroke in 191 patients. In publications

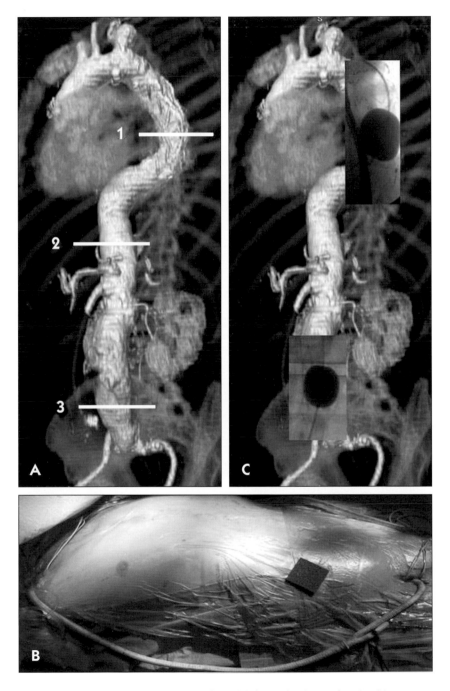

FIGURE Patient with thoracic stent-graft and infrarenal tube graft. A - Diameter at level 1 (38 millimeters), level 2 (80 millimeters) and level 3 (32 millimeters) permitted endovascular treatment. B - An external axillofemoral bypass served as distal aortic perfusion during the operation. C - Motor-evoked potentials were measured during proximal and distal aortic balloon occlusion.

reporting on perioperative stroke, incidence varies from 3% to 20% [22,23,36-44]. The recently published data from the combined experience of the EUROSTAR and United Kingdom thoracic endograft registries indicate postoperative stroke in: 2.8% in atherosclerotic aneurysms; 1.5% in aortic dissections; 2.0% in traumatic ruptures; and 0% in false aneurysms [45].

Although intra-arterial trombolysis and mechanical trombectomy are treatment options used in spontaneous stroke [46,47], there are no reports in the literature describing this approach in stroke following stent grafting of the thoracic aorta. Conservative management - including maintenance of vital signs, patency of airway, fluid and electrolyte balance, and prevention of complications like pulmonary aspiration, seizures and bedsores - are mandatory.

PARAPLEGIA

The combined experience of the EUROSTAR and United Kingdom thoracic endograft registries report postoperative paraplegia or paresis in: 4.0% in atherosclerotic aneurysms; 0.8% in aortic dissections; and 0% in traumatic ruptures and false aneurysms [45]. Most cases of paraplegia after endovascular treatment of the thoracic aorta develop after several hours up to ten weeks [18,21,22,24,48-50]. Early paraplegia is described only in cases with intraoperative complications and conversion to open repair [19,22,23]. Postoperative periods of hypotension are the main causes of delayed paraplegia in open [51] and endovascular repair of the thoracic aorta [24]. CSF-drainage can, often successfully, reverse delayed onset paraplegia [18,21,49,50,52,53]. In addition, blood pressure management after paraplegia develops can alter the outcome. A 50-year-old patient with a lower thoracic aortic rupture of his acute type B dissection was treated endovascularly. Under local anesthesia, the thoracic aorta was covered from the subclavian artery down to the level T12 using perioperative CSF-drainage and steroid administration. Four hours after the operation, the patient had a complete bilateral paraplegia of his legs. The paraplegia resolved after raising his mean blood pressure up to 160 mmHg. In a period of relative hypotension, bilateral paraplegia occurred again during the night. However, elevation of the blood pressure only improved his neurological status to the level of a unilateral paraparesis.

Conversion to open repair with reattachment of intercostal arteries is the last available option.

Again, time between the decision to convert and the moment of reestablished flow to the segmental arteries can be several hours, which is probably too long for a successful outcome. However, one case of successful conversion for delayed paraplegia after thoracic stent grafting has been reported [32].

PERSONAL EXPERIENCE

In our experience of 40 endovascular thoracic stent-graft procedures, we treated 29 thoracic aortic aneurysms, 9 acute dissections, 1 aorto esophageal fistula and 1 aorto bronchial fistula. We experienced two cases of delayed paraplegia both of which did not resolve completely. The first case concerned a 70-year-old woman with a saccular aneurysm distal to the subclavian artery. An iliac conduit was necessary because of atherosclerotic lesions in the iliac arteries. The left subclavian artery was not covered. Three days after the operation, she developed paraplegia which ultimately improved to bilateral paresis. The second patient was mentioned above.

One case of direct postoperative stroke occurred in a 71-year-old man with a saccular aneurysm directly distal to the left subclavian artery. Preoperative duplex scanning of his cerebral circulation showed no stenosis in the carotid and vertebral arteries, without dominancy. The left subclavian artery was covered during the procedure. The patient had postoperative bilateral cortical blindness. There was evidence for bilateral occipital infarction on MRI. No postoperative improvement was noted.

Conclusion

Stroke after endovascular treatment of the diseased descending thoracic aorta is not an infrequent complication. Identification of patients with higher risk is an important first step in reducing the postoperative stroke rate. Intraoperative manipulations in the aortic arch and adequate blood pressure control can further decrease stroke rate.

The risk of paraplegia after treatment of thoracic aortic pathology varies extensively and is associated with several risk factors. For patients at low risk of developing spinal cord ischemia, eventual paraplegia rarely occurs (approximately 1%). However, in patients with a compromised spinal cord collateral circulation, paraplegia risk probably compares to the risks following open thoracoabdominal repair (approximately 10%). Adjunctive measures, such as perioperative CSF drainage and blood pressure control, can improve outcome. Postoperative blood pressure control has an important role in the prevention of delayed paraplegia. Assessing spinal cord function by means of MEP potentials during stent placement can guide the application of adjunctive measures and can even influence the timing for conversion to open repair with intercostal artery reattachment.

REFERENCES

1 Safi HJ, Campbell MP, Ferreira ML et al. Spinal cord protection in descending thoracic and thoracoabdominal aortic aneurysm repair. *Semin Thorac Cardiovasc Surg* 1998; 10: 41-44.

2 Coselli JS, LeMaire SA, Miller CC, 3rd et al. Mortality and paraplegia after thoracoabdominal aortic aneurysm repair: a risk factor analysis. *Ann Thorac Surg* 2000; 69: 409-414.

3 Svensson LG, Crawford ES, Hess KR et al. Experience with 1509 patients undergoing thoracoabdominal aortic operations. *J Vasc Surg* 1993; 17: 357-368.

4 Kawachi Y, Nakashima A, Toshima Y et al. Stroke in thoracic aortic surgery: outcome and risk factors. *Asian Cardiovasc Thorac Ann* 2003; 11: 52-57.

5 Macleod MR, Amarenco P, Davis SM, Donnan GA. Atheroma of the aortic arch: an important and poorly recognised factor in the aetiology of stroke. *Lancet Neurol* 2004; 3: 408-414.

6 Konig M. Brain perfusion ct in acute stroke: current status. *Eur J Radiol* 2003; 45: S11-22.

7 Carpenter JP, Holland GA, Golden MA et al. Magnetic resonance angiography of the aortic arch. *J Vasc Surg* 1997; 25: 145-151.

8 Guo Y, Jiang X, Zhang S et al. Application of transesophageal echocardiography to aortic embolic stroke. *Chin Med J (Engl).* 2002; 115: 525-528.

9 Weinberger J, Azhar S, Danisi F et al. A new noninvasive technique for imaging atherosclerotic plaque in the aortic arch of stroke patients by transcutaneous real-time b-mode ultrasonography: an initial report. *Stroke* 1998; 29: 673-676.

10 Riambau V, Caserta G, Garcia-Madrid C et al. When to revascularize the subclavian artery in thoracic aortic stenting? In: Branchereau A, Jacobs M (eds). *Hybrid vascular procedures.* Malden, Massachusetts, Futura, Blackwell Publishing; 2004: pp 85-90.

11 Tiesenhausen K, Hausegger KA, Oberwalder P et al. Left subclavian artery management in endovascular repair of thoracic aortic aneurysms and aortic dissections. *J Card Surg* 2003; 18: 429-435.

12 Schoning M, Walter J, Scheel P. Estimation of cerebral blood flow through color duplex sonography of the carotid and vertebral arteries in healthy adults. *Stroke* 1994; 25: 17-22.

13 Reivich M, Holling HE, Roberts B, Toole JF. Reversal of blood flow through the vertebral artery and its effect on cerebral circulation. *N Engl J Med* 1961; 265: 878-885.

14 Amar AP, Levy ML, Giannotta SL. Iatrogenic vertebrobasilar insufficiency after surgery of the subclavian or brachial artery: review of three cases. *Neurosurgery* 1998; 43: 1450-1457.

15 Jeng JS, Yip PK. Evaluation of vertebral artery hypoplasia and asymmetry by color-coded duplex ultrasonography. *Ultrasound Med Biol* 2004; 30: 605-609.

16 Lambrechts D, Casselman F, Schroeyers P et al. Endovascular treatment of the descending thoracic aorta. *Eur J Vasc Endovasc Surg* 2003; 26: 437-444.

17 Heijmen RH, Deblier IG, Moll FL et al. Endovascular stent-grafting for descending thoracic aortic aneurysms. *Eur J Cardiothorac Surg* 2002; 21: 5-9.

18 Tiesenhausen K, Amann W, Koch G et al. Cerebrospinal fluid drainage to reverse paraplegia after endovascular thoracic aortic aneurysm repair. *J Endovasc Ther* 2000; 7: 132-135.

19 Greenberg R, Resch T, Nyman U et al. Endovascular repair of descending thoracic aortic aneurysms: an early experience with intermediate-term follow-up. *J Vasc Surg* 2000; 31: 147-156.

20 Carroccio A, Marin ML, Ellozy S, Hollier LH. Pathophysiology of paraplegia following endovascular thoracic aortic aneurysm repair. *J Card Surg* 2003; 18: 359-366.

21 Gravereaux EC, Faries PL, Burks JA et al. Risk of spinal cord ischemia after endograft repair of thoracic aortic aneurysms. *J Vasc Surg* 2001; 34: 997-1003.

22 Bell RE, Taylor PR, Aukett M et al. Mid-term results for second-generation thoracic stent-grafts. *Br J Surg* 2003; 90: 811-817.

23 Dake MD, Miller DC, Mitchell RS et al. The "first generation" of endovascular stent-grafts for patients with aneurysms of the descending thoracic aorta. *J Thorac Cardiovasc Surg* 1998; 116: 689-703.

24 Kasirajan K, Dolmatch B, Ouriel K, Clair D. Delayed onset of ascending paralysis after thoracic aortic stent-graft deployment. *J Vasc Surg* 2000; 31: 196-199.

25 Weigand MA, Schumacher H, Allenberg JR, Bardenheuer HJ. Adenosine-induced heart arrest for endovascular reconstruction of thoracic aneurysms of the aorta. *Anasthesiol Intensivmed Notfallmed Schmerzther* 1999; 34: 372-375.

26 Kahn RA, Moskowitz DM, Marin ML et al. Safety and efficacy of high-dose adenosine-induced asystole during endovascular AAA repair. *J Endovasc Ther* 2000; 7: 292-296.

27 von Knobelsdorff G, Hoppner RM, Tonner PH et al. Induced arterial hypotension for interventional thoracic aortic stent-graft placement: impact on intracranial haemodynamics and cognitive function. *Eur J Anaesthesiol* 2003; 20: 134-140.

28 Coselli JS, Lemaire SA, Koksoy C et al. Cerebrospinal fluid drainage reduces paraplegia after thoracoabdominal aortic aneurysm repair: results of a randomized clinical trial. *J Vasc Surg* 2002; 35: 631-639.

29 Jacobs MJ, de Mol BA, Elenbaas T et al. Spinal cord blood supply in patients with thoracoabdominal aortic aneurysms. *J Vasc Surg* 2002; 35: 30-37.

30 Watanabe Y, Ishimaru S, Kawaguchi S et al. Successful endografting with simultaneous visceral artery bypass grafting for severely calcified thoracoabdominal aortic aneurysm. *J Vasc Surg* 2002; 35: 397-399.

31 Ishimaru S, Kawaguchi S, Koizumi N et al. Preliminary report on prediction of spinal cord ischemia in endovascular stent graft repair of thoracic aortic aneurysm by retrievable stent graft. *J Thorac Cardiovasc Surg* 1998; 115: 811-818.

32 Reichart M, Balm R, Meilof JF et al. Ischemic transverse myclopathy after endovascular repair of a thoracic aortic aneurysm. *J Endovasc Ther* 2001; 8: 321-327.

33 Midorikawa H, Hoshino S, Iwaya F et al. Prevention of paraplegia in transluminally placed endoluminal prosthetic grafts for descending thoracic aortic aneurysms. *Jpn J Thorac Cardiovasc Surg* 2000; 48: 761-768.

4

43

34 Bafort C, Astarci P, Goffette P et al. Predicting spinal cord ischemia before endovascular thoracoabdominal aneurysm repair: monitoring somatosensory evoked potentials. *J Endovasc Ther* 2002; 9: 289-294.

35 Buffolo E, da Fonseca JH, de Souza JA, Alves CM. Revolutionary treatment of aneurysms and dissections of descending aorta: the endovascular approach. *Ann Thorac Surg* 2002; 74: S1815-1817.

36 Bergeron P, De Chaumaray T, Gay J, Douillez V. Endovascular treatment of thoracic aortic aneurysms. *J Cardiovasc Surg* 2003; 44: 349-361.

37 Criado FJ, Clark NS, Barnatan MF. Stent-graft repair in the aortic arch and descending thoracic aorta: a 4-year experience. *J Vasc Surg* 2002; 36: 1121-1128.

38 Ishida M, Kato N, Hirano T et al. Endovascular stent-graft treatment for thoracic aortic aneurysms: short- to midterm results. *J Vasc Interv Radiol* 2004; 15: 361-367.

39 Lepore V, Lonn L, Delle M et al. Endograft therapy for diseases of the descending thoracic aorta: results in 43 high-risk patients. *J Endovasc Ther* 2002; 9: 829-837.

40 Lonn L, Delle M, Falkenberg M et al. Endovascular treatment of type B thoracic aortic dissections. *J Card Surg* 2003; 18: 539-544.

41 Lopera J, Patino JH, Urbina C et al. Endovascular treatment of complicated type-B aortic dissection with stent-grafts: midterm results. *J Vasc Interv Radiol* 2003; 14: 195-203.

42 Neuhauser B, Perkmann R, Greiner A et al. Mid-term results after endovascular repair of the atherosclerotic descending thoracic aortic aneurysm. *Eur J Vasc Endovasc Surg* 2004; 28: 146-153.

43 Scharrer-Pamler R, Kotsis T, Kapfer X et al. Complications after endovascular treatment of thoracic aortic aneurysms. *J Endovasc Ther* 2003; 10: 711-718.

44 Scheinert D, Krankenberg H, Schmidt A. Endoluminal stent-graft placement for acute rupture of the descending thoracic aorta. *Eur Heart J* 2004; 25: 694-700.

45 Leurs LJ, Bell R, Degrieck Y et al. Endovascular treatment of thoracic aortic diseases: combined experience from the EUROSTAR and United Kingdom thoracic endograft registries. *J Vasc Surg* 2004; 40: 670-679.

46 Ng PP, Higashida RT, Cullen SP et al. Intra-arterial thrombolysis trials in acute ischemic stroke. *J Vasc Interv Radiol* 2004; 15: S77-85.

47 Berlis A, Lutsep H, Barnwell S et al. Mechanical thrombolysis in acute ischemic stroke with endovascular photoacoustic recanalization. *Stroke* 2004; 35: 1112-1116.

48 Chuter TA, Gordon RL, Reilly LM et al. An endovascular system for thoracoabdominal aortic aneurysm repair. *J Endovasc Ther* 2001; 8: 25-33.

49 Fleck T, Hutschala D, Weissl M et al. Cerebrospinal fluid drainage as a useful treatment option to relieve paraplegia after stent-graft implantation for acute aortic dissection type B. *J Thorac Cardiovasc Surg* 2002; 123: 1003-1005.

50 Hutschala D, Fleck T, Czerny M et al. Endoluminal stent-graft placement in patients with acute aortic dissection type B. *Eur J Cardiothorac Surg* 2002; 21: 964-969.

51 Maniar HS, Sundt TM 3rd, Prasad SM et al. Delayed paraplegia after thoracic and thoracoabdominal aneurysm repair: a continuing risk. *Ann Thorac Surg* 2003; 75: 113-119.

52 Fuchs RJ, Lee WA, Seubert CN, Gelman S. Transient paraplegia after stent grafting of a descending thoracic aortic aneurysm treated with cerebrospinal fluid drainage. *J Clin Anesth* 2003; 15: 59-63.

53 Oberwalder PJ, Tiesenhausen K, Hausegger K, Rigler B. Successful reversal of delayed paraplegia after endovascular stent grafting. *J Thorac Cardiovasc Surg* 2002; 124: 1259-1260.

5

ANATOMIC ANOMALIES ENCOUNTERED DURING AORTIC SURGERY

PIERRE JULIA, CHARLES PIERRET
CHRISTIAN LATRÉMOULLE, JEAN-NOËL FABIANI

The most important anatomic anomalies encountered during aortic surgery are venous and renal variations. If unnoticed during preoperative assessment, these anomalies can be the cause of major intraoperative complications, such as massive bleeding due to venous injury.

At present, anatomic anomalies are most often identified by computer tomography (CT) scanning and are preoperatively analyzed, even resulting in modified surgical strategies and adapting surgical access. Sometimes, these anomalies are discovered during the procedure, either because preoperative assessment was limited or the radiologists and surgeons did not notice the abnormalities. In these cases, immediate analysis is necessary and the procedure must be modified according to differences in anatomy.

Venous anomalies

EMBRYOLOGY

The development of the inferior vena cava system is a complex process which arises between the sixth and eighth weeks of gestation. Three distinct venous systems develop and subsequently regress partially, leading to the constitution of the final venous system: the posterior cardinal veins are followed by the more interior subcardinal veins and then, located between the previous sets, the supra

cardinal veins. The connections form and develop between these three systems: intercardinal, intersubcardinal, cardino-subcardinal and sub-supracardinal anastomoses. The latter forms a periaortic venous circle and, subsequently, the renal veins. Two renal veins develop at each site: a ventral and dorsal vein. The retro-aortic dorsal vein most frequently degenerates and the final renal vein develops from the ventral vein. The posterior cardinal veins which develop behind the aorta will regress and only persist as part of the ilio-caval confluence. If the left supra cardinal vein regresses, the right supra cardinal vein increases its caliber to form the infrarenal portion of the inferior vena cava (IVC), located at the right side of the aorta. Its cranial portion forms the azygos vein. The main venous anomalies encountered during aortic surgery are attributable to alterations in this embryologic development.

ANOMALIES OF THE INFERIOR VENA CAVA

Two principle types can be distinguished: the double IVC and the left IVC. The double IVC results from a defect regression of the left supracardinal system and leads to formation of two infrarenal IVC, the incidence of which is approximately 0.2% to 3% (Fig. 1) [1]. The right IVC usually has the greatest diameter and the left IVC lies anterior to the aorta (in rare occasions, posterior to the aorta) at the level of the renal veins [2]. The left IVC results from the persistence of the left supra cardinal vein with regression of the right supra cardinal vein, the incidence of which is between 0.2% and 0.5% (Figs. 2, 3). Following an ascending route left to the infrarenal aorta, the left IVC most often crosses the anterior side of the abdominal aorta at the level of the renal veins after connection of the left renal vein. Thus, it finds a normal position at the right side of the aorta, after the connection of the right renal vein. In very rare cases, the left IVC can cross the posterior side of the aorta with substantial risks of venous injury during surgery. In patients with a left IVC, the iliac venous confluence is located behind the left common iliac artery rather than behind the right common iliac artery as in a normal situation. This anatomic variant is important if iliac artery clamping is performed.

Different but rarer anomalies might be encountered, such as a retrocaval ureter, occurring with a prevalence of 1/1000 [2]. In this case, a right ureter initially descends behind the IVC, crosses posteriorly at the level of L2 and reroutes at its left position, finally at its anterior side [3].

A preaortic iliac venous confluence can be due to a left IVC crossing the aorta anteriorly just above its bifurcation and immediately rejoining the right IVC [4], or at the union of both common iliac veins anterior to the aortic bifurcation (Fig. 4) [5,6].

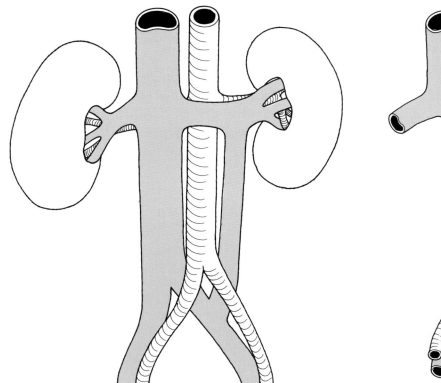

FIG. 1 Duplication of the inferior vena cava.

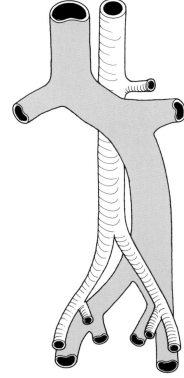

FIG. 2 Left inferior vena cava

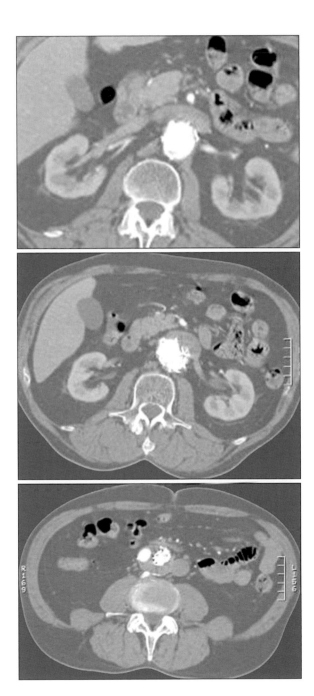

FIG. 3 Patient with a left inferior vena cava and aortic endograft.

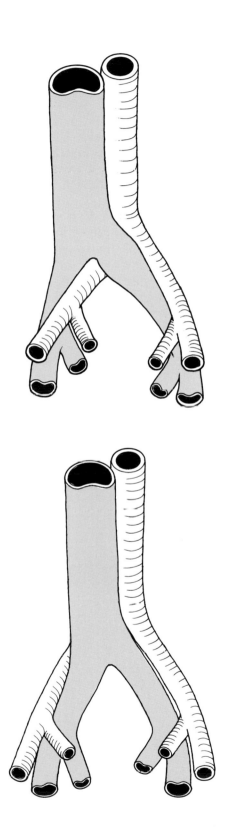

FIG. 4 Schematic drawing of two types of preaortic venous confluence.

5

47

Finally, the extension of the azygos or hemiazygos of the IVC corresponds to the absence of the suprarenal IVC and has been associated with cardiac malformations and disorders in venous return [7]. Isolated forms, however, occur very rarely. The renal segment of the IVC drains the renal venous blood and crosses the diaphragm behind the fibrous portion to enter the thorax as the azygos vein [8]. This anomaly is especially important to detect prior to surgery with extra corporeal circulation or cardiac catheterization.

ANOMALIES OF RENAL VEINS

These anomalies are caused by disorders in the development of the initial venous aortic neck (Fig. 5). The latter is formed by anastomoses between the subcardinal veins located in front of the aorta and the posterior supracardinal veins located behind the aorta. The definitive renal veins are formed from these transversal anastomoses.

The retro-aortic position of the left renal vein occurs in 2% to 3% of patients and represents an important variant. Two main types are distinguished [9,10]:
- type I is due to the persistence of the left sub-supracardinal and inter-supracardinal anastomoses with disappearance of the ventral renal vein. Therefore, a left renal vein crosses behind the aorta at the level L2;
- type II is caused by the persistance of the left sub-supracardinal and left supracardinal vein anastomoses. The renal vein crosses behind the abdominal aorta at the level of L4/L5 and receives the gonadic vein and the ascending lumbar vein.

The existence of two left renal veins, one in a normal anterior position and one behind the aorta, is due to the persistence of the two portions of the venous periaortic neck (Fig. 6). The incidence of this anomaly is variable, depending on the size of the retro-aortic vein: in fact, if all vessels (even the

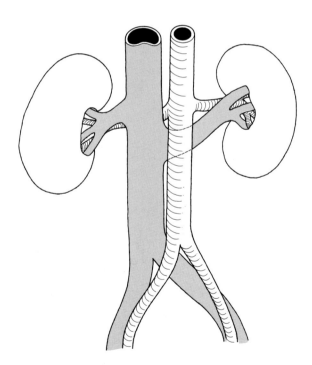

FIG. 5 Left retroaortic renal vein.

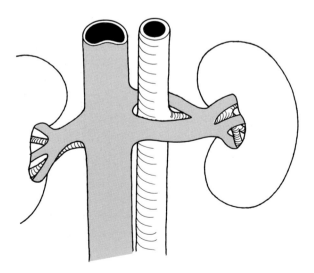

FIG. 6 Persistance of periaortic venous neck.

smaller ones) are included it can reach 16% whereas it only occurs in 8% if only the major veins are considered. The anomaly is caused by the persistance of the inter-supracardinal and left supracardinal anastomoses as one part and of the left dorsal vein as another part. The retro-aortic vein usually follows a right-sided and low oblique route, to connect to the IVC below the ostium of the right renal vein.

Prior to routine preoperative CT scanning, the major risk of these venous anomalies was the intraoperative discovery at the moment that a severe and dangerous bleeding occurred [11,12]. Currently, the accurate preoperative CT images should allow one to identify the majority of these anomalies (Fig. 7) [13]. Contrast enhanced spiral CT scanning is highly accurate to visualize these anomalies [14], but is not systematically performed prior to all aortic surgical procedures, especially in occlusive lesions. Duplex scanning might be insufficient to detect such venous variants [15].

Two large retrospective studies have used CT scanning to analyze congenital venous anomalies and found that the observed anomalies were in concordance with those described in the classic autopsy studies [16,17]. The only important difference concerned the double IVC, which can be explained by the small diameter of the left IVC, less visible at CT scanning. However, CT scanning (even without contrast) is not systematically performed prior to all aortic procedures, especially occlusive lesions, and duplex scanning is not sensitive enough to detect these anomalies [18]. Finally, most patients presenting with a ruptured aneurysm being hemodynamically instable are operated on without preoperative CT scan and such venous anomalies are, therefore, discovered during surgery. It is also possible that the venous anomaly remains unrecognized on CT scanning because the surgeon's and radiologist's attention is focused on the aneurysm and hematoma [6].

In all these cases, knowledge of these anomalies and careful surgical dissection will reduce the incidence of venous injuries [19].

A retro-aortic left renal vein should be suspected if dissection shows absence of the left renal vein at the anterior site of the aorta. The danger is causing venous injury when encircling the aortic neck in aneurysm surgery or the infrarenal aorta in occlusive lesions. The rule is that if the left renal vein is not visualized at its normal position, a venous anomaly should be suspected and the surgeon should avoid blind maneuvers at the posterior side of the aorta. Simple dissection at the lateral borders of the aorta down to the spine will normally be enough to place a cross-clamp. This limited access reduces the risk of venous injury considerably because the retro-aortic vein usually crosses the aorta much lower (L4-L5) than the site of clamping.

There are, however, cases in which the retro-aortic vein is located at the level of clamping, especially in ruptured aneurysms. Serious venous injury can occur with subsequent dramatic results [12,20]. Adequate venous repair is only possible after complete transection of the infrarenal aorta, which obviously requires a rapid decision. Control and hemostasis

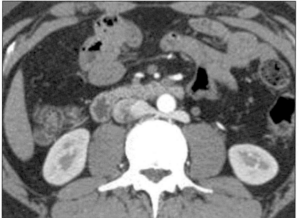 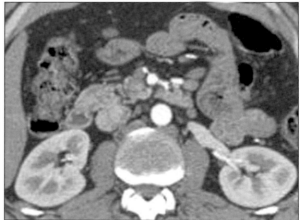

FIG. 7   CT scan showing a left retro-aortic renal vein at th level L4.

can be obtained by proximal and distal venous compression. The risk of injuring a left retro-aortic vein increases in surgical procedures of inflammatory aneurysms [21] because of the associated dissection problems in the fibrous tissue.

A double left renal vein is more misleading because the surgeon will find a left renal vein at its orthotopic position. However, the small diameter of this vein and its adherence to the aorta should alert the surgeon. Infrarenal aortic control should be performed proximal or distal to this venous circle, realizing that the posterior vein is often located lower. These details can be assessed at preoperative CT scanning. However, if this is not performed, an increased risk in injuring the posterior branche is evident [22].

A double IVC does not cause specific problems because it is often recognized at preoperative CT scanning. The left IVC can be transected before its junction with the left renal vein. The latter drains into the right IVC. Another option can be to transect the left renal vein anterior to the aorta; it will subsequently drain in the distal left IVC [20].

The left IVC can cause more complex technical problems if it crosses the aorta at an aneurysm neck [23]. Sufficient access to the aortic neck can be achieved by extensive dissection of these large venous structures [24]. In inflammatory aneurysms, a left IVC is more dangerous because it can be fused in the fibrous process and, therefore, unrecognizable during preoperative CT scanning. Accidental injury can occur when the aneurysm is opened, which is even more difficult to repair because of the fibrous shell [25]. Sometimes the left IVC and left renal vein can be partially mobilized in order to obtain sufficient access to clamp the aorta. In other cases, the simplest solution consists of transecting the right renal vein flush to the IVC (equivalent to transecting the left renal vein in normal situations). As in normal procedures, repairing the renal vein at the end of the procedure is recommended. However, the vein can be ligated if there is no renal failure and all collateral branches are preserved.

Renal anomalies

Renal anatomic anomalies likely to interfere with abdominal aortic surgery can basically be devided in two types: ectopic kidneys (especially pelvic and iliac kidneys) and horseshoe kidneys.

Ectopic kidneys result from disturbed ascension of the kidney between the fourth and eighth gestational weeks [26]. The incidence is 1/2000 to 1/3000 and these are more frequently located at the left side. Associated renal fusion anomalies do not occur but arterial variations are numerous: one or two arteries originating from the distal aorta or iliac arteries (Fig. 8). Because of this, additional arterial reimplantation during aortic repair is often required [27]. The ureters are short and enter the bladder without crossing the mid-line. A crossed ectopic kidney is a rare anomaly (1/7000) and is defined by a kidney which is located opposite to insertion of its ureter in the bladder [28] and associated kidney fusion anomalies frequently occur.

The main risks of ectopic kidneys are intraoperative vascular or ureter injury due to inadequate preoperative imaging. Assessment should, therefore, be completed using CT scanning, arteriography and, if necessary, intravenous urography. These investigations do not guarantee complete information but unidentified abnormal arteries at arteriography might be discovered during the procedure [28,29].

The most dangerous postoperative complication is renal failure, caused by insufficient renal protection during aortic cross-clamping. Several protective measures have been described. The most frequently applied technique at present is described by Lacombe [30], in which double proximal clamping is combined with infusion of cold Ringer's lactate [26] (Fig. 9). Efficient results can be obtained if ischemia is reduced to less than one hour. Double aortic clamping can also be combined with a temporary shunt in case of distal ectopic kidney revascularization [29]. These renal protection techniques for pelvic kidneys are similar to those applied in aortoiliac reconstructions in patients with kidney transplants. Horseshoe kidneys result from anomalies in the process of rotation and ascension of the metarenal masses, associated with a fusion of both kidneys, most frequently of the inferior lobe [31]. The isthmus fusing both kidneys can be rather fibrous but often contains viable parenchyma. The ureters cross anterior to this isthmus. The renal pelvis can have an asymmetric development and come in contact with the isthmus. For some surgeons, the risk of injury and subsequent urinary fistula represents a contraindication to transect the isthmus [32]. Arterial anomalies frequently occur (60%-80% of cases) and are ideally depicted by contrast enhanced scanning or selective arteriography

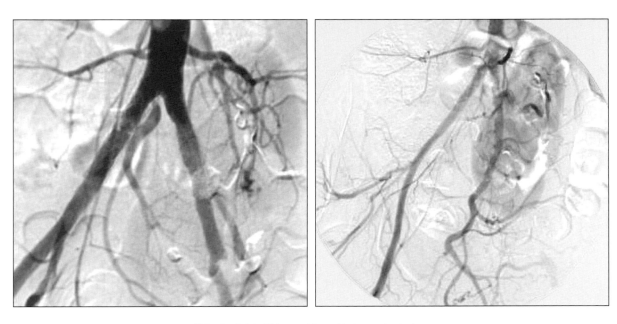

FIG. 8   Pelvic kidney with multiple renal arteries.

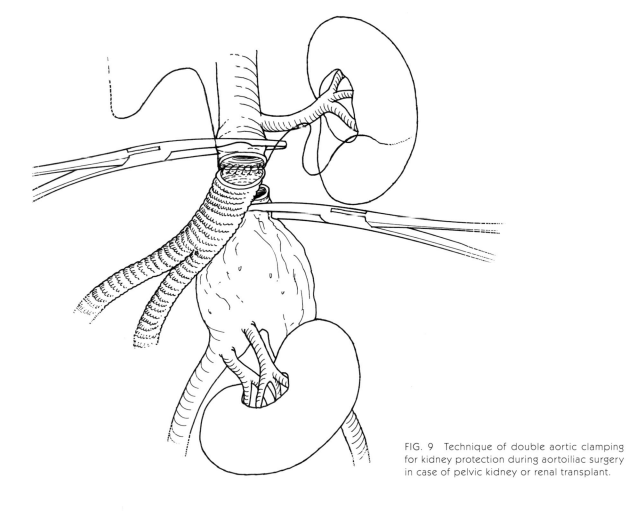

FIG. 9   Technique of double aortic clamping for kidney protection during aortoiliac surgery in case of pelvic kidney or renal transplant.

in order to visualize the territories of each individual branche.

In abdominal aortic aneurysm (AAA) surgery, accurate preoperative assessment of this vascularization is essential to define the operative strategy. A simplified classification has been proposed by Lesage et al. [33]:
- Group I: all renal arteries originate above the aneurysm;
- Group II: two dominant renal arteries originate from the aneurysm and are associated with polar arteries or arteries from the isthmus;
- Group III: one or two dominant renal arteries originate from the aneurysm.

Patients in Group I should be operated via anterior transperitoneal access whereas patients in Groups II and III should be treated by the retroperitoneal approach. In cases where the horseshoe kidney is discovered during surgery (most frequently in ruptured AAA), transection of the isthmus and ligation of the accessory renal arteries seem to reduce morbidity by making the vascular repair easier.

Arterial anomalies

Separate from the renal artery anomalies described above, one may be confronted with iliac artery anomalies during aortic surgery. Two cases have been described in which the iliac artery was located behind the psoas muscle [34,35]. One of these was associated with a preaortic confluence, possibly due to an anomaly between the umbilical artery and the fourth lumbar artery. Preoperative CT scanning should allow one to notice this anomaly, but this variation should be considered during surgery if the common iliac artery is not at its usual position.

Conclusion

Knowledge of the different anatomic anomalies which can be encountered during aortic surgery is essential in order to reduce the incidence of complications. Current practice is determined by preoperative CT scanning, which has substantially diminished the risk of venous injury, as compared to the historical series of Brener et al. [12]. Intraoperative discoveries, however, still exist, mainly in urgent procedures. In these cases, prudent and limited dissection, associated with knowledge of the possible anomalies should allow the surgeon to avoid serious complications.

REFERENCES

1 Giordano JM, Trout HH 3rd. Anomalies of the inferior vena cava. *J Vasc Surg* 1986; 3: 924-928.
2 Mathews R, Smith PA, Fishman EK, Marshall FF. Anomalies of the inferior vena cava and renal veins: embryologic and surgical considerations. *Urology* 1999; 53: 873-880.
3 Shindo S, Kobayashi M, Kaga S et al. Retrocaval ureter and preaortic iliac venous confluence in a patient with an abdominal aortic aneurysm. *Surg Radiol Anat* 1999; 21: 147-149.
4 Ruemenapf G, Rupprecht H, Schweiger H. Preaortic iliac confluence: a rare anomaly of the inferior vena cava. *J Vasc Surg* 1998; 27: 767-771.
5 Baldridge ED Jr., Canos AJ. Venous anomalies encountered in aortoiliac surgery. *Arch Surg* 1987; 122: 1184-1188.
6 Schiavetta A, Cerruti R, Cantello C et al. Marsupial cava and ruptured abdominal aortic aneurysm: a case report and review of the literature. *J Vasc Surg* 1998; 28: 719-722.
7 Pillet J, Chevalier JM, Enon B et al. Les variations d'origine embryologique de la veine cave inférieure. In: Kieffer E (ed). *Chirurgie de la veine cave inférieure et de ses branches*. Paris, Expansion Scientifique Francaise 1985: pp 105-116.
8 Bass JE, Redwine MD, Kramer LA et al. Spectrum of congenital anomalies of the inferior vena cava: cross-sectional imaging findings. *Radiographics* 2000; 20: 639-652.
9 Karkos CD, Bruce IA, Thomson GJ, Lambert ME. Retroaortic left renal vein and its implications in abdominal aortic surgery. *Ann Vasc Surg* 2001; 15: 703-708.
10 Hoeltl W, Hruby W, Aharinejad S. Renal vein anatomy and its implication for retroperitoneal surgery. *J Urol* 1990; 143: 1108-1114.
11 Bartle EJ, Pearce WH, Sun JH, Rutherford RB. Infrarenal venous anomalies and aortic surgery: avoiding vascular injury. *J Vasc Surg* 1987; 6: 590-593.
12 Brener BJ, Darling RC, Frederick PL, Linton RR. Major venous anomalies complicating abdominal aortic surgery. *Arch Surg* 1974; 108: 159-165.
13 Gomes MN, Choyke PL. Assessment of major venous anomalies by computerized tomography. *J Cardiovasc Surg* 1990; 31: 621-628.
14 Kudo FA, Nishibe T, Miyazaki K et al. Left renal vein anomaly associated with abdominal aortic aneurysm surgery: report of a case. *Surg Today* 2003; 33: 609-611.
15 Rispoli P, Ortensio M, Cassatella R et al. Anomalies of the inferior vena cava in patients treated with surgical vascular procedures in the aorto iliac area. Report of 2 cases and review of the literature. *Minerva Cardioangiol* 2001; 49: 141-146.

16 Aljabri B, MacDonald PS, Satin R et al. Incidence of major venous and renal anomalies relevant to aortoiliac surgery as demonstrated by computed tomography. *Ann Vasc Surg* 2001; 15: 615-618.

17 Trigaux JP, Vandroogenbroek S, De Wispelaere JF et al. Congenital anomalies of the inferior vena cava and left renal vein: evaluation with spiral CT. *J Vasc Interv Radiol* 1998; 9: 339-345.

18 Hingorani A, Ascher E. Dyeless vascular surgery. *Cardiovasc Surg* 2003; 11: 12-18.

19 Nonami Y, Yamasaki M, Sato K et al. Two types of major venous anomalies associated with abdominal aneurysmectomy: a report of two cases. *Surg Today* 1996; 26: 940-944.

20 DeLaurentis DA, Calligaro KD, Savarese RP. Anomalies veineuses compliquant la chirurgie des anévrysmes de l'aorte abdominale. In: Kieffer E (ed). *Les anévrysmes de l'aorte abdominale sous-rénale.* Paris, AERCV 1990: pp 287-294.

21 Shindo S, Kubota K, Kojima A et al. Anomalies of inferior vena cava and left renal vein: risks in aortic surgery. *Ann Vasc Surg* 2000; 14: 393-396.

22 Toda R, Iguro Y, Moriyama Y et al. Double left renal vein associated with abdominal aortic aneurysm. *Ann Thorac Cardiovasc Surg* 2001; 7: 113-115.

23 Bastounis E, Maltezos C, Kaponis A et al. Abdominal aortic aneurysm and left sided inferior vena cava. A case report. *Int Angiol* 1995; 14: 229-232.

24 Tsukamoto S, Shindo S, Obana M et al. Operative management of abdominal aortic aneurysm with left-sided inferior vena cava. *J Cardiovasc Surg* 2000; 41: 287-290.

25 Gargiulo M, Stella A, Caputo M et al. Anomalies of the subrenal inferior vena cava in the surgery of non-specific and inflammatory abdominal aortic aneurysms. *Phlebologie* 1993; 46: 489-495.

26 Hollis HW, Rutherford RB, Crawford GJ et al. Abdominal aortic aneurysm repair in patients with pelvic kidney. Technical considerations and literature review. *J Vasc Surg* 1989; 9: 404-409.

27 Glock Y, Blasevich R, Laghzaoui A et al. Abdominal aortic aneurysm and congenital pelvic kidney. A rare association. *Tex Heart Inst J* 1997; 24: 131-133.

28 Yano H, Konagai N, Maeda M et al. Abdominal aortic aneurysm associated with crossed renal ectopia without fusion: case report and literature review. *J Vasc Surg* 2003; 37: 1098-1102.

29 Schneider JR, Cronenwett JL. Temporary perfusion of a congenital pelvic kidney during abdominal aortic aneurysm repair. *J Vasc Surg* 1993; 17: 613-617.

30 Lacombe M. Abdominal aortic aneurysmectomy in renal transplant patients. *Ann Surg* 1986; 203: 62-68.

31 O'Hara PJ, Hakaim AG, Hertzer NR et al. Surgical management of aortic aneurysm and coexistent horseshoe kidney: review of a 31-year experience. *J Vasc Surg* 1993; 17: 940-947.

32 Faggioli G, Freyrie A, Pilato A et al. Renal anomalies in aortic surgery: contemporary results. *Surgery* 2003; 133: 641-646.

33 Lesage R, Vignes B, Bahnini A et al. Anévrysmes de l'aorte abdominale et anomalies rénales congénitales. In: Kieffer E (ed). *Les anévrysmes de l'aorte abdominale sous-rénale.* Paris, AERCV 1990: pp 319-335.

34 Vohra R, Leiberman DP. An anomalous right iliac artery presenting as iliac stenosis. *Eur J Vasc Surg* 1991; 5: 209-211.

35 Sonneveld DJ, van Dop HR, van der Tol A. Anomalous retropsoas iliac artery in a patient with an abdominal aortic aneurysm. *Eur J Vasc Endovasc Surg* 1998; 16: 85-86.

6

CROSS-CLAMPING OF THE DISEASED THORACIC AND ABDOMINAL AORTA

ROBERTO CHIESA, GERMANO MELISSANO
ENRICO MARIA MARONE, YAMUNE TSHOMBA, CHIARA BRIOSCHI
EFREM CIVILINI, FRANCESCO SETACCI, LUCA BERTOGLIO
FABIO MASSIMO CALLAIRI, LUCA DEL GUERCIO, GABRIELE DUBINI

The development of vascular surgery has been made possible by several technological breakthroughs such as the introduction of heparin, vascular grafts and also through the manufacturing of appropriate instruments, most importantly vascular clamps. We owe the idea of instruments suitable for clamping vessels with the least possible damage to the tissues to the ingenuity of surgeons such as DeBakey, Dardick, Dubost, Fogarty and many others.

In spite of several decades of continuous efforts in order to improve the design and the materials of vascular clamps, we must admit that even the most atraumatic instrument may still be traumatic at some level, especially on the diseased vessels that occur in our surgical practice. It was only at the end of the last century that techniques were developed for reconstructing and anastomosing arteries [1]. Atraumatic vascular clamps were, therefore, required to prevent arterial lesions.

Until 1897, there had been only occasional, often unsuccessful, reports dealing with vascular sutures when John B. Murphy published his invagination technique requiring clamping of the vessel on both sides. In 1902, Alexis Carrel published his work dealing with vessel anastomosis with a circular non-interrupted vascular suture. In 1903, Edmund Hopfner developed the first atraumatic clamp specifically developed for vascular surgery. This instrument was about 15 centimeters long and its spring steel jaws were separated in the middle, graduated towards the ends and rubber-coated. Hopfner used this clamp during his studies at the University of Berlin for clamping of arteries temporarily to perform end-to-end anastomoses in dogs. His atraumatic vascular clamps were copied, commonly used and sold by various companies until the 1960s. Erns Jeger and Rudolf Stitch later modified the shape of this vascular clamp [2].

The construction of tangential holding vascular clamps for the partial occlusion of vessels to allow partial blood flow for reconstruction or side-to-side anastomosis of large vessels started only after the development of atraumatic straight vessel clamps at the beginning of this century. The first surgeon who developed a tangential holding vascular clamp was Friedrich Trendelenburg in 1907. He used it during pulmonary artery embolectomy. After removal of the pulmonary embolus via arteriotomy, tangential clamping allowed arterial repair [3]. In 1925, Arthur W. Meyer observed that the Trendelemburg vascular clamp was too broad and allowed only insufficient blood flow and, therefore, he modified its angle. The tangential vascular clamp developed by Trendelemburg and later modified by Meyer is the ancestor of modern side clamps (Satinsky, Derra, Cooley and DeBakey).

The introduction of new materials and technologies borrowed from the military and space industries in more recent years allowed the development of new high quality surgical instruments.

Injury from vascular clamps

Temporary local vascular control may be achieved by occluding tapes, intra-arterial balloons or clamps. Although these methods are designed to prevent morphological damage, unfortunately none of them is entirely atraumatic. Intimal lesions may determine success or failure of an otherwise technically successful surgical procedure. Traumatic disruption of the intima can result in thrombosis, embolization, flap formation, dissection, accelerated local atherosclerosis, fibroproliferative stenosis and pseudoaneurysm formation. Therefore it is prudent to seek the least traumatic means of vascular occlusion. Conventional vessel clamps and snares often compress the vessel wall more than is needed and subsequently cause tissue injury [4,5].

Occlusive devices have been classified according to Moore and Bunt [6] in six classes:
1 - crossmembered metallic clamps (non-serrated jaws, non-coiciding serrated jaws and interdigitating serrated jaws),
2 - spring-loaded opposing clamps,
3 - crossmembered metallic clamps with protective surfaces,
4 - loop tourniquets,
5 - intraluminal balloon occluders,
6 - miscellaneous (Berlin clamp, Dunn inflatable occluder and Adler).

These authors also classified arterial injury in six classes [7]:
0 - no injury,
1 - endothelial imprint without disruption,
2 - separation of endothelium, 3 millimeter intimal flap,
3 - endothelial denudation, exposed subendothelium, endothelial shredding,
4 - medial laceration, medial hemorrhage and necrosis,
5 - adventitial laceration or crush,
6 - arterial disruption, dissection and pseudoaneurysm.

Class I vascular clamps exert strong forces at the jaws with steadily increasing forces as the size of the vessel increases. The serration of the jaws necessary for accurate holding is often associated with deep medial penetrations and medial injuries. Often the holding pressure is adequate at the lowest ratchet closure and, therefore, it should be utilized. Use of these clamps should be restricted to situations in which holding power is mandatory or large vessels where other methods may not provide control.

Class II vascular clamps are relatively non-damaging. The clamp should be used with the least applied force to obtain reliable occlusion. The use of these clamps is limited by elastic resilience, or the fibrous resistance of larger or diseased vessels that may prevent adequate occlusion.

Class III clamps have a low injury potential because of decreased applied force without concentration at discrete sites. The disadvantage of these instruments is the reduced holding power.

Class IV occluders provide adequate occlusion of small to medium size vessels with little injury because the loop is sufficiently wide to disperse the applied force. Their use is simple but if control cannot be obtained gently it is better to use another occlusive device.

Class V occluders are appropriate for the rapid and easy intraluminal control of aneurysm or pseudoaneurysm and obviating the proximal and distal dissection for standard circumferential control in redo surgery. The major problem of these devices is the difficult direct control over potential arterial injury by the surgeon. Dobrin defined six potential lesions from balloon catheters: puncture of the distal artery; arterial disruption by overdistention of the vessel wall; antegrade dissection of an atherosclerotic plaque with flap, thrombosis or dissection; intimal flap raised during retrograde introduction of the catheter; balloon rupture with embolization; and detachment of the balloon. Care in introduction of the catheter, direct visualization of the lumen of the vessel and non-forceful advancement are critical to avoid lesions.

From the pathological point of view, the effects of placing a variety of vascular clamps have been extensively studied.

Henson and Rob in 1956 studied the effects of crossmembered vascular clamps and loops tourniquets. They observed that all class I clamps and 2-0 silk looped as a tourniquets inflicted severe medial and endothelial injury to the vessels and theorized that arterial injury was related to concentration of applied force on a small surface area of the vessel.

Hickman and Mortenson in 1981 observed how increased severity of injury was caused by increasing closure of the clamp. Harvey and Gough in 1981 noted that the holding pressure with some class I clamps was obtained at minimal ratchet closure, while class III clamps required maximal occlusive pressure to obtain adequate holding pressure. They confirmed, however, the severe patterns of injury associated with class I clamps but not with class III clamps.

Successive studies of Guidoin et al. [8] observed how initial endothelial injuries were accompanied by fibrin and platelet deposition, medial necrosis, hemorrhage and inflammatory exudates.

In 1999, Moore et al. [9] observed how fundamental clamp design dictates the magnitude of applied transmural force required for cessation of flow and how intensity and the vectors of that force are directly responsible for the degree of resultant intimal injury. The intima appears to possess an injury threshold of approximately $5 \times 10e4$ dynes/cm^2.

In conclusion, clamp geometry, closing force, holding ability, type of vessel and duration of clamping are important factors determining vascular trauma.

Computational finite element study of arterial clamping

Arterial compression during clamping may lead to injuries of the vessel wall with different short- and long-term complications. We performed a computational finite element study in order to evaluate the different behavior between a healthy and a calcified artery during clamping and to understand how the variation of the aortic state pressure, the internal aortic diameter and the size of the clamp could lead to a stress change (Fig. 1).

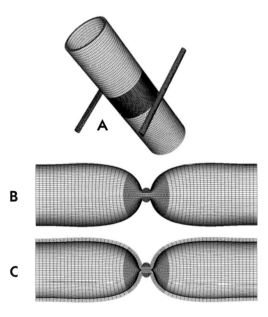

FIG. 1 Geometry of computational model of the aorta in its initial configuration (A) and following aortic clamping in front view (B) and sectional view (C).

In the first phase of this study, the aim was to analyze the stress change on the arterial wall using different pressures (Fig. 2) and to evaluate the difference between a healthy and a calcified aorta (Fig. 3). For this group, an aorta with an internal diameter of 25 millimeters a thickness of 3 millimeters and a length of 150 millimeters was considered. The clamp size was 6 millimeters.

In the second phase we analyzed the influence of the aortic diameter (from 15 to 40 millimeters). For this group a physiological vessel with a thickness of 3 millimeters, a length of 150 millimeters, and a clamp dimension of 6 millimeters were considered.

In the third phase we analyzed the influence of the dimension of the clamp (from 3 to 6 millimeters). For this group, a physiological vessel with a thickness of 3 millimeters, a length of 150 millimeters, a diameter of 25 millimeters and a vessel pressure of 100 mmHg were considered.

Computational simulations have been performed by the commercial finite element code ABAQUS/Explicit *(ABAQUS Inc., RI, USA)* [10].

The area subjected to the most stress is the part compressed by the clamp, as expected. In the first phase, it appeared that in a calcified aorta, the arterial wall is more stressed when compared to a healthy aorta (Fig. 2). The highest stresses are on the internal aortic surface. By increasing the pressure, the stress state increases (Fig. 3). The second phase showed that the greater the diameter, the greater the wall stress at the same internal pressure (Fig. 4). In the third phase, reduction of the clamp's dimension resulted in wall stress increase (Fig. 5).

These preliminary results show the value of computational simulations with regard to better understanding of these complex problems. Further analysis will include evaluation of the shape, size and material of the vascular clamps and the amount of pressure exerted on the instrument.

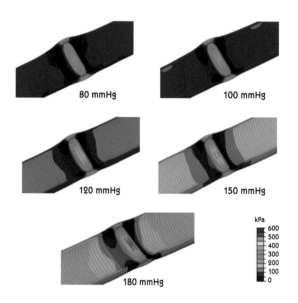

FIG. 2 Contour maps of calcified aortic models loaded at different pressures.

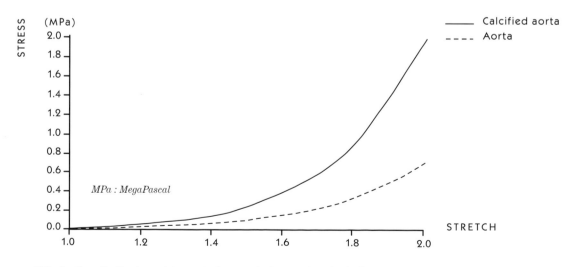

FIG. 3 Constitutive laws *(stress-strain curve)* of normal and calcified aorta utilized in the simulations.

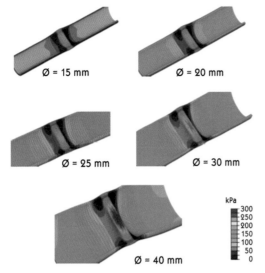

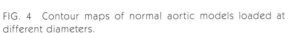

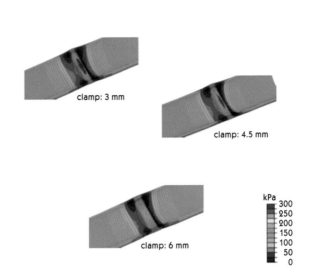

FIG. 4 Contour maps of normal aortic models loaded at different diameters.

FIG. 5 Contour maps of normal aortic models loaded at different clamp sizes.

Problems in the aortic arch

Aortic arch cross-clamping may be required in several situations during thoracic and thoracoabdominal aortic repair (Fig. 6). This is a dangerous area for cross-clamping. In fact, even an undiseased aorta has a large diameter, presents a curvature, experiences incessant movements with every heartbeat and is exposed to high fatigue loads.

Surgical dissection and cross-clamping of the aortic arch may not be feasible in large aneurysms of the distal arch, frozen chest, severely calcified aorta and aortic dissective disease.

6

59

FIG. 6 Thoracoabdominal aortic aneurysm operated with atrio-femoral left heart bypass. The proximal clamp (arrow) is positioned between the left common carotid and the left subclavian artery with the encircling tapes around the left subclavian artery and the vagus nerve.

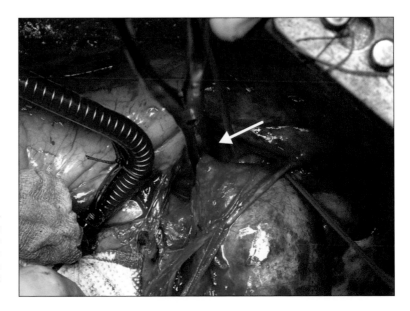

Hypothermic circulatory arrest may be the only alternative (Fig. 7). With this method, aortic cross-clamping is avoided and both the risk of visceral and neurological injuries related to aortic neck dissection and the risk of aortic clamping-related complications are eliminated. However, hypothermic circulatory arrest presents significant morbidity and mortality rates related to coagulopaty and multiple organ failure [11] and the time limitation is still considerable [12].

When the aorta is clamped at the distal arch level, problems may be related to both surgical dissection and cross-clamping.

SURGICAL DISSECTION OF THE AORTIC ARCH

The aortic arch represents a very unsafe region to dissect. A lesion of the aorta or other greater vessels in this area may be fatal. A circumferential dissection of the distal arch and aortic arch encircling should be avoided because of the significant risk of injuries in the bordering structures. The dissection should be performed until the trachea may be reached with a finger. In an aortic arch aneurysm with a large amount of thrombus, the mobilization of the aortic arch to achieve control of the proximal neck should be weighted against the increased risk of distal embolization.

A neck of at least 2 centimeters below the left subclavian artery is usually required to clamp the vessel safely and to perform the anastomosis comfortably. If the neck is shorter or absent, the aorta may be clamped between the left common carotid and the left subclavian artery or proximal to the left common carotid artery after extra-anatomic supra-aortic vessel revascularization. In these cases, the origin of the left subclavian and left common carotid artery is identified and the aortic arch is mobilized, bluntly separating the mediastinum between the supra-aortic arteries. The remnant of the ductus arteriosus is divided close to the aortic wall. The vagus nerve may be divided distal to the recurrent laryngeal nerve to allow for additional mobility of the aortic arch. To reduce the risk of aortic rupture and embolization, these maneuvers may be performed under systemic heparinization with a systolic arterial blood pressure lowered to about 80-100 mmHg.

AORTIC ARCH RUPTURE

In order to control the proximal aortic neck during the dissection phase in cases of minor aortic hemorrhage, aortic sutures with polypropilene 4-0 and teflon felt may be carefully applied at the bleeding site with the systolic arterial blood pressure lowered as much as possible. If major hemorrhage occurs, the bleeding site should be compressed and cardiopulmonary bypass (usually via the femoral vessels) instituted in order to repair the damage in hypothermic circulatory arrest. If a temporary hemostatic compression is not possible, the aortic site of lesion should be preferably side-clamped or, if it is not possible, the aortic segment immediately proximal to the lesion should be carefully cross-clamped and a rapid repair performed. If these maneuvers are not possible due to the site of the lesions or due to massive bleeding, the hemostatic procedures are performed with the heart beating and aorta unclamped. If, during this phase, cardiac arrest occurs, this time may be used to perform a rapid repair before the resuscitation procedures start.

AORTIC ARCH CLAMPING

Great attention is paid when cross-clamping the aorta at the level of the arch in order to avoid damage of the pulmonary artery and the esophagus. Malleable handled clamps may be useful in this region (Fig. 8).

When clamping the aortic arch, left heart bypass and appropriate pharmacological treatment may be used in order to reduce the blood pressure, the cardiac overload and peripheral ischemic complications. However, the risk of rupture remains significant.

In case of arch clamping proximal to the origin of supra-aortic vessels, extra-anatomic supra-aortic artery revascularization may be required. In particular, when clamping the aortic arch between the left carotid and subclavian arteries, the left upper limb revascularization is recommended only in selected cases or if postoperative symptoms develop.

In cases of aortic clamping between the innominate artery and left common carotid artery, the latter must be revascularized with either a cervical right carotid-to-left common carotid, or an intrathoracic innominate artery-left common carotid bypass.

Nowadays endovascular techniques, in many cases, avoid proximal aortic arch cross-clamping. In spite of eliminating cross-clamping, fatal lesions of the neck have also been reported with the use of endovascular techniques, especially using endografts with proximal bared stents [13].

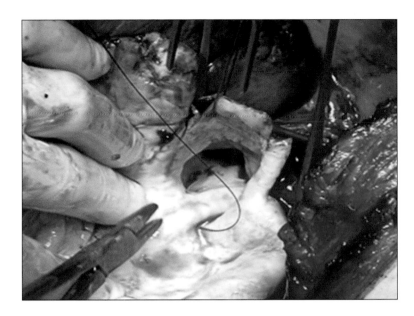

FIG. 7 Thoracoabdominal intramural hematoma operated with hypothermic circulatory arrest.

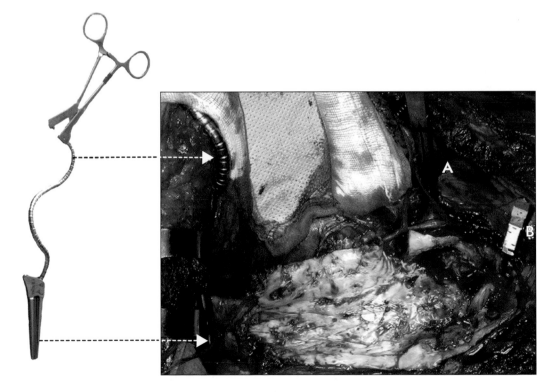

FIG. 8 Malleable handle clamp *(left)* with its intraoperative use *(arrows)* during descending thoracic aneurysm repair. A - Proximal aortic clamp. B - Bulldog on the left subclavian artery.

Problems in the thoracoabdominal aorta

Thoracoabdominal aortic aneurysms are often associated with severe and extensive atherosclerosis or connective tissue pathology usually involving the whole aortic wall, also at the proximal and distal aortic necks. Clamping-related problems are magnified by the poor quality of aortic necks that are usually friable, tortuous, large, calcified and prone to embolization or dissection. Additional problems are related to the surgical technique of repair. The preferred technique for surgical repair of the more extensive thoracoabdominal aortic aneurysms is distal aortic perfusion and sequential aortic clamping; in other words, moving the clamps downwards, as the more proximal anastomoses are accomplished, in order to limit the region of the aorta excluded from circulation. This technique pioneered by Crawford and mastered by Coselli also implies the revascularization of renal, visceral and, if necessary, intercostal arteries by anastomosing to the tube graft an aortic patch from which the aortic side branches arise [14,15]. This inclusion technique allows acceptable results for this extensive operation. Beside the well-known and feared ischemic complications, particularly of the spinal cord and kidneys, problems specifically related to sequential clamping and the visceral aortic patch do exist.

SEQUENTIAL CLAMPING-RELATED PROBLEMS

The problems related to proximal aortic neck cross-clamping and rupture have been described previously. The sequential clamping technique also involves direct cannulation and clamping of the aneurysmatic aorta which is often very large and contains the thrombus (Fig. 9). This implies two significant problems: the first one is related to the risk of rupture of the clamped aneurysm; and the second is related to the risk of embolization to the lower limb, renal and visceral arteries. To reduce the risk of aneurysm rupture at the clamping site, the left heart bypass should always be temporarily interrupted during the aneurysm clamping maneuver: the larger clamps designed by Fogarty with rubber-shod jaws may be helpful in this area.

In case of renal and visceral embolization related to aortic clamping and to distal aortic perfusion, selective thrombectomy with Fogarty catheters or alternative perioperative thromboaspiration and renal and visceral arteries stenting may be employed (Fig. 10). Several problems related to embolization, atherosclerotic plaque rupture and dissection may arise at the level of distal aortic or iliac clamping.

VISCERAL AORTIC PATCH-RELATED PROBLEMS

A specific aortic neck problem after thoracoabdominal aortic repair may occur at the level of aortic patches that are anastomosed to the tube graft for the revascularization of renal, visceral and, if required, intercostal arteries. Patients with extensive thoracoabdominal aortic aneurysms generally exhibit a tendency to aneurysmal degeneration and all the remaining aortic segments, as with these aortic patches, may dilate and complications may occur, especially in young patients or when using larger grafts [16].

The original repair must be as extensive as possible and theoretically no amount of pathological tissue must be left untreated. The size of the aortic patches should be as small as possible and, if anatomically possible, separate reimplantation of the left renal artery should be performed, directly or by means of an interposition graft [16].

Some running suture bites could be placed intentionally in the orifices of visceral arteries both to reduce the size of aortic patch and to benefit from the greater strength of the aortic tissues near side branches [17]. This maneuver, however, may sometimes be hazardous because of the risk of focal ostial plaque disruption and dissection. This may lead to visceral and/or renal artery malperfusion which subsequently has to be corrected with selective visceral bypasses or stenting. Primary endarterectomy of visceral or intercostal aortic patches should always be avoided because of the significant risk of uncontrollable anastomotic bleeding, aortic patch rupture and aortic branch dissection following aortic unclamping. An open stenting (Fig. 11) is preferential in severe stenotic pathology of visceral artery ostia.

Separate reimplantation of each visceral artery is a time consuming strategy because of the increased number of anastomoses and the risk of bleeding. This method should be reserved for patients with a higher risk of aortic patch aneurysmatic evolution, as seen in cases of connective tissue, dissection and/or widely displaced visceral ostia.

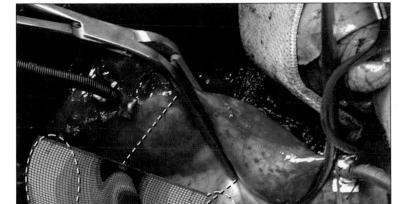

FIG. 9 First phase of sequential clamping at the level of the aneurysm during a type III thoracoabdominal aortic aneurysm repair. Computational finite element model shows a stress value of 230 KPa in the internal aortic surface of the 50 millimeter diameter aneurysm at a pressure of 100 mmHg.

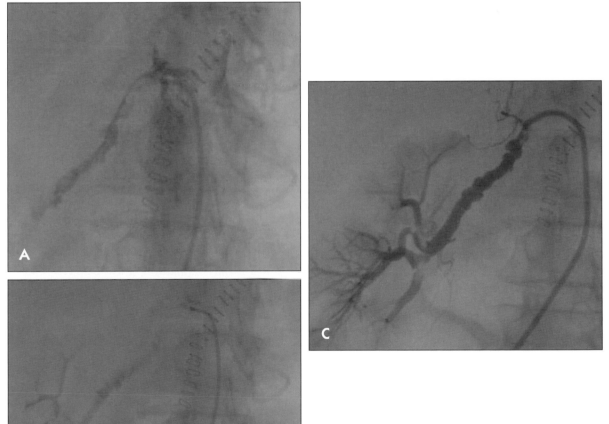

FIG. 10 A - Perioperative angiography showing partial embolic occlusion of the right renal artery following descending thoracic aortic grafting. B - Angiographic result following transfemoral partial thromboaspiration. C - Completion angiography.

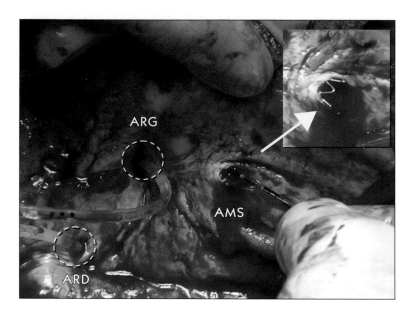

FIG. 11 Open stenting of stenotic ostium of the superior mesenteric artery (SMA) during a type III thoracoabdominal aortic aneurysm repair. Cold perfusion catheters are inserted in the right renal (RRA) and left renal arteries (LRA). Arrow indicates a detail of open stent in the ostium of SMA.

Problems in aortic dissection

ACUTE PATTERN

The management of the majority of patients with acute type B aortic dissection consists of aggressive hypotensive treatment, pain control and careful follow-up. Early surgical treatment is generally indicated only in presence of persistent and uncontrollable pain, medically uncontrollable hypertension, rapid expansion of a dissecting aneurysm, blood leakage, rupture and distal organ or limb ischemia. In these cases, the thoracic aortic repair is reserved for patients with high risk of imminent massive bleeding; in other cases peripheral open or endovascular procedures are preferred.

AORTIC CLAMPING

Clamping of an acutely dissected aorta is dangerous due to its friability (Fig. 12). In order to minimize this risk, proximal aortic clamping between the left subclavian artery and common carotid is usually preferred over clamping the descending aorta. The intimal layer may tear at the site of clamping, converting a type B dissection into a non-A non-B retrograde arch dissection or into a type A dissection.

The aorta is dissected distally. In order to avoid distal aortic injuries caused by the clamp, an *open distal anastomosis* or endovascular balloon occlusion may be performed.

AORTIC REPAIR

Prior to performing the anastomosis, a glue aortoplasty may be carried out to obliterate the false lumen and teflon felts may be placed both outside and inside the lumen to protect the aortic wall *(sandwich technique)*. If, following aortic isthmus cross-clamping after aortotomy, the dissection appears unexpectedly to involve the aortic arch proximally to the left common carotid artery, hypothermic arrest is required to allow appropriate treatment. Alternatively, thoracic endovascular grafting represents an appealing treatment option. However, results have to be assessed.

CHRONIC PATTERN

Aortic clamping. In chronic dissection the aortic wall is thicker, allowing a less dangerous aortic cross-clamping and thoracic and thoracoabdominal inclusion techniques are usually performed in case of large dissecting aneurysms. In these cases, the distal anastomosis is carried out to the outer aortic layer after surgical fenestration to allow perfusion of all the distal aortic channels.

Aortic repair. In these cases, resection of the intimal septum as distally as possible should be performed to improve distal organ perfusion (Fig. 13). In chronic dissection, the true and false lumen generally communicate through several entry and re-entry tears and both may be important for distal organ perfusion.

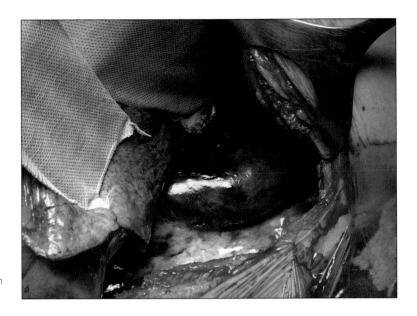

FIG. 12 Acute type B aortic dissection with a large subadventitial hemorrhage.

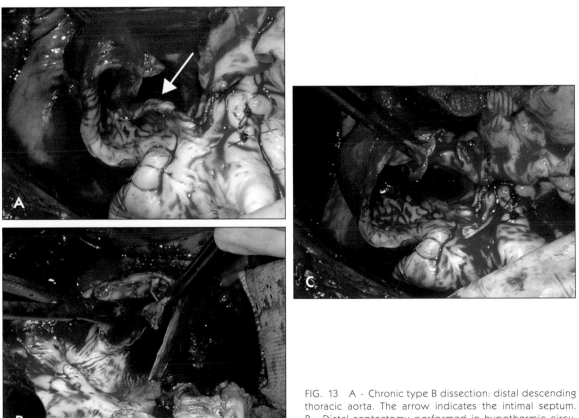

FIG. 13 A - Chronic type B dissection: distal descending thoracic aorta. The arrow indicates the intimal septum. B - Distal septectomy performed in hypothermic circulatory arrest. C - Result following septectomy.

Problems in the abdominal aorta

The infrarenal abdominal aorta is clamped during the treatment of abdominal aortic aneurysms (AAA) and aortoiliac or aortofemoral bypass for lower limb ischemia. These two situations present different problems and will be discussed separately.

Aortic Clamping in the Treatment of Abdominal Aortic Aneurysms

Most infrarenal AAA can be repaired safely with infrarenal clamping, but unusual lesions make infrarenal clamping difficult or even impossible (Table). In these cases, neck dissection may result in injury to the duodenum, renal arteries or the neck itself. Moreover, excessive aneurysm manipulation may dislodge atheromatous debris with subsequent embolization and severe end-organ damage. For aneurysms that are close to the origin of the renal arteries, suprarenal clamping is mandatory to substitute the entire infrarenal aorta. However, some surgeons [18] prefer clamping the infrarenal aorta and performing to anastomose on an ectasic and fragile neck to avoid the risks associated with this maneuver. Frequently, in these cases, infrarenal clamping does not allow a radical treatment of juxtarenal aneurysms, with a high risk of renal embolization, intraoperative bleeding, early anasto-

motic failure, false aneurysm and supra-anastomotic aneurysm formation.

Since endovascular repair has become feasible in an increasing number of infrarenal abdominal aneurysms, open surgery is nowadays frequently reserved for anatomically complex cases and, in particular, for juxtarenal aneurysms. In fact, the absence of an adequate proximal neck to anchor the endoprosthesis is one of the major contraindications for an endovascular procedure and vascular surgeons will have to face this challenge with increasing frequency.

Suprarenal cross-clamping. Suprarenal aortic cross clamping in AAA surgery is actually used with a frequency varying from 2% to 20% according to the various series reported in literature [19]. This heterogeneity reflects both the different anatomy of the treated lesions and the personal preference of the surgeon. Deciding the optimal level of proximal aortic control in the treatment of abdominal aneurysms is still controversial. Suprarenal clamping (Fig. 14) has a limited additional hemodynamic impact but is associated with a high rate of renal and gastrointestinal complications, probably because of the greater likelihood of dislodging atherosclerotic debris from the pararenal aorta (usually severely diseased) and because of distortion of the ostia of the visceral vessels (especially of the superior mesenteric artery) caused by the clamp. This kind of clamping requires careful dissection of the visceral aorta with risk of injury to the pancreas, duodenum and renal or superior mesenteric arteries. The mobilization and the section of the left renal vein may often be necessary to achieve control of the pararenal aorta (Fig. 15A). This procedure is often perceived as harmless, though others [20] have reported that ligation of the left renal vein increases the risk of postoperative renal failure and recommend reanastomosis, especially in case of collateral vessel ligation and stump venous pressure above 60 centimeters of water. In these cases, when direct reconstruction (Fig. 15B) is not possible for excessive tension of the venous segments, interposition of a reinforced PTFE graft may be helpful (Fig. 15C).

Supraceliac cross-clamping. The supraceliac aorta is less likely affected by significant atherosclerotic disease than the infrarenal and visceral aorta. Cross-clamping of the supraceliac aorta avoids clamp encroachment next to the aortic disease process and distortion of the ostia in the renal arteries.

Table	PATHOLOGIES AND CHARACTERISTICS OF THE AORTIC NECK THAT MAY COMPLICATE AORTIC CLAMPING

- ✔ Aneurysm associated with renal or visceral arterial disease
- ✔ Pararenal aneurysm
- ✔ Excessive calcification/atherosclerosis of juxtarenal aorta
- ✔ Aortic tearing or dissection
- ✔ Incomplete inflow control
- ✔ Para-anastomotic pseudoaneurysm
- ✔ Aneurysm of the residual neck

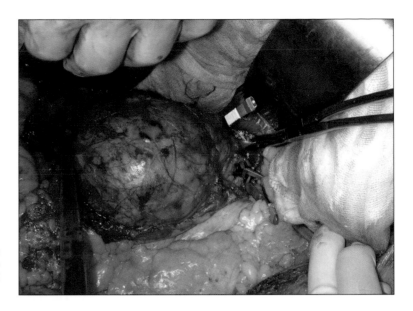

FIG. 14 Suprarenal aortic clamping with bilateral clamping of renal arteries to reduce the risk of embolization. Left renal vein is retracted cranially.

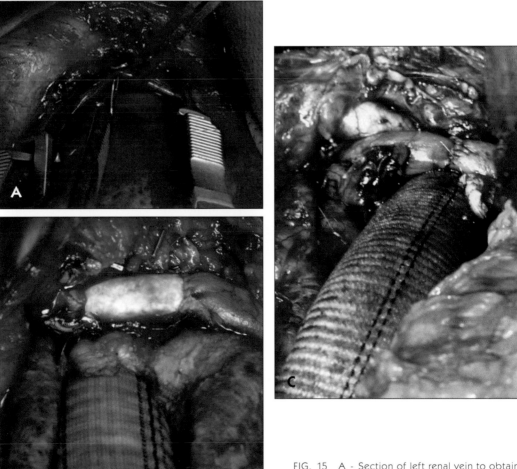

FIG. 15 A - Section of left renal vein to obtain proximal control in pararenal aortic aneurysm. B - Direct reconstruction of the left renal vein. C - Reconstruction of the left renal vein with interposition of ePTFE graft.

When renal artery repair is not necessary, it is easier to approach the aorta at the diaphragm and to work inside the neck to remove debris and sew the anastomosis. Supraceliac clamping also avoids the need for retraction and manipulation of large aneurysms and might reduce the risk of embolization during dissection. Division of the left renal vein is not necessary. This kind of clamping facilitates the repair of difficult and ruptured abdominal aortic aneurysms since aortic control may be achieved simply and rapidly through either a transperitoneal or retroperitoneal approach. In the transperitoneal method the gastro-hepatic ligament and the peritoneum overlying the supraceliac aorta are sectioned exposing the diaphragmatic crus. Careful blunt dissection of the fibers of the crus allows the surgeon to clamp the aorta. In the retroperitoneal approach, section of the left fibers of the diaphragmatic crus allows the surgeon to control the supraceliac aorta. Complete circumferential control of the aorta is dangerous and must be avoided.

Despite fears of cardiac morbidity, paraplegia, renal failure and intestinal or hepatic ischemia, favorable experiences are reported with supraceliac clamping [21] as compared to clamping of the visceral aorta. Supraceliac clamping is theoretically associated with a higher cardiac stress. Anesthetic management including use of vasodilator drugs, intravascular volume loading, correction of acid-base abnormalities and hemodynamic monitoring during unclamping are fundamental to minimizing cardiac morbidity. Despite the increased hemodynamic stress, several series in the literature report that supraceliac clamping is associated with similar operative mortality rates, comparable renal function and frequency of cardiac events as compared to infrarenal clamping. The incidence of vital organ ischemic complications during supraceliac clamping is related to the level of preoperative renal or mesenteric insufficiency, the severity of pararenal atherosclerosis, the extent of the operative procedure and the duration of proximal aortic cross-clamping.

Visceral ischemia. Duration of visceral ischemia has been recognized as the primary determinant of subsequent multiple organ failure. Acute ischemia during aortic cross-clamping, as well as reperfusion after unclamping, results in disorders in organ systems both proximal and distal to the aortic occlusion and may complicate the outcome with induced regional ischemia as well as remote organ dysfunction after reperfusion. When neck dis-

section is hazardous, suprarenal or supraceliac clamping must be considered for proximal control of the infrarenal aorta. Selection of the best approach to gain the required arterial exposure, careful dissection and proper sequences for clamping and unclamping the aorta and visceral branches are of paramount importance and may be even more crucial than the actual cross-clamping position.

Thromboembolism. Thromboembolism is a well-known complication of aortic clamping and unclamping and its prevention represents an interesting area of research for vascular surgeons. Aortic clamping during AAA repair exposes the patient to the risk of distal (lower limb ischemia and trash foot) and proximal embolization (trash kidney, renal insufficiency and intestinal ischemia).

The presence of distal embolism can easily be detected during the intraoperative period by observing the absence of adequate back flow from the vessels concerned. In the perioperative period, the evaluation of pulses, doppler flow and the status of perfusion of the extremities allow prompt diagnosis and treatment.

The incidence of limb ischemia due to distal embolism during infrarenal aneurysms repair is estimated to be around 3.3% [22]. The incidence of proximal embolism to renal and visceral branches is not precisely assessed because diagnosis is difficult and less well defined; the effects of proximal emboli from other causative factors of renal and visceral ischemia are not easy to distinguish. Traditional wisdom states that distal clamps should be applied prior to the proximal clamps in order to avoid distal embolism during infrarenal aneurysm repair, but this recommendation does not take into account the risk of proximal embolism that, although rare, may be devastating. In their study in dogs, Lipsitz et al. [23] observed that initial distal clamping minimizes distal embolization but may result in renal or visceral embolism, whereas initial proximal clamping prevents proximal embolization and does not promote distal embolism. The probable mechanism of this phenomenon is that the occlusion of the iliac arteries causes a pressure wave which generates a turbulent flow and a retrograde movement of embolic material towards the suprarenal aorta, thus promoting visceral embolism. Webster et al. [24], in a randomized analysis of 40 patients undergoing AAA repair, have not noticed a difference in the number of emboli passing to the lower limbs when the first vascular clamp was applied to the proximal aorta or iliac arteries. The major risk factor for distal embolization from the aneurysm sac remains aortic manipulation. Therefore, careful handling of the aneurysmal sac and gentle but decisive clamping may minimize embolic complications.

Aortic fracture. Aortic fracture is a rare but severe complication of aortic clamping. Causes of transmural fracture of the aortic wall are extensive calcification, porcelain aorta and malacic aorta due to previous retroperitoneal irradiation for gynecologic and genitourinary malignancies. Aortic fracture results in dramatic hemorrhage and necessitates immediate control by moving the clamp above the lesion. In infrarenal aortic lesion, suprarenal or supraceliac clamping allows the bleeding to stop. Fractures localized at the visceral aorta can require control of the thoracic aorta. The use of endoluminal devices, such as Foley's catheters or Pruitt's aortic balloons, for aortic clamping may be helpful in case of unclampable aorta.

JUXTARENAL AORTIC OCCLUSION

Juxtarenal aortic occlusion may present as an acute event or as chronic lower limb ischemia. Atherosclerotic occlusion of the infrarenal aorta can produce gangrene, rest pain, claudication and, in rare cases, can progress to involve the renal arteries' origins. In 1963, Bergan and Trippel [25] described juxtarenal occlusion as a terminal stage of Leriche syndrome and the extension of continued proximal thrombosis. They also described the techniques for juxtarenal thrombo-endo-atherectomy and bypass grafting. They already advised renal cross-clamping before aortic manipulation to avoid embolization, renal hypothermia and mannitol infusion. Although new solutions have been developed (embolectomy, thrombolytic therapy and extra-anatomic bypass) and, despite progress in materials and techniques, surgical treatment of this condition is still challenging.

The surgical approach to the abdominal aorta is performed through a transperitoneal access with an adequate dissection of the infrarenal aorta, mobilization of the left renal vein and exposure of the pararenal aorta and the renal arteries. The renal arteries are clamped first to reduce the risk of embolization and then the aorta is occluded at the suprarenal level. The aortic endarterectomy is performed through an infrarenal aortotomy with a direct view of the renal ostia. After abundant irrigation and removal of debris, the aortic clamp can be transferred at an infrarenal level and the aorto-

bifemoral bypass performed (Figs. 16,17). In cases of intraoperative oligo/anuria, renal embolization must be suspected. Intraoperative angiography offers a quick diagnosis and helps to plan the treatment, as either surgical or endovascular. Despite the added operative complexity associated with manipulation of the visceral aorta and its branches and the need for extended infrainguinal revascularization, satisfactory clinical outcomes can be achieved [26].

Older patients and patients with severe comorbidity can benefit from minimally invasive procedures such as extra-anatomic bypasses. These techniques offer satisfactory results but are complicated by lesser patency of the graft and do not avoid the risk of proximal spread of the thrombus towards renal and visceral branches.

PROBLEMS DURING LAPAROSCOPIC AORTIC SURGERY

Videoscopic surgical techniques have been developed to reduce morbidity of open aortic reconstructions, but widespread application of totally laparoscopic aortic reconstruction is limited by three troublesome issues: exposure of the aorta, videoscopic clamping of the aorta, and extensive cross-clamping times required to perform the aortic anastomosis. Aortic neck problems during laparoscopic vascular surgery are essentially a result of limited availability of efficient instruments to approach ectasic or calcified aortic necks. A major leak occurring during the anastomosis phase can result in prompt surgical conversion. As demonstrated by Geier et al. [27], laparoscopic aortic clamps need further careful planning and testing to develop a safe and effective laparoscopic vascular clamp.

Killewich et al. [28] tried the Da Vinci robotic system (developed to allow the surgeon to suture in the same manner as in open procedures) to perform an aortic reconstruction for occlusive disease. The procedure was successful but it lasted 8 hours with a clamping time of 62 minutes. Elkoury et al. [29] have experimented on sheep and tested a new intraluminal stapler for vascular reconstruction. It allowed an aorta to graft anastomosis through a minimally invasive approach with short clamping times. However, reliability of this technique is still low and further improvements are needed. The development of intraluminal stapler devices for aortic anastomosis may increase the applicability of techniques in aortic surgery in the future.

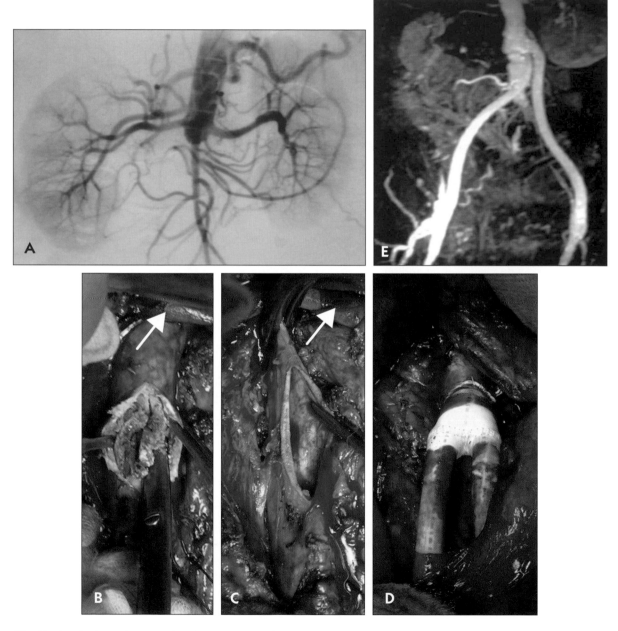

FIG. 16 A - Angiography scan showing occlusion of infrarenal aorta. B - Intraoperative image of infrarenal longitudinal aortotomy and endarterectomy with suprarenal aortic clamping *(arrow indicates left renal vein)*. C - Infrarenal aortic clamping after aortic endarterectomy *(arrow indicates left renal vein)*. D - Aorto-bifemoral bypass with ePTFE graft. E - Six months postoperative angioMR.

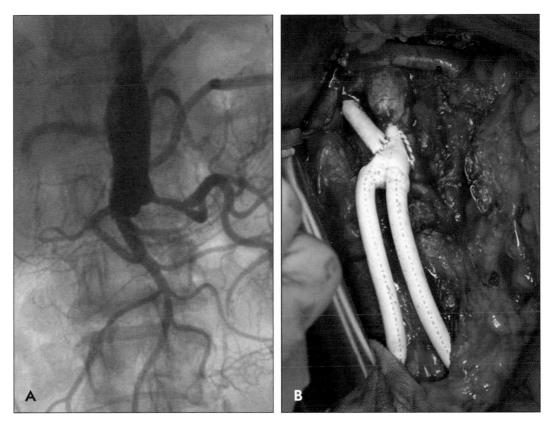

FIG. 17   A - Angiography of an occlusion of the infrarenal aorta associated with occlusion of the right renal artery.   B - Aorto-bifemoral bypass associated with a bypass to the right renal artery with an ePTFE graft.

Laparoscopic hand assisted abdominal aortic surgery combines the advantages of minimally invasive surgery and the reliability of established open procedures. In various series, this approach allowed for successful aortic surgery within acceptable operating and clamping times [30].

Conclusion

Aortic neck problems during aortic surgery can cause complications which are more difficult than the planned procedure. Adequate preoperative evaluation is essential to evaluate extensive calcification, thrombus, dissection, blistering or the presence of aberrant arteries in the aortic neck. Careful intraoperative neck assessment allows the surgeon to plan the best surgical approach and to reduce clamping lesions. Systemic heparinization, pressure control and gentle handling of the aneurysm reduces the risk of thromboembolism. Experience with circulatory arrest and extracorporeal circulation can resolve very complex situations. Endovascular skills may be helpful for the treatment of embolic complications.

REFERENCES

1 Riles TS. Presidential address: the next quarter. *J Vasc Surg* 2004; 39: 275-278.

2 Sachs M, Auth M, Encke A. Historical development of surgical instruments exemplified by hemostatic forceps. *World J Surg* 1998; 22: 499-504.

3 Friedman S. *The history of vascular surgery*. Mount Kisco, NY: Futura Publishing Company, Inc.; 1989; pp 1-14.

4 Darcin OT, Cenzig M, Ozardali L, Andac MH. Pressure controlled vascular clamp: a novel device for atraumatic vessel occlusion. *Ann Vasc Surg* 2004; 18: 254-256.

5 Margovsky AI, Chambers AJ, Lord RS. The effect of increasing clamping forces on endothelial and arterial wall damage: an experimental study in the sheep. *Cardiovasc Surg* 1999; 7: 457-463.

6 Bunt TJ, Manship LL, Moore WM. Iatrogenic vascular injury during peripheral revascularization. *J Vasc surg* 1985; 2: 491-498.

7 Manship LL, Moore WM, Bynoe R, Bunt TJ. Differential endothelial injury caused by vascular clamps and vessel loops. II. Atherosclerotic vessels. *Am Surg* 1985; 51: 401-406.

8 Guidoin R, Doyon B, Blais P et al. Effects of traumatic manipulations on grafts, sutures, and host arteries during vascular surgery procedures. Experiments on dogs. *Res Exp Med* 1981; 179: 1-21.

9 Moore WM, Bunt TJ, Hermann GD, Fogarty TJ. Assessment of transmural force during application of vascular occlusive devices. *J Vasc Surg* 1988; 8: 422-427.

10 Salunke NV, Topoleski, LD, Humphrey JD, Mergner WJ. Compressive stress-relaxation of human atherosclerotic plaque. *J Biomed Mater Res* 2001; 55: 236-241.

11 Hirotani T, Kameda T, Kumamoto T, Shirota S. Aortic arch repair using hypothermic circulatory arrest technique associated with pharmacological brain protection. *Eur J Cardiothorac Surg* 2000; 18: 545-549.

12 Immer FF, Lippeck C, Barmettler H et al. Improvement of quality of life after surgery on the thoracic aorta: effect of antegrade cerebral perfusion and short duration of deep hypothermic circulatory arrest. *Circulation* 2004; 14; 110 (11 Suppl 1): II 250-255.

13 Hansen CJ, Bui H, Donayre CE et al. Complications of endovascular repair of high-risk and emergent descending thoracic aortic aneurysms and dissections. *J Vasc Surg* 2004; 40: 228-234.

14 Coselli JS. The use of left heart bypass in the repair of thoracoabdominal aortic aneurysms: current techniques and results. *Semin Thorac Cardiovasc Surg* 2003; 15: 326-332.

15 Chiesa R, Melissano G, Civilini E et al. Ten years experience of thoracic and thoracoabdominal aortic aneurysm surgical repair: lessons learned. *Ann Vasc Surg* 2004; 18: 514-526.

16 Tshomba Y, Melissano G, Civilini E et al. Fate of visceral aortic patch after thoracoabdominal aortic repair. *Eur J Vasc Endovasc Surg*, in press.

17 Lee D, Chen JY. Numerical simulation of steady flow fields in a model of abdominal aorta with its peripheral branches. *J Biomech* 2002; 35: 1115-1122.

18 Lipski DA, Ernst CB. Natural history of the residual infrarenal aorta after infrarenal abdominal aortic aneurysm repair. *J Vasc Surg* 1998; 27: 805-811.

19 Giulini SM, Bonardelli S, Portolani N et al. Suprarenal aortic cross clamping in elective abdominal aortic aneurysm surgery. *Eur J Vasc endovasc Surg* 2000; 20: 286-289.

20 AbuRhama AF, Robinson PA, Boland JP, Lucente FC. The risk of ligation of left renal vein in resection of the abdominal aortic aneurysm. *Surg Gynecol Obstet* 1991; 173: 33-36.

21 El-Sabrout RA, Reul GJ. Suprarenal or supraceliac aortic clamping during repair of infrarenal abdominal aortic aneurysms. *Tex Heart Inst J* 2001; 28: 254-264.

22 Johnston KW. Multicenter prospective study of non ruptured abdominal aortic aneurysm. Part II: variables predicting morbidity and mortality. *J Vasc Surg* 1989; 9: 437-447.

23 Lipsitz EC, Veith FJ, Ohki T, Quintos RT. Should initial clamping for abdominal aortic aneurysm repair be proximal or distal to minimise embolisation? *Eur J Vasc Endovasc Surg* 1999; 17: 413-418.

24 Webster SE, Smith J, Thompson MM et al. Does the sequence of clamp application during open abdominal aortic aneurysm surgery influence distal embolisation? *Eur J Vasc Endovasc Surg* 2004; 27: 61-64.

25 Bergan JJ, Trippel OH. Management of juxtarenal aortic occlusions. *Arch Surg* 1963; 87: 230-238.

26 Back MR, Johnson BL, Shames ML, Bandyk DF. Evolving complexity of open aortofemoral reconstruction done for occlusive disease in the endovascular era. *Ann Vasc Surg* 2003; 17: 596-603.

27 Geier B, Neuking K, Mumme A et al. Comparison of laparoscopic aortic clamps in a pulsatile circulation model. *J Laparoendosc Adv Surg Tech A* 2002; 12: 317-326.

28 Killewich LA, Cindrick-Pounds LL, Gomez G. Robot-assisted laparoscopic aortic reconstruction for occlusive disease-a case report. *Vasc Endovascular Surg* 2004; 38: 83-87.

29 Elkouri S, Noel AA, Gloviczki P et al. Stapled aortic anastomosis: a minimally invasive, feasible alternative to videoscopic aortic suturing? *Vasc Endovascular Surg* 2004; 38: 321-330.

30 Kolvenbach R, Da Silva L, Deling O, Schwierz E. Video-assisted aortic surgery. *J Am Coll Surg* 2000; 190: 451-457.

7

AORTIC NECK PROBLEMS DURING EVAR

MARTIN MALINA, BJÖRN SONESSON, KRASSI IVANCEV

In endovascular aneurysm repair (EVAR), the proximal and distal aneurysm necks have two separate functions, namely fixation of the stent-graft and sealing of the aneurysm. The challenge of EVAR is to select a suitable stent-graft that provides fixation and sealing and to deploy the device adequately. Unexpected challenges occur due to erroneous selection of stent-graft and inaccurate deployment. This chapter deals with some aspects of the proximal and distal landing sites of thoracic and subsequently abdominal aortic aneurysms.

Proximal neck of thoracic lesions

REACHING THE NECK

The aortic arch provides a curved and inherently challenging proximal neck. Reaching it is an *unexpected problem* in itself. The remote distance from the femoral access site combined with the tortuosity of the elongated arch and descending aorta often inhibit insertion of the sheath (Fig. 1).

Recently developed kink-resistant and flexible large bore sheaths greatly facilitate insertion. The sheaths offer improved pushability and flexibility. Updating the stock of emergency stent-grafts with the last generation of introducer sheaths is recommended in order to avoid failed device insertion or deployment. Most stiff dilators soften considerably upon heating. Submerging the dilator briefly in boiling water prior to insertion is helpful. The Gore device does not require passing the sheath into the arch and is also highly capable of negotiating severe tortuosity.

An ultrastiff guide wire is always a prerequisite. The wire should be curved by the physician prior to insertion. Both the soft tip and the adjacent stiff portion of the wire that is aimed at the arch need to be precurved. The soft tip is curled up against the aortic valve in order to ensure that the stent-graft is only supported by the stiff portion of the wire inside the arch (Fig. 2 A). The Lunderkvist wire is the stiffest wire available but carries a suboptimal transition zone that may kink between the soft tip and the body of the wire.

Additional wire support for the extremely angulated arch can be accomplished with a brachial *through-and-through* wire with a loop in the ascending

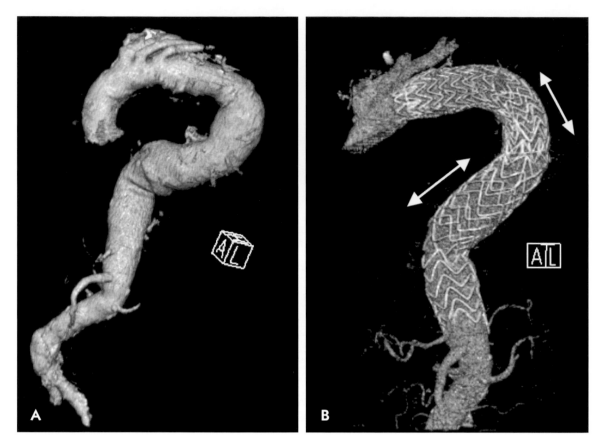

FIG. 1 Preoperative 3D reconstruction of tortuous thoracic aortic aneurysm. Note that a lateral projection is required for the arch branches. B - Postoperative reconstruction illustrates the stent-graft extending from the horizontal portion of the arch to the celiac trunk with generous overlap zones between stent-graft components *(arrows)*.

aorta (Fig. 2B). Although the stiff loop is traumatic, it seems to be gentler than passing the wire from the arm straight into the descending aorta because the latter approach requires the dilator tip to be passed into the brachiocephalic trunk (Fig. 2C).

Whenever substantial difficulties to pass the sheath are encountered in the descending aorta or iliac arteries, stretching the wire and pulling the sheath from the arm rather than pushing it from the groin should be attempted. Snaring the sheath from the arm in order to pull the sheath into the arch may also be attempted.

Any maneuvering inside the arch determines a risk for cerebral complications. Aggressive heparinization is therefore recommended. Once the device reaches the arch, deployment must not be delayed. An angiographic catheter should be placed in the ascending aorta and connected to a power injector beforehand. The motion of a mobile C-arm might be obstructed by the patient's arms, the operating table or anesthetic equipment and ought to be tested in advance while positioning the patient. Left anterior oblique projection of at least 60 degrees is required in most patients to visualize the origin of the arch branches.

DEPLOYMENT

Deployment of the thoracic stent-graft is less accurate than abdominal stent-grafting. The curved device is under tension and may move unexpectedly. The physician should hold it firmly throughout deployment. Visualizing all the arch branches in one single projection is often impossible. There is significant motion of the target area due to systodiastolic pulsatility and breathing.

Arterial blood flow is most forceful in the aortic arch. Hypotension during deployment is therefore recommended and close collaboration with the anesthetist is mandatory [1].

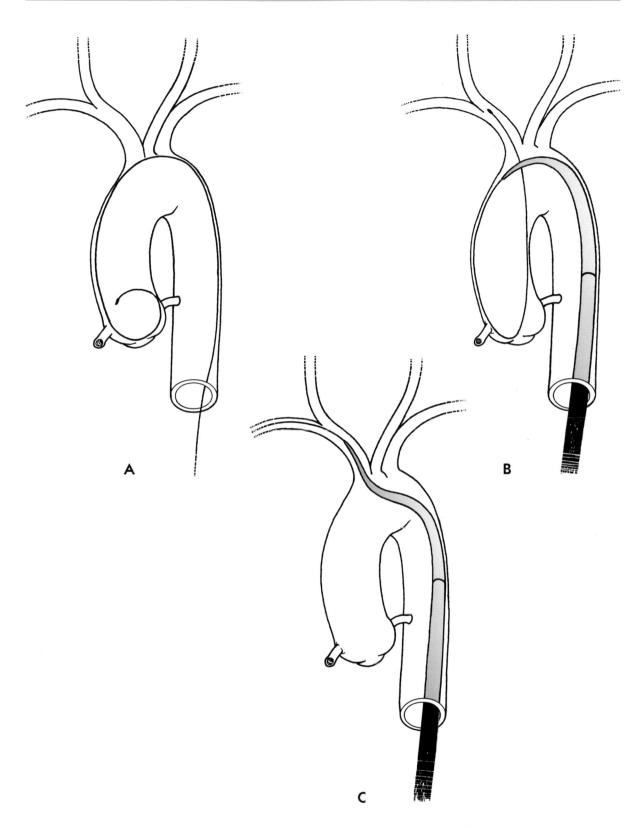

A

B

C

FIG. 2 Guide wire in the arch. A - Soft tip curled up against the aortic valve to offer rigid support in the arch. B - Loop in the ascending aorta to allow the dilator to be passed beyond the brachiocephalic trunk. C - Through-and-through brachial wire requires that the dilator enters the brachiocephalic trunk.

Simple *pull-back* deployment is hazardous because the stent-graft may be swept away downstream (Fig. 3). Most stent-grafts can be repositioned distally during the early stage of deployment. Advancing the stent-graft is, on the other hand, impossible after the first stent has been released. We therefore routinely start deployment one centimeter proximal to the intended landing site and pull the device distally after the top stent has been released but not yet fully deployed. Contrary to abdominal stent-grafts, thoracic devices should not carry a bare top stent as it may erode the arch or cause retrograde type A dissection.

The pull-back technique deploys the stent-graft along the lesser curvature of the arch (Fig. 4). The ensuing angulation of the stent-graft at the vertex of the arch is rather acute and kinking and, therefore, excessive stent motion or leakage may arise. The stent-graft should be placed along the outer curvature by advancing both the sheath and the pusher after half the length of the stent-graft has been deployed.

The Gore device allows a predictable placement thanks to its extremely rapid release that is initiated from the mid portion of the stent-graft. The *umbrella* is thereby constrained until free flow is

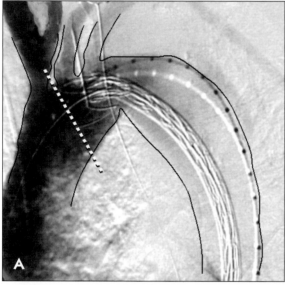

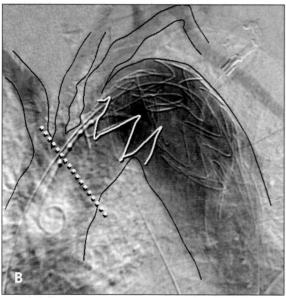

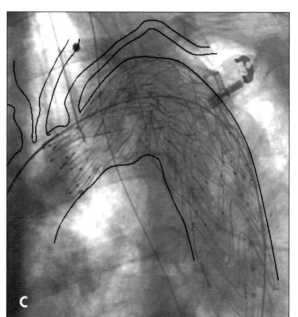

FIG. 3 The hazards of pull-back deployment. A - Starting deployment *(broken line)*. B - End result (proximal stent has been emphasized). C - Proximal extension into the safer horizontal portion of the arch.

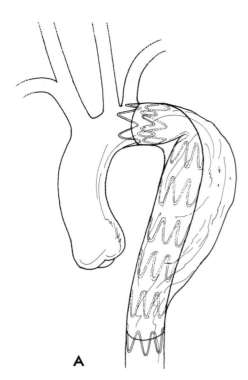
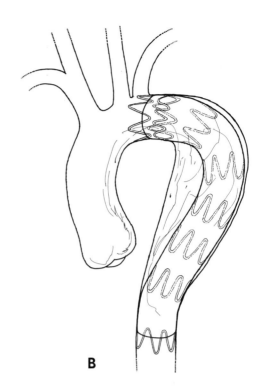

FIG. 4 A - Unfavorable acute angulation of a stent-graft that was deployed along the minor curvature. B - Correctly deployed stent-graft.

established. The disadvantage of the Gore technique is that no repositioning can be made after deployment has been initiated.

A proximal safety wire to release the top stent after the rest of the device has been deployed allows the most accurate placement in our hands. Significant repositioning can be made until the safety wire is withdrawn. Despite this, minor displacement does occur during the final release of the proximal stent.

MALPOSITIONING

Accidental overstenting of the arch branches is not always deleterious. The left subclavian artery can be covered at low risk except in patients with known contraindications [2]. Whenever preservation of the left subclavian artery is vital, a catheter ought to be passed from the arm into the arch before placing the stent-graft. The proximal edge of the stent-graft can then be pushed aside with a stent if necessary. The approach from the left arm is also helpful whenever an overstented subclavian artery may cause a type II endoleak. In this case, the proximal subclavian stump is coil embolized instantly. Aggressive stent-graft deployment in the vicinity of the left common carotid artery or the brachiocephalic trunk should be carried out in readiness to stent the orifices from a retrograde approach similar to that described for the subclavian artery (Fig. 5). Retrograde puncture of the common carotid artery, however, requires surgical cut down for hemostasis.

Accidental distal slippage of the stent-graft during deployment should be corrected immediately (Fig. 3C). Short proximal body extensions are available but more difficult to deploy accurately. The ensuing short overlap may not offer a durable telescopic anastomosis. We prefer placing an additional full-length stent-graft whenever proximal extension is required. Stent-grafts shorter than 15 centimeters are rarely indicated in the thoracic aorta and the overlap between stent-grafts should exceed 5-7 centimeters.

Durability of the proximal fixation of thoracic stent-grafts remains an issue and primary anchoring in the horizontal, or even ascending, portion of the arch is increasingly advocated (Fig. 3C). Attempts to anchor the stent-graft at the vertex of the arch may lead to proximal leakage or pulsatile pivoting

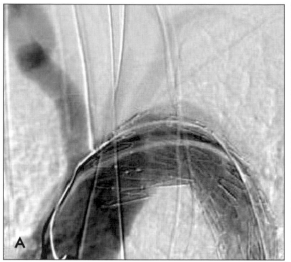

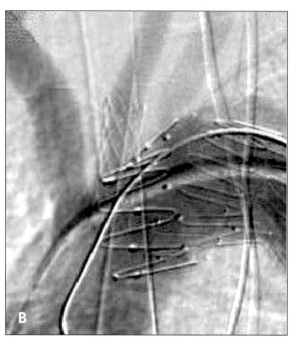

FIG. 5   A - Left common artery accidentally covered by the thoracic stent-graft. B - The patency of the carotid artery is reestablished by a stent that pushes aside the edge of the stent-graft.

motion of the uppermost stent (Fig. 6) with high risk for early material fatigue and collapse. Molding the stent-graft with large balloons or stents is hazardous in the arch and must be avoided if possible. Accurate proximal deployment in an acutely angulated arch may be facilitated by placing a more distal component that barely reaches the apex first. This stent-graft may support the final, most proximal piece.

Distal neck of thoracic lesions

The most common "unexpected" problems associated with the distal neck of thoracic lesions include underestimated length, inaccurate distal landing and poor distal fixation with subsequent cranial migration of the caudal stent.

LENGTH
The length of a thoracic lesion is notoriously underestimated. The tortuosity and large diameter of the descending aorta make it difficult to appreciate the length even with a calibrated catheter that tends to follow a straight course along the inner curves.

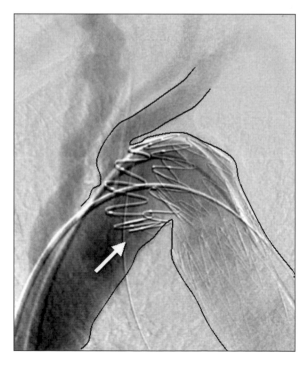

FIG. 6   Stent-graft pivoting at the vertex of the arch. There is risk from stent fracture and endoleak due to the excessive pulsatile motion as the blood stream hits the outside of the stent-graft *(arrow)*.

Some stent-grafts are only 10 centimeters long. Considering the aforementioned need for overlap between stent-grafts of more than 5-7 centimeters it is hardly surprising that problems will arise when each component adds only a few centimeters to the overall length. We therefore recommend the use of stent-grafts longer than 20 centimeters except in extremely short lesions such as ulcers or transection in an otherwise healthy aorta. We also recommend the routine use of two long stent-grafts in order to allow accurate deployment both proximally and distally. Generous overlap between stent-graft components makes it possible to vary the length liberally and offers a very stable anastomosis. It allows the physician to pay all their attention exclusively to the landing sites.

MISPLACEMENT

The horizontal portion of the elongated descending aorta above the diaphragm is frequently mistaken for a durable neck. This aortic segment, however, tends to undergo continuous dilation and offers poor stent-graft fixation. Unless the supradiaphragmatic aorta is evidently healthy, the stent-graft ought to be extended below the diaphragm to the vertical aortic segment right above the celiac axis.

Inaccurate placement of the distal end of the stent-graft at the celiac trunk is common. The origin of the celiac trunk is poorly visualized on AP-view aortography. The distal end of the stent-graft should, therefore, be deployed in lateral projection. Again, lateral projection is difficult to obtain in the operating room with a mobile C-arm for the same reasons as adequate oblique projections are cumbersome to obtain in the arch.

A selective catheter can be used to indicate the level of the celiac trunk. It is difficult to discern the precise level of the celiac origin even with a selective catheter in place because the vertex of the catheter may protrude above the orifice by several centimeters. Furthermore, the selective catheter tends to be dislodged by the large thoracic sheath passing by.

Accidental obliteration of the celiac trunk is not entirely safe although it is tolerated by most patients. The predictive value of selective injection into the superior mesenteric artery in order to visualize collateral hepatic flow is uncertain. The long-term outcome of bail out celiac stenting is jeopardized by mechanical compression of the stent by the aortic crura.

CRANIAL MIGRATION OF THE DISTAL END

Even seemingly accurate distal deployment of a thoracic stent-graft is often disappointing. The rigid introducer sheath straightens out the aorta at the level of the diaphragm but the vessel resumes its tortuous course upon deployment, rendering the stent-graft too short. *Unexpected* distal extension is therefore frequently required and extensions need to be kept on the shelf. Short extension pieces are avoided even in this setting.

The horizontal portion of the elongated descending aorta above the diaphragm produces so called vector forces that pull the distal end of the stent-graft cranially. We advocate the use of a bare distal stent for improved mechanical fixation in patients with a poor distal neck. A stent-graft with a bare bottom stent carrying cranially orientated barbs is now commercially available *(Cook Inc.)*. The most stable aortic segment is at the level of the visceral arteries. The bare stent is deployed across the visceral vessels in a similar manner as the bare top stent of some abdominal stent-grafts. The bare bottom stent should be avoided in dissections because the stent may pierce the dissection membrane creating undesired re-entries.

Proximal neck of the abdominal aortic aneurysm

AVOIDING MISPLACEMENT

The neck of the infrarenal aortic aneurysm is often short. Highly accurate deployment is necessary and, indeed, fully feasible with present technology [3]. Instant release should be avoided in the short neck because readjustments are needed during deployment. Particularly in tortuous vessels, the final tilting of the proximal graft edge is difficult to predict. The graft should be gently laid against the aortic wall rather than being *released*.

The bare top stent improves fixation. There is substantial experimental data to demonstrate the mechanical benefit of a bare top stent. During the last few years, the attachment between the top stent and the stent-graft itself has been necessarily strengthened because the axial forces may pull the device downstream, ripping it off from the top stent entirely.

The use of a bare top stent not only improves fixation but also facilitates accurate deployment. Several stent-grafts offer the option of repositioning after the top stent has been partially released (Fig. 7).

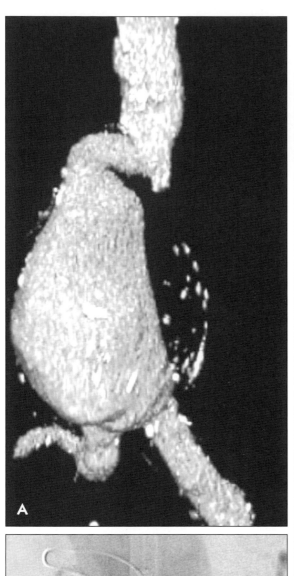

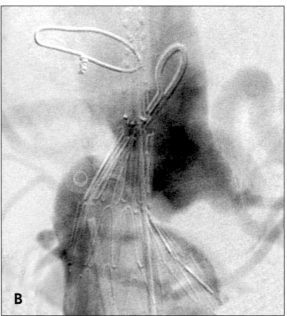

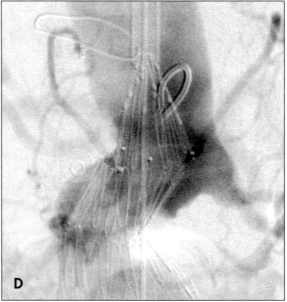

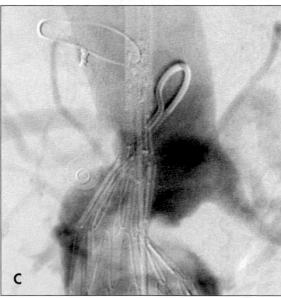

FIG. 7 Careful stent-graft deployment in the angulated neck. A - 3D reconstruction. B - The stent-graft is released while the top stent remains constrained. Position is too cranial. C - Repositioned stent-graft. D - Most of the bare top stent has been released. It becomes evident where the edge of the graft will end up. *(E, F, G)* ▶

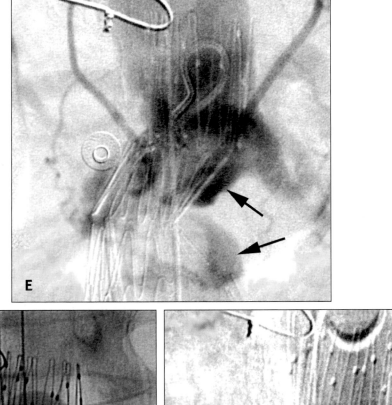

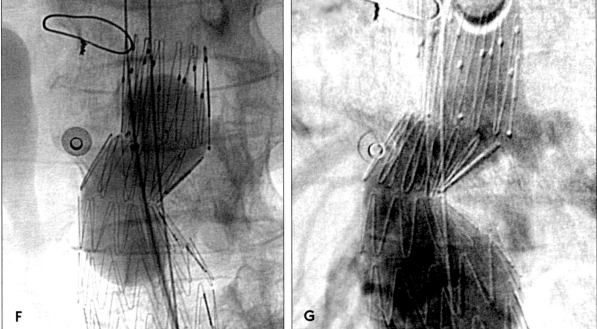

FIG. 7   E - The stent-graft is fully released but the apposition is poor and there is a type I leak *(arrows).*   F - Moulding the stent-graft with a compliant latex balloon.   G - Final result.

The bony landmarks are not reliable for orientation during repositioning of a partially deployed stent-graft. The stent-graft may already have engaged the aortic wall to some extent and repositioning will pull the entire aorta up or down without moving the stent-graft relative to the renal arteries. Multiple angiographies therefore need to be carried out to confirm adjustments. The contrast volume is reduced by injecting 5-10 ml of contrast at 20 ml/s through a multiple side hole catheter.

MISPLACEMENT

Distal misplacement of the abdominal stent-graft is corrected with an extension, as in the thorax. Extending a bifurcated abdominal stent-graft is difficult because there is only room for a short extension piece above the bifurcation of the primary stent-graft. Insertion of an aortouniiliac device is often the safest option. The bare top stent of the primary stent-graft may prevent adequate aposition between the extension piece and the aortic wall and the type I leak may persist.

Aggressive juxtarenal placement of the primay stent-graft avoids these problems but the renal artery may need stenting if it is accidentally covered. Unless the stent-graft has been grossly misplaced, the renal arteries can be salvaged with a stent that pushes down the upper edge of the fabric (Fig. 8). Passing the stent into the renal artery over the edge

of the fabric requires substantial pushability. A pre-curved Amplatz *Superstiff* wire with a short tip has proven beneficiary on these occasions. A large latex balloon inflated above the renal arteries may support the wire and facilitate access to the renal access from below. Brachial approach is rarely needed.

TYPE I LEAKS FROM POOR SEALING

A primary type I endoleak occurs frequently in the angulated or irregular neck. The significance of a minor type I leak is debatable but in our experience there is persistent pressurization of the sac with risk for rupture. We try to avoid type I leaks by oversizing the stent-graft generously in the angulated or irregular neck. Thereby, the sealing zone is extended by 1 or 2 centimeters into the wider distal portion of the neck.

Primary type I endoleaks can be treated with a Palmaz 4014 stent (Fig. 9). The stent is expandable up to 30 millimeters. It straightens out the neck, improves graft aposition to the aortic wall and compresses the graft folds. The only adverse event encountered in our series of 40 patients is one neck rupture in a female patient of extremely high age. Although the primary success rate of this technique is high, the long-term durability remains to be proven.

Fenestrated stent-grafts are used in patients with very short necks [4]. The fenestrated stent-graft may

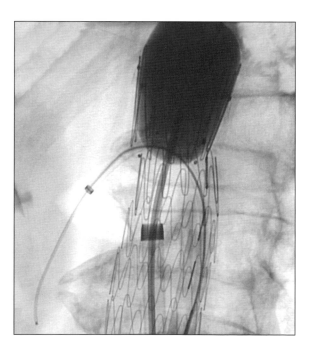

FIG. 8 Salvage of a graft covered renal artery. A sheath has been advanced into the renal artery over an Amplatz wire in order to allow stenting. A latex balloon inflated in the supra-renal aorta supports the wire.

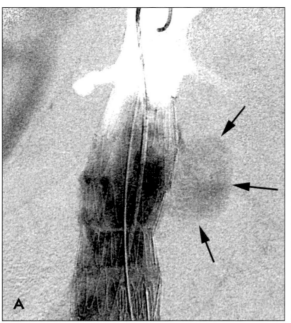
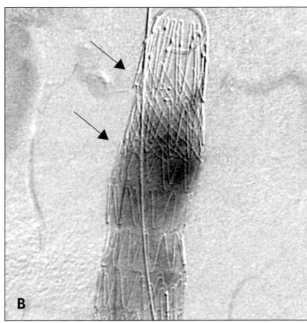

FIG. 9 A - Accurately deployed stent-graft with proximal type I endoleak *(arrows)* due to neck irregularities. B - The leak has been sealed with a Palmaz 4014 stent deployed at the level of the arrows.

reduce the risk for type I leakage but inadvertent obliteration of a renal artery does occur. Treating a type I endoleak with a fenestrated stent-graft is challenging. Friction between the stent-grafts may hinder accurate repositioning of the fenestrated body.

Distal neck of the abdominal aorta

Tubular aorto-aortic stent-grafts are avoided in abdominal aortic aneurysm repair because the distal neck above the aortic bifurcation is a poor landing site [5]. An adequate distal neck is sometimes present in short aortic lesions such as ulcers or pseudoaneurysms. Whenever in doubt about the distal neck, we prefer placing a bifurcated or aortouniiliac device.

It should be kept in mind that large percutaneous transluminal angioplasty balloons have long shoulders. The shoulder may injure the common iliac artery if attempts are made to inflate a balloon expanded stent right above the aortic bifurcation. Aortic dilation next to the bifurcation should be carried out with *kissing balloons*.

REFERENCES

1 Alric P, Berthet JP, Branchereau P et al. Endovascular repair for acute rupture of the descending thoracic aorta. *J Endovasc Ther* 2002; 9: II 51-59.

2 Hausegger KA, Oberwalder P, Tiesenhausen K et al. Intentional left subclavian artery occlusion by thoracic aortic stent-grafts without surgical transposition. *J Endovasc Ther* 2001; 8: 472-476.

3 Ibertini J, Kalliafas S, Travis S et al. Anatomical risk factors for proximal perigraft endoleak and graft migration following endovascular repair of abdominal aortic aneurysms. *Eur J Vasc Endovasc Surg* 2000; 19: 308-312.

4 Verhoeven EL, Prins TR, Tielliu IF et al. Treatment of short-necked infrarenal aortic aneurysms with fenestrated stent-grafts: short-term results. *Eur J Vasc Endovasc Surg* 2004; 27: 477-483.

5 Chuter TA, Green RM, Ouriel K, DeWeese JA. Infrarenal aortic aneurysm structure: implications for transfemoral repair. *J Vasc Surg* 1994; 20: 44-49.

PROBLEMS AND SOLUTIONS TO DIFFICULT REPAIRS OF THE AORTIC NECK IN RUPTURED ANEURYSMS

MARCUS BROOKS, JOHN WOLFE

Rupture of an abdominal aortic aneurysm is currently the thirteenth most common cause of death in men in the western world (25-30/100 000). Rupture is rare before the age of fifty and more common in men (4: 1). The strict definition of aortic rupture is leak of blood from the aorta into either the peritoneum (free rupture) or retroperitoneum (contained rupture). In patients who reach the hospital, mortality from rupture of an abdominal aortic aneurysm is 30% to 60%. The aim of management is therefore prompt diagnosis, rapid transfer to the operating theater, control of hemorrhage by aortic cross-clamp placement and exclusion of the aneurysm.

This chapter examines the problems encountered in gaining proximal control of the aneurysm and performing the proximal anastomosis in an emergency setting. We would hope that in patients undergoing elective aneurysm repair these problems would have been detected preoperatively and the approach to the aneurysm modified accordingly. In aneurysm rupture, transfer for CT scan is unnecessary and may be dangerous.

Proximal aortic control

While speed is important during dissection onto the aortic neck, damage to the lumbar, gonadal and left renal veins or mesenteric or colic vessels at this stage may subsequently prove fatal. It is important that the entire small bowel mesentry is taken over to the patients right and that the colic mesentry is protected (Fig. 1). The inferior mesenteric vein can safely be divided if needed to improve proximal

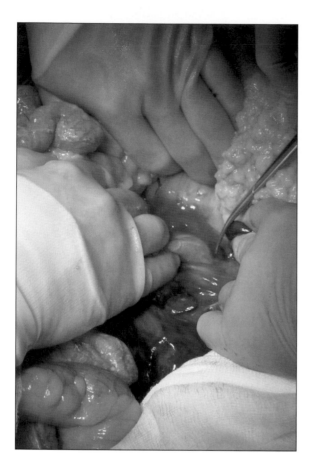

FIG. 1 Evisceration of the intestines to the right side, supported by the surgical assistant: the surgeon is at the left side of the patient.

neck or left renal vein are encountered. The aorta is then palpated to determine if the neck is suitable for cross-clamping; if so, the dissection is continued at each side of the aorta to the lumbar spine and a cross-clamp applied. If an infrarenal clamp cannot be applied, the Foley catheter is left in-situ and the aortic graft passed over it to perform the proximal anastomosis. Alternatively, the neck can be clamped in the lesser sac. For a ruptured aneurysm the safe proximal occlusion of the aorta is the key to success, whereas the prior application of distal clamps to avoid embolic complications is less important in these circumstances. The aortic clamps commonly used are designed to apply either anterior-posterior or transverse compression. The latter type necessitates dissection posterior to the aorta, which we believe is associated with a high risk of injury to either lumbar arteries or para-aortic veins. We therefore advocate vertical application of a straight clamp with no retro-aortic dissection (Fig. 2).

If clamping is not possible at an infrarenal level, then control can be gained at the level of the diaphragm. The peritoneum is divided over the esophagus and right crus of the diaphragm and the crus partially divided with diathermy. The esophagus is retracted to the left and the aorta identified and clamped. The disadvantage of this technique is that the viscera and kidneys are rendered ischemic. The clamp should be re-applied distally once either the infrarenal aneurysm neck has been adequately exposed and clamped or the proximal anastomosis has been performed.

exposure. Ideally the aorta is controlled distal to the renal artery orifices so as to avoid renal ischemia. However, in an unstable hypotensive patient it may be necessary, at least initially, to control the aorta at a higher level. This is achieved most simply by the assistant surgeon manually compressing the suprarenal aorta against the lumbar spine using pressure from a fist or a Langenbeck-type retractor. This technique is unreliable; a better alternative is to open the aneurysm sac, if the rupture point is not already visible, and that the surgeon uses the thumb to "cork" the neck of the aneurysm. A large (24 French) Foley catheter connected to a 50 ml syringe of saline is then passed by the same route into the suprarenal aorta and inflated. The infrarenal aortic neck can then be dissected out proximally until either the aneurysm

Anastomotic technique

Once the proximal aorta and iliac arteries have been controlled, the aneurysm sac is opened and thrombus removed. Where possible a straight tube graft is used. It is important that this is sized correctly as the proximal anastomosis is more likely to leak if distance has had to be made up on either the native aorta or the graft. The end of the graft can be cut obliquely or beveled to match the aortic diameter. The anastomosis is performed using a 1.2 m 3.0 monofilament suture with assistants maintaining tension of the suture and adequate exposure by retraction of the bowels and left renal vein. The surgeon should stand on the patient's left in order to have both hands free for the suturing. The anastomosis is started at the nine o'clock position with six or seven deep bites securing the posterior wall. These bites ideally incorporate the anterior spinal ligament as the aortic wall is often deficient posteriorly. Once the suture line has reached the three o'clock position it is useful to place a corner stitch to pull the graft up into the native aorta. This is achieved by taking the suture inside out right through the aortic wall, re-entering the aortic wall more distally and then going inside to out on the graft. The stitch is performed with the stitch at the nine o'clock position and the anterior wall can then simply be overrun.

The graft is clamped and the proximal aortic clamp removed slowly to test the proximal anastomosis. If there are areas that bleed, these should only be stitched after the clamp has been reapplied. If there is concern regarding the quality of the aortic wall this can be buttressed with teflon pledgets. If the bleeding is coming from the posterior wall then it may help to overrun the entire wall with a new suture. The most important factor in performing the anastomosis is to be aware that there is only one good chance to get it right. It is better to take time and ensure that each stitch is correctly placed and pushed through the tissues vertically and cleanly rather than a speedy leaking anastomosis.

If an anastomosis is insecure or attempts at pledgeted sutures have been unsuccessful the only, and final option, is to cut it out and resuture at a higher level. While the technique for medial visceral rotation is described later in this chapter for the repair of suprarenal aneurysms, we would avoid its use where possible; it is usually possible to get higher by pulling down on the aneurysm and moving the clamp to a suprarenal position. Glue will not make an anastomosis secure and tends to be lifted away from a leaking suture line by the bleeding.

Left-sided inferior vena cava Retro-aortic left renal vein

A retro-aortic left renal vein is the most common anomaly and has been identified in 2% of aortic aneurysms. It crosses the aorta by passing behind the aneurysm neck and frequently has an associated anterior branch. The inferior vena cava (IVC) may also cross to the left side of the aorta at the level of the neck and similarly may have both anterior and posterior branches. When the aorta is approached anteriorly, a left-sided IVC should not present problems and with vertical anterio-posterior clamping the same applies to a retro-aortic renal vein.

Horseshoe kidney

This is a congenital abnormality of renal development observed in 1 in 500 to 1000 patients. Fusion of the upper poles (90%) or lower poles (10%) of the kidneys produces a horseshoe-shaped structure running across anterior to the aorta (Fig. 3). If the abnormality is picked up preoperatively, there is the option of using a retroperitoneal approach. If the abnormality is discovered intraoperatively, it is preferable to control the aorta

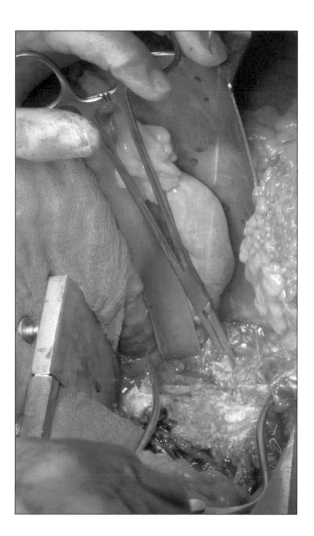

FIG. 2 The aorta is clamped in an anterior-posterior plane by means of a straight clamp.

proximally and the iliac artery orifices with balloons from within the sac, leaving the aneurysm sac. The proximal and distal anastomoses can both be per-

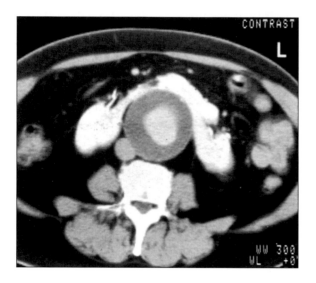

FIG. 3 CT-scan image of a horseshoe kidney.

formed from within the aneurysm sac. If there are multiple low renal arteries then these will need to be revascularized using an inlay technique.

Inflammatory aortic aneurysm

Between 2% and 10% of infrarenal abdominal aortic aneurysms are inflammatory. If an inflammatory aneurysm is diagnosed preoperatively it is better repaired via a retroperitoneal approach (see below) as the inflammatory process encases the duodenum and left renal vein. The CT-scan will show an abnormal soft tissue lying anterior to the aneurysm wall; this wraps posteriorly in a horseshoe and may extend laterally to involve the retroperitoneum and ureters. Intraoperatively, the aortic wall appearance is glistening pearly white (Fig. 4). The duodenum is firmly applied to the aneurysm wall and attempts to separate it may result in duodenal perforation. Some surgeons dissect the aneurysm neck using sharp dissection with a knife through the layers of the aortic wall. We do not believe that this is advisable. The aorta can be controlled proximally

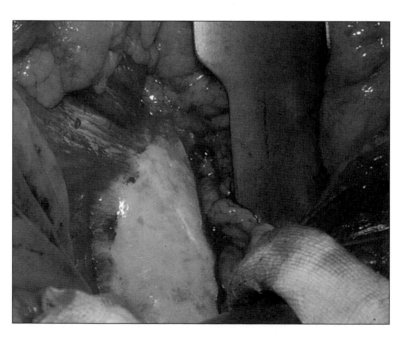

FIG. 4 Intraoperative picture of an inflammatory aneurysm with its typical glistening pearly white appearance.

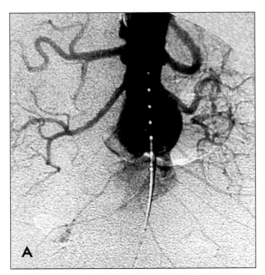

from within the lesser sac; the aneurysm can then be opened and the iliac arteries can be controlled with balloon catheters. The aneurysm is then repaired in the standard way using an inlay graft.

Suprarenal aneurysm

In approximately 5% of aortic aneurysms, disease extends proximally into the juxta- or suprarenal aorta. More frequently, anterior angulation of the aortic neck under the left renal vein masquerades as a suprarenal aneurysm (Fig. 5).

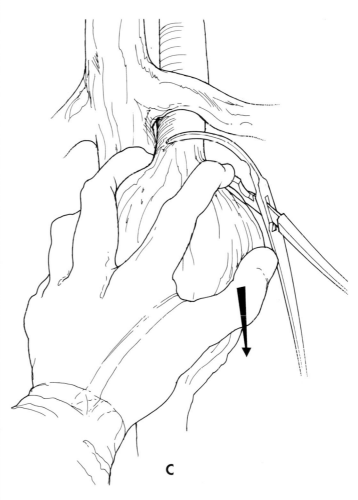

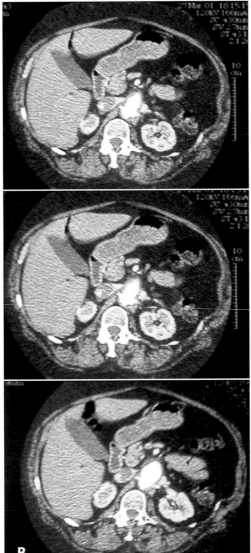

FIG. 5 Large aneurysm with horizontal aortic neck. A - Angiography, suggesting that the renal artery would originate from the aneurysm. B - CT scan showing the horizontal neck. C - Schematic drawing showing how the hand of the surgeon pulls down the aneurysm in order to present the neck to cross-clamp.

Such angulation will also result from a posterior aneurysm rupture. In these cases it is often necessary to pull down on the aneurysm and mobilize the left renal vein proximally. If the vein is to be divided it is important to preserve its side branches. One therefore needs to make an early decision whether to ligate the renal vein and maintain the adrenal and gonadal side branches or to sacrifice the gonadal vein to facilitate mobilization. Ligation of the gonadal vein followed by ligation of the left renal vein leads to left renal venous hypertension and a deterioration in renal function.

If the aneurysm is truly suprarenal then there may be no option but to use a retroperitoneal approach with medial visceral rotation. It is possible to convert to this approach intraoperatively by controlling the supra-celiac aorta and extending the midline laparotomy incision beneath the left costal margin. It may also be necessary to position the left arm across the patient's body on a support and place a sand bag under the left flank to improve exposure. The reflection of the peritoneum is divided lateral to the sigmoid mesocolon and the avascular plane developed along the anterior surface of the psoas muscle. It is important to extend this dissection as high as the left crus of the diaphragm. The spleen is then mobilized as the final stage of the dissection. This dissection exposes the left diaphragmatic crus which is divided using diathermy to allow access to the aorta at the hiatus. The aneurysm sac is opened accepting that there will be mild back bleeding from the visceral and renal ostia. These arteries should not be clamped. An aortic graft is then sewn in with a beveled proximal anastomosis incorporating the celiac axis, superior mesenteric artery and right renal origins (Fig. 6). The left renal artery can be either included in this anastomosis or separately re-implanted.

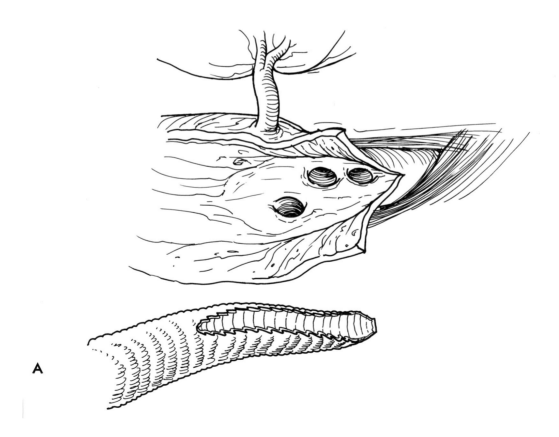

A

FIG. 6 Beveled proximal anastomosis. A - Opening of the aorta at the left-posterior side, beyond the level of the renal arteries, giving access to the visceral arteries. Clamping is performed at the diaphragm and a beveled anastomosis is constructed.

(to be continued)

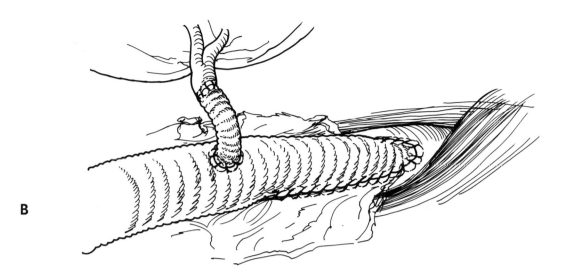

B

FIG. 6 B - Completed anastomosis. The left renal artery is repaired by means of a prosthetic graft.

It is essential that a cell saving device is used as blood loss is considerable and that patients are given adequate infusions of fresh frozen plasma and platelets. The visceral and renal arteries will back bleed during the procedure. This can be controlled by pressure down on the mesentry. We would avoid occluding these vessels with balloon catheters due to the risk of dissection and distal embolization.

Conclusion

A careful planned approach to the proximal aortic neck in patients with aortic aneurysm rupture is vital if success is to be achieved. Success is unlikely if the anastomosis is not performed correctly first time. The surgeon must be able to gain access and control of the aorta rapidly without disrupting adjacent structures. This necessitates an awareness of both the normal anatomy and common variants as described. The anastomosis must achieve adequate fixation without further disrupting the aortic wall. The help of an experienced assistant in ensuring adequate light, exposure and suture tension is vital. The anastomosis must be adequate at first attempt. While the technique for the management of suprarenal aneurysms has been described in the emergency setting, an anterior approach is preferred, even if this means leaving a proximal dilated aortic segment.

9

RECONSTRUCTION OF A COMPLETELY CALCIFIED AORTA

ALAIN BRANCHEREAU, GABRIELLE SARLON, NICOLAS VALERIO

Reviewing this problem for all aortic locations would imply considering all possible aortic reconstruction techniques. We will restrict ourselves to the calcified lesions of the infrarenal aorta, which comprise the most commonly occurring problems.

When discussing a completely calcified aorta, two questions should be raised: first, what is the importance and sometimes the specificity of this lesion in relation to other atherosclerotic lesions; and second, how should we treat it? Given that the topic of this book is the difficult and unexpected problems a vascular surgeon should resolve, we will focus in particular on the second question, even though the first is covered in a separate paragraph.

Anatomical and pathophysiological aspects

PATHOPHYSIOLOGY

Atherosclerosis is characterized by a chronic inflammation of the arterial wall, initiated and sustained by disturbances of the lipid metabolism, and is frequently associated with calcium deposits. The arterial calcification process, as it occurs in atherosclerosis, starts early in life and increases with age, in parallel with the degree of atherosclerosis.

In the literature two types of arterial calcification have been described [1]: intimal calcifications in the atheromatous plaque; and media calcifications (Mönckeberg sclerosis or media sclerosis), which can develop in the presence or absence of atherosclerosis. Calcifications of the atheromatous plaque mostly occur deep in the intima, close to the internal elastic layer. They are localized particularly in areas with hemodynamic stress and fibromuscular proliferation, where the intima tends to become more rigid (Fig. 1).

In contrast, media calcifications occur independently of the atherosclerosis and are often associated with metabolic disorders, such as hypervitaminosis D, chronic terminal renal insufficiency, or diabetes.

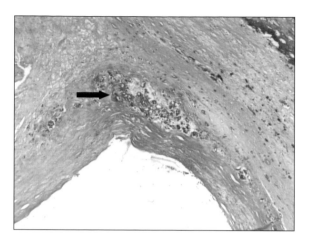

FIG. 1 Arterial specimen showing intimal calcifications.

These usually occur in arteries that are less frequently affected by atheroma, such as the abdominal visceral, thyroid, and mammarian arteries. They may also appear in the aorta, except for the coronary arteries. A genetic factor, independent of diabetes or atherosclerosis, appears to be related to this process. This media sclerosis is associated with an elevated cardiovascular risk profile in diabetic patients. In renal insufficiency, it is due to secondary hyperparathyroidism, which changes the calcium and phosphor metabolism. It is strongly associated with the duration of hemodialysis and the severity of the disturbance in the calcium and phosphor metabolism.

MOLECULAR ASPECTS

Many studies have demonstrated the similarity between the development of calcifications and osteogenesis. Recently, cellular and molecular components involved in osteogenesis have been identified in atheromatous plaques at the level of the calcified areas. Two models of formation and inhibition of the calcification process have been described [2].

The active model is based on the existence of arterial cells that are phenotypically similar to cells involved in osteogenesis. Cytokines and proteins resembling those found in osseous tissue interfere with the intercellular signaling routes, leading to the appearance of calcifications. Thus, the calcium containing deposits of osseous hydroxyapatite are very like those found in arterial calcifications.

The passive model is based on abnormal deposits of calcium which are fostered by a reduction of proteins usually present in a healthy arterial wall that inhibit the deposition of serum calcium. This model is in agreement with the calcification process of the media. Furthermore, it is known that certain cytokines are produced by inflammatory atheromatous plaques and play a facilitating role in osteogenesis.

ENDOCRINE AND PHARMACOLOGICAL ASPECTS

Physiological and pathophysiological circumstances, as well as therapeutical interventions, may modify the calcification of an atheromatous plaque. Parathormone and vitamin D are the main factors in the homeostasis of osseous calcium. Hyperparathyroidism or hypervitaminosis D may cause arterial calcifications. Estrogens [3] possess an anti-atherogenic effect and could inhibit the development of calcifications when atherosclerotic lesions are present. Statins and serum lipids (LDL and HDL cholesterol) might also play an as yet unclear role in the occurrence of calcifications [4].

GENETIC ASPECTS

The use of animal models has allowed us to discover genetic factors that play a role in atherosclerosis. The existence of a genetic predisposition helps to understand the interindividual variation in the atherosclerotic process and arterial calcifications.

Ongoing research focuses on osteoclast-like arterial cells, which appear to be a promising therapeutic option to counteract the growth of arterial calcium deposits.

MECHANICAL PROPERTIES

Arterial calcifications [5] lead to rigidity of the arterial wall, which reduces arterial compliance. The subsequent increase of the afterload results in an elevation of systolic blood pressure, which is deleterious to the cardiovascular system.

How to avoid surprises

Nowadays it is astonishing and questionable when a vascular surgeon is confronted with major aortic calcifications without having identified these preoperatively. Modern imaging techniques [6], in particular CT-scanning, should enable surgeons to identify these lesions, guide preoperative investigations, and choose an appropriate therapeutic strategy.

PLAIN X-RAY

This is a simple, well-tolerated and reliable method. It is not routinely performed and if its quality is mediocre with a considerable amount of abdominal air, the calcifications may be overlooked. If requested in order to find calcifications, it is nearly always possible to diagnose this on a plain X-ray (Fig. 2).

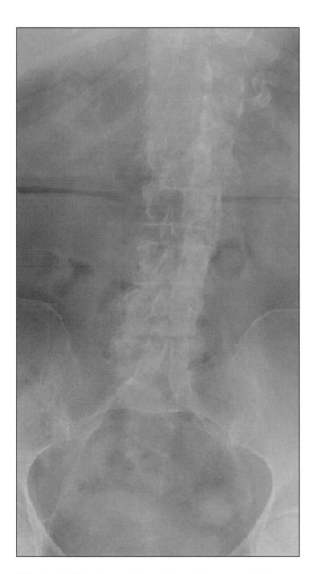

FIG. 2 Calcifications of the abdominal aorta visible on a plain abdominal X-ray.

DUPLEX SCANNING

Arterial calcifications can be detected as a hyperdensity on duplex scanning. Because calcified plaques cannot be penetrated by ultrasound, no image can be derived from structures below the plaque, resulting in a shadowed cone underneath (Fig. 3). Beyond the image itself, it is the investigator's interpretation that is important and should detect the presence and localization of calcifications. The presence of calcium deposits makes quantification of the size of an arterial stenosis hard, or even impossible, and only hemodynamic quantification can be done by calculating the peak systolic velocity in the stenosis. Recognized limitations of this method are its operator dependency and poor reproducibility.

CT-SCANNING

CT-scanning is the most reliable, reproducible and noninvasive technique to detect the presence of calcifications in the form of a varying hyperdensity of the arterial wall. Currently, this technique is the investigation that most commonly leads to the diagnosis of a calcified aorta. It enables visualization of all calcifications: their thickness, extent, regularity, homogeneity, and involvement with the visceral arteries (Fig. 4). Moreover, it allows visualization of frequently related intraluminally burgeoning calcified lesions (Fig. 5). The calcifications may be difficult to discern from the enhanced arterial lumen on a contrast-enhanced CT-scan. In order to differentiate these lesions, performing a CT-scan before and after injection of a contrast agent is recommended (Fig. 6).

A recent technique, electron beam CT-scan (EBCT), measures the calcium content of the plaque to use as a marker of the atheromatous disease and to deduce the associated cardiovascular risk from it [6].

MAGNETIC RESONANCE IMAGING (MRI)

Gadolinium-enhanced magnetic resonance angiography shows only the arterial lumen and does not enable analysis of the arterial wall. The classic MRI with weighed T1 and T2 sequences cannot show wall calcifications, but can detect their presence by means of a hypodense signal [7].

High-resolution MRI analyzes the biochemical composition of the wall, in particular its lipid compound. It should enable the detection of calcifications. However, it can only be performed by means of low-penetration detectors, which precludes its

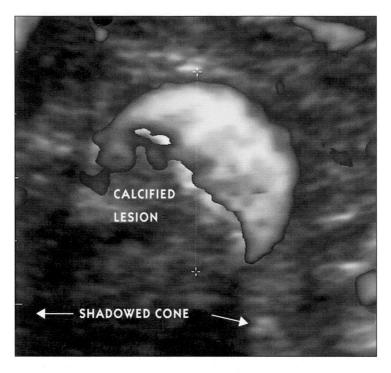

FIG. 3 Ultrasound image of shading generated by calcifications in the abdominal aorta.

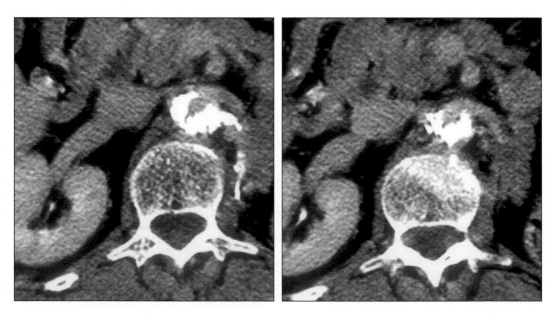

FIG. 4 CT-scan showing calcifications of the abdominal aorta and renal arteries.

use for the abdominal aorta. In general, the MRI technique does not contribute substantially to the investigation of aortic calcifications.

INVESTIGATION STRATEGY

This comprises two phases: first, recognition of the calcified aorta; and second, preoperative assessment of how to manage the calcified aorta. Elective surgery of the infrarenal aorta is being performed more frequently for an abdominal aortic aneurysm (AAA) than for an occlusive lesion. In our experience of the last three years, 72% of the aortic reconstructions were because of an AAA (204 AAAs vs. 79 aortoiliac occlusive lesions). If the presence of a

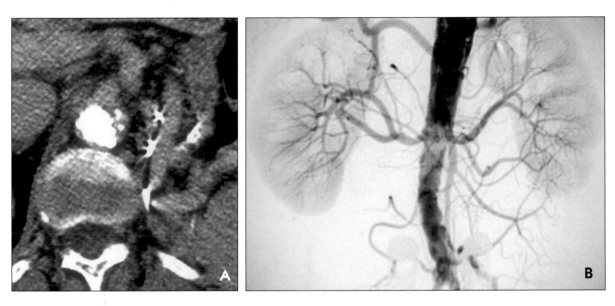

FIG. 5 A - CT-scan showing aortic calcifications with a calcified intraluminal protrusion. B - Digital subtraction angiography. Calcified intraluminal protrusion, manifested by a clear defect in the contrast column.

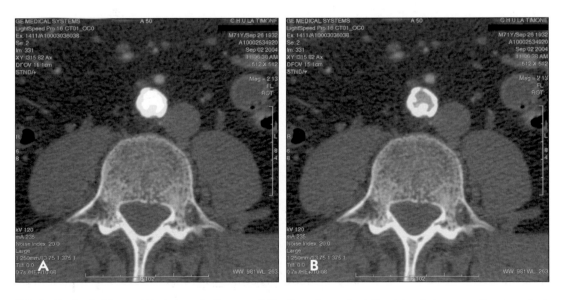

FIG. 6 Contrast CT-scan (A) does not discern calcifications from circulating blood. Images without contrast injection (B) are required.

totally calcified aorta *(porcelain aorta)* is specific to occlusive lesions, then the same incidence of major calcifications occupying the whole circumference of the aorta at a certain level is seen in occlusive and aneurysmatic lesions. If the indication is based on a digital angiography, the calcifications are usually visible and major calcifications should not be overlooked while interpreting the negatives, even the subtracted ones (Fig. 7). If the indication is based on a CT-scan, calcifications are not to be missed. It is more problematic to base the indication for operation on duplex scanning. The scanned images are at best poorly informative and it is the investigator who should indicate the presence of calcifications. Their detection depends on the operator.

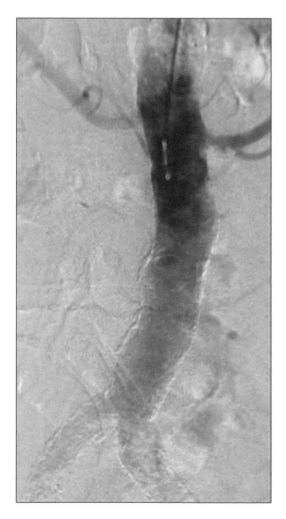

FIG. 7 Digital subtraction angiography shows the presence of calcifications, due to the subtraction mask.

Therefore, it is the task of the surgeon who operates merely on these data to establish an investigation protocol and communication method with the vascular technician, in order that severe calcifications are not missed before the intervention. When both surgeon and technician are unsure, an additional CT-scan should be performed or at least a plain abdominal X-ray to ascertain an accurate result. In the case of severe calcifications, the whole aorta should be explored in order to find a proximal aortic area that is sufficiently unaffected to place a clamp. This exploration can best be done by means of a CT-scan. Routinely, a plain X-ray gives the best information. It is also essential to evaluate the vessel wall and the degree of calcification of the arteries that may be involved in the same procedure, for example: the renal arteries (Fig. 4), if a simultaneous aortic and renal surgical procedure is anticipated; the inferior mesenteric and hypogastric arteries, if there is a risk of colic ischemia; the iliac arteries, in case of AAA surgery; and the femoral arteries, in the case of occluding lesions. CT-scanning offers the best information in these instances. If the femoral trifurcation is not included, ultrasound can be used as a means of investigation, if the aim is specified.

ASSESSMENT OF THE RISK AND PREOPERATIVE STRATEGY

The question is whether the finding of a calcified aorta is a manifestation of a particularly severe location of generalized atherosclerosis, which should determine a specific preoperative assessment, especially regarding the cardiac risk. Wilson et al. [8] have shown that arterial calcifications are a preclinical marker of atheromatous disease, as well as an independent risk factor for cardiovascular morbidity and mortality, and coronary disease. In a similar study, Walsh et al. concluded that calcium deposits of the abdominal aorta are an independent risk factor for congestive heart failure [9]. Furthermore, the presence of aortic calcifications increases the risk of calcifications in the coronaries and aortic valves.

Thus, the detection of major aortic calcifications should incite a more thorough cardiac evaluation than is common before infrarenal aortic surgery. At least some functional tests, such as stress ultrasound or myocardial thallium scintigraphy, should be performed in all these patients. A coronary angiography is performed by many centers in these patients as a routine or if the functional tests are positive.

Clamping techniques

MECHANICAL ASPECTS

The possibility of clamping the aorta and its effectiveness are the first problems in surgery in case of a calcified aorta. The existence of calcifications has several mechanical consequences. A so-called *lead pipe aorta* or *porcelain aorta* may be totally impossible to clamp because of its rigidity (Fig. 8). In other cases, the pressure exerted by the clamp leads to the breaking of the calcifications, which allows general compression of the aorta by squeezing two plaques against each other. The danger in the latter case is that the areas of the plaque that have been fractured during squeezing may perforate the aortic wall sideways (Fig. 9). A last hurdle, which may lead to ineffective clamping, is related to calcified protrusions that are frequently associated with wall calcifications (Fig. 5). In this case, a clamping that has succeeded in squeezing the aorta may be insufficient because of a calcified protrusion, which leaves the aortic lumen partly unoccluded (Fig. 10).

ENDOVASCULAR OCCLUSION

Occlusion of the aorta by means of an intraluminal balloon may at first seem appealing, but it is usually inapplicable in practice. One cannot use the standard 14F Fogarty occlusion catheters *(Edwards Lifescience Corporation)* to occlude the iliac arteries during AAA surgery. When the corresponding balloon is inflated and reaches a sufficient diameter to fill the aortic lumen, its form and pressure on the wall are inadequate to resist the arterial pressure, because this type of balloon is invariably displaced after a few minutes by the systemic arterial pressure. For aortic occlusion, one should use a specific catheter, whose balloon reaches a diameter of 45 millimeters after inflation, i.e. a 22F Fogarty occlusion catheter. Figure 11 shows these two balloons for iliac and aortic occlusion.

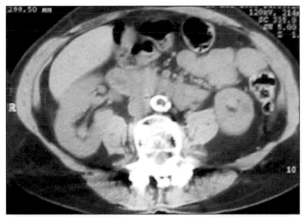

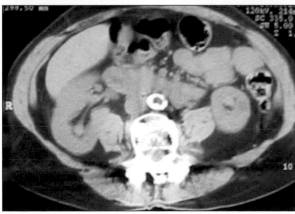

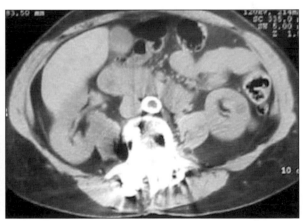

FIG. 8 CT-scan image of a completely calcified aorta. These so-called *lead tube* or *porcelain aorta* lesions completely prevent clamping.

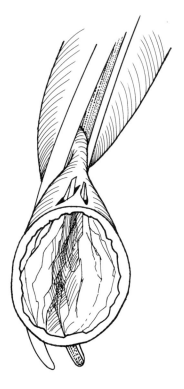

FIG. 9 Scheme showing clamping allowed by fracturing the calcifications and squeezing the two plaques together. The danger is creating a wall perforation with the spikes of the broken calcified plaque.

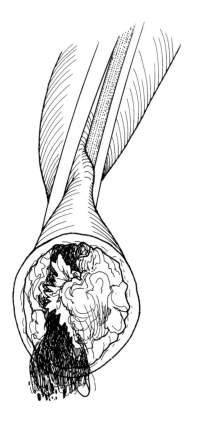

FIG. 10 Scheme showing how a calcified protrusion may result in ineffective clamping.

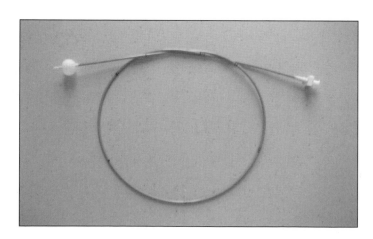

FIG. 11 Fogarty occlusion catheters: 14F for iliac occlusion (diameter when inflated: 28 millimeters); 22F for aortic occlusion (diameter when inflated: 45 millimeters).

The technique for endoluminal occlusion from the infrarenal level was described and proposed in the surgical treatment of ruptured aortic aneurysms [10]. When a completely calcified aorta is present, this technique has two major drawbacks: catheterization difficulties due to endoluminal lesions; and the risk of incomplete occlusion or balloon rupture due to the presence of calcified, coral-like protrusions in the aortic lumen.

Other aortic occlusion techniques by means of a balloon, introduced preoperatively from a distance and under endoscopic control, are theoretically possible. However, catheterization through a femoral artery is problematic when these lesions are present, and catheterization via an upper limb requires leaving the sheet in-situ during the whole access and reconstruction procedure, with the associated risk of vertebro-subclavian thrombosis.

In total, these endoluminal aortic occlusion techniques are more theoretical than practical. We do not have any experience with them and did not find any study in the literature presenting a patient series operated with such a device.

AORTIC OCCLUSION USING EXTERNAL COMPRESSION

Under extreme and unexpected circumstances, in which standard clamping appears impossible or ineffective, one may obtain an aortic occlusion "by chance", by means of a clamp that compresses the aorta against the spine (Fig. 12). This clamp may be positioned without dissection, guided by the palpation of the aortic pulsations. For this purpose, however, a directly suprarenal or supraceliac area needs to be present where the calcifications can be compressed. The clamp is held by an assistant as long as the surgeon needs to find a solution for regular clamping. In general, this solution is found

by desobstructing an infrarenal aortic segment, which is then supported by means of pladgets (see below) and enables the placement of an infrarenal clamp. One should realize that such clamping by compression is often incomplete as it relies on the complete immobility of the assistant and the possibility to completely squeeze the aortic lumen. This may not be achieved continuously. This solution should not be used on purpose during elective surgery and should be considered as a rescue option.

SUPRACELIAC AORTIC CLAMPING VIA MEDIAN LAPAROTOMY

This is the classic technique and widely used in the treatment of juxtarenal aneurysms [11]. Minimal access to the supraceliac aorta will suffice as it is not necessary to dissect the aorta on all its sides. This is obtained after transection of the triangular hepatic ligament, on the right of the esophagus and after transection of the right pillar of the diaphragm [12]. Subsequently, the lateral sides of the aorta are released digitally, an open clamp is introduced (the beak of which is strongly supported by the underlying vertebra) and the clamping is performed. This clamping method is simple, quick, and well known by all vascular surgeons. Because the clamp cannot be moved up or down, it has the inconvenience of allowing clamping at a single aortic level only. The clamp is always positioned proximal to the celiac trunk and causes hepatic, intestinal and renal ischemia.

In case of a calcified aorta, one should make sure that the calcifications do not reach the supraceliac aorta, as this may hinder the clamping. If no preoperative CT-scan is made and the maneuver is used during the operation, one should preferably check by palpation that the aorta does not have major calcifications at that level.

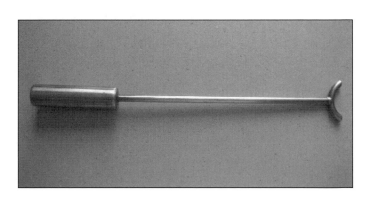

FIG. 12 Aorta squeezing clamp.

EXTRAPERITONEAL AORTIC CLAMPING

Access to the aorta is obtained via a left lateral thoracoabdominal approach. An incision in the tenth intercostal space with transection of the left pillar of the diaphragm opens the access to the visceral and supraceliac aorta [13]. An incision at the level of the ninth intercostal space, which implies opening of the pleural cavity and partial resection of the diaphragm, enables access to the distal 5 to 10 centimeters of the descending aorta. The advantages of this approach are: an excellent window to the visceral aorta and, if required, the descending aorta; a continuous exposition of the suprarenal and infrarenal aorta; the opportunity to choose the best clamping site; and, in particular at the level of the visceral arteries, the preservation of part of the abdominal viscera during the clamping.

Techniques for aortic reconstruction

BYPASS PROCEDURES FROM THE INFRARENAL ARTERY

When the aorta is clamped, an end-to-side anastomosis may always be attempted using firm needles and a Wylie perforator for calcified walls (Fig. 13). When the aorta is completely calcified, this technique seems hazardous to us and is dissuaded. It may lead to irreversible damage to the aortic wall, inexorable bleeding, or may simply be impossible to perform. An innovative technique has been proposed by a Japanese group to achieve an end-to-side anastomosis on a porcelain aorta [14]. This technique consists of creating a window in the anterior side of the aorta that has been desobstructed and reinforced, to which the prosthesis can be anastomosed (Fig. 14). It is interesting to note that with their technique the authors achieve the aortic desobstruction by means of a rotating cutter.

Our technique is an end-to-end anastomosis after preparation of the proximal aorta. After clamping, always above the renal arteries, the aorta is opened transversely, leaving an infrarenal aortic segment of 3 to 5 centimeters. Bleeding from the proximal aorta should be stopped or the blood saved. In this case, it is possible to stop the bleeding by means of a balloon catheter that is not exposed to the systemic blood pressure. However, its introduction is not always easy. Another solution, especially when the bleeding is moderate, is to place a suction tube, connected with the cell saver, in the aortic lumen (Fig. 15). This has the advantage of not hampering the exposed area and not immobilizing the assistant's hands. The distal aortic segment is shortened 3 to 4 centimeters to allow for a correct positioning of the prosthesis. It is then desobstructed for 1 to 2 centimeters to be able to close the distal aorta by means of a double transverse suture. Subsequently a 1 to 2 centimeter desobstruction of the proximal aorta is performed, while taking care not to extend the aortic desobstruction to the orifices of the renal arteries (Fig. 16). If a pair of lumbar arteries originate from that level, they are oversewn. In this way, a 1 to 2 centimeter segment of desobstructed and smooth aorta is obtained. It is possible to anastomose the prosthesis directly to this aortic segment. However, the wall is thin and fragile. One may use 4x0 stitches, but this induces the risk of bleeding from the needle holes, or a 5x0 su-

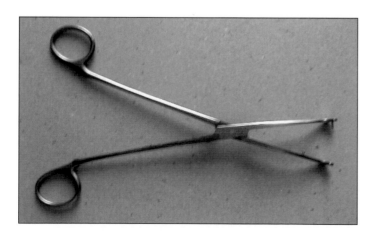

FIG. 13 Wylie perforator for calcified wall.

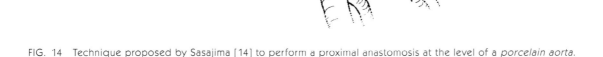

FIG. 14   Technique proposed by Sasajima [14] to perform a proximal anastomosis at the level of a *porcelain aorta*.

ture, which is rather thin for an aortic suture. For these reasons, we routinely apply a teflon reinforcement band for the aortic wall, placed around the aorta with a four-point fixation with monofilament 5x0. One may also reinforce the wall by injecting a small amount of biological glue between the desobstructed aortic wall and the teflon felt collar (Fig. 17). The suture between the prosthesis and the aorta prepared in this manner may be achieved by means of monofilament 4x0 or 3x0 at large intervals. When this suture is tested, usually the supraceliac aortic clamp is removed and a clamp is placed over the aortic prosthesis. The rest of the procedure does not cause specific problems to this area.

Bypass Procedure from the Descending Aorta

The site of the proximal anastomosis of the bypass depends on the extent and the localization of the calcifications. If these stop at the level of the visceral arteries, an extraperitoneal approach via the ninth intercostal space allows control over the distal end of the descending aorta to perform the aortic clamping and anastomosis directly proximal to the origin of the celiac trunk. This two-pronged solution, comprising wide access to the infrarenal and visceral aorta, requires a large and rather aggressive dissection but has no advantage if a revascularization from the descending aorta has been planned. If so, the best option is to use the revascularization technique from the descending aorta as has been described extensively [15] and of which several series have been reported with satisfactory results [16]. The special feature of this technique is to avoid access to the abdominal aorta and to gain a minimal access to the descending aorta by means of a short thoracotomy at the level of the seventh or eighth intercostal space. The general impact is less than that of a laparotomy and much less than a thoracophrenicolaparotomy. The tunneling of the prosthesis is completed extraperitoneally and extraanatomically (Fig. 18).

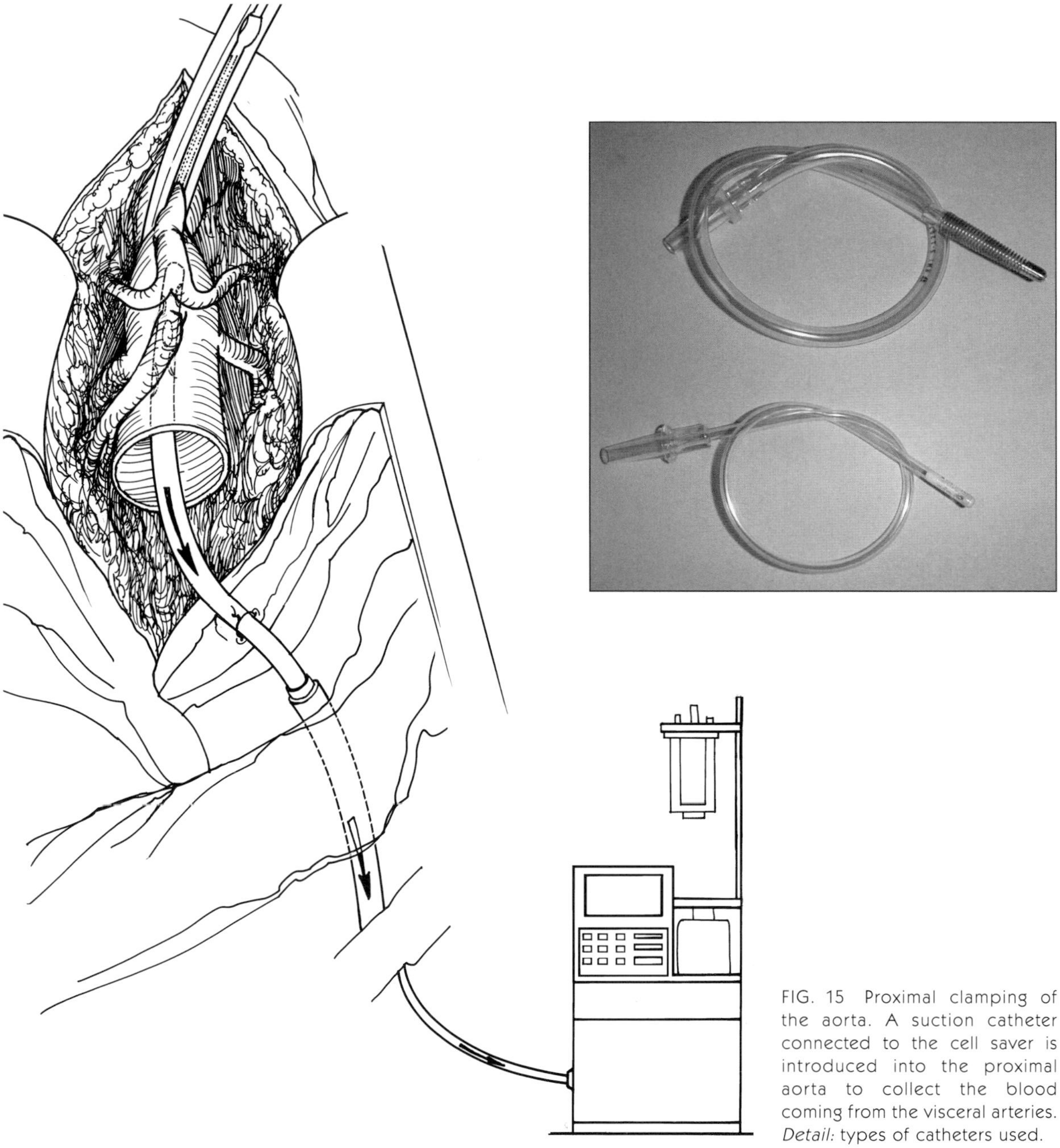

FIG. 15 Proximal clamping of the aorta. A suction catheter connected to the cell saver is introduced into the proximal aorta to collect the blood coming from the visceral arteries. *Detail:* types of catheters used.

BYPASS PROCEDURE FROM THE ASCENDING AORTA: VENTRAL AORTA

This is the last-resort technique, to be combined with an axillobifemoral bypass, if the whole descending and abdominal aorta is calcified. This technique is applied especially to treat diffuse aortic lesions, as seen in Takayasu's disease. We have used it to revascularize the limbs and renal arteries in two patients presenting with an aortic hypoplasia [17]. In two other cases we have used the ascending aorta to revascularize the digestive arteries in two patients presenting with chronic abdominal angina and a completely calcified descending and abdominal aorta. This requires a sternolaparotomy. The proximal anastomosis is carried out by lateral clamping of the ascending aorta under systemic arterial

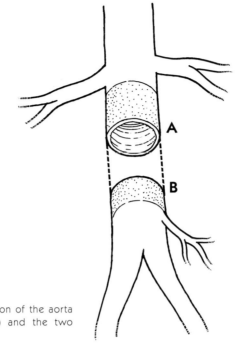

FIG. 16 Scheme showing the transaction of the aorta (A), the resection of the aorta (AB) and the two desobstructed areas *(shaded)*.

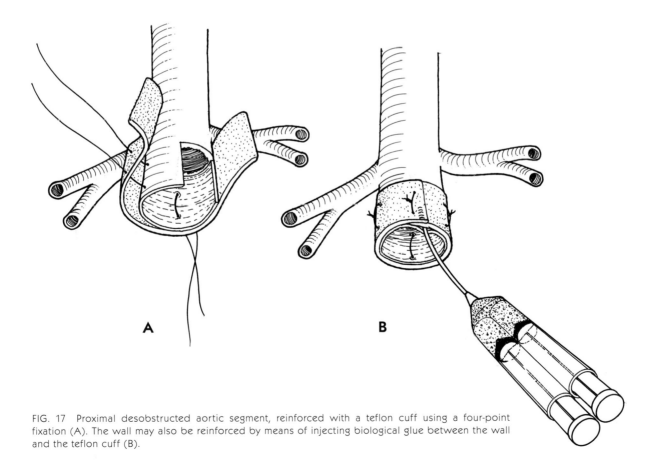

A

B

FIG. 17 Proximal desobstructed aortic segment, reinforced with a teflon cuff using a four-point fixation (A). The wall may also be reinforced by means of injecting biological glue between the wall and the teflon cuff (B).

hypotension. The tunneling of the prosthesis is S-shaped with a proximal right convexity and a convexity to the left in the distal part. It crosses the diaphragm through a window in the right diaphragmatic arch and passes behind the left lobe of the liver into the retroperitoneal region (Fig. 19). The prosthesis then joins the infrarenal aorta and the iliac vessels according to a standard technique.

Therapeutic strategy

AORTIC ANEURYSM

The insertion of an endoprosthesis in case of a totally calcified aorta cannot often be accomplished. A circular calcification is not a contraindication for an endoprosthesis, but is undoubtedly a limiting factor. If such a collar has an angulation, a length below

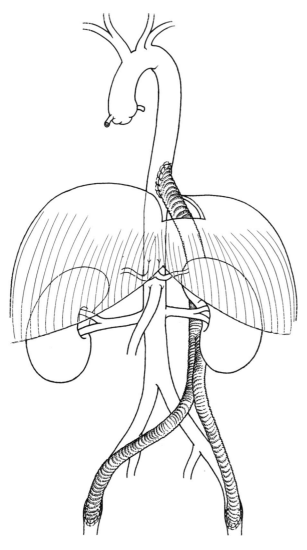

FIG. 18 Revascularization technique of the femoral arteries from the descending aorta.

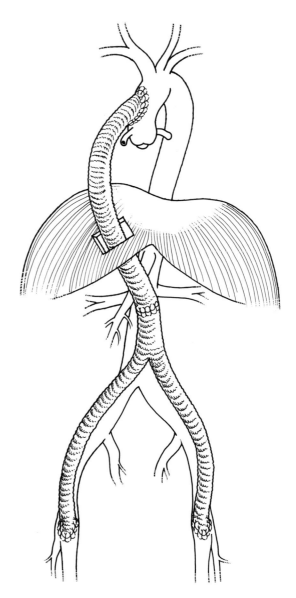

FIG. 19 Revascularization technique of the femoral arteries from the ascending aorta: *ventral aorta*.

10 to 15 millimeters, or anomalies such as calcified protrusions, it should not be considered feasible to perform endovascular treatment. Moreover, a circular calcification is generally associated with major calcifications of the iliac arteries, which usually means that introducer's tunneling of the endoprosthesis is impossible.

Conventional surgery necessarily implies access to the AAA in order to exclude the aneurysm either by closure at the aortic neck or by means of the inlay technique. It requires suprarenal or supraceliac aortic clamping at the level of the descending aorta. It is therefore important to assess the extent of the calcifications from the preoperative investigations exactly, in order to determine the precise level of clamping and to choose the approach to this level. Preferably, the aorta should be transected completely in order to perform the proximal anastomosis. As seen earlier, in some cases this may be done across the calcifications, if not after desobstruction of the aorta and reinforcement of the remaining wall by a teflon cuff. Under these circumstances, one can rarely implant an aorto-aortic tube or a bifurcated prosthesis at the level of the common iliac arteries, as this may compromise flow in the hypogastric arteries. A simple solution might be to desobstruct the distal end of the aorta, which is roughly resutured, and then to implant a bifurcated prosthesis to the common femoral arteries, in order to restore the hypogastric flow in a reverse direction.

OCCLUSIVE LESIONS

The choice is first and foremost determined by the possible clamping sites. If suprarenal or supraceliac clamping is an option, reconstruction from the abdominal aorta is the simplest solution. We prefer to use a left retroperitoneal approach, which seems to have a smaller impact than a median laparotomy and facilitates a better choice of the level of clamping between the directly suprarenal aorta and the distal descending aorta. The bypass procedure is then performed from the infrarenal aorta after transecting it as previously described.

If the supraceliac aorta is completely calcified and clamping at that level is thought to be problematic, one should preferably aim at revascularizing from the descending aorta with extraperitoneal extra-anatomical tunneling. The best approach is a limited thoracotomy, the level of which depends on the localization of the calcifications. This technique is less aggressive than a transperitoneal or extraperitoneal laparotomy. This is favorable in patients with an elevated operation risk. Some cases of revascularization from the descending aorta by means of video-assisted thoracoscopy have been described [18]. The technique is under evaluation and may be a promising option for this type of patient.

Finally, in cases where the complete descending aorta is calcified, revascularization from this level, as well as from the abdominal aorta, is impossible. One option is revascularization from the ascending aorta, after having ascertained by means of CT-scanning that there are no calcifications at that level. This comprises a more aggressive technique and requires a sternolaparotomy. If necessary, it allows for a simultaneous revascularization of the visceral arteries. Another alternative is an axillobifemoral bypass procedure, which is much less aggressive and suitable for high-risk patients. However, elevated complication rates are known for this type of bypass procedure, which should be reserved for critically ischemic patients [19].

Conclusion

The main point is to identify a calcified aorta preoperatively and to undertake a morphological assessment, preferably a CT-scan, which establishes the extent of the calcifications. These patients appear to have a higher-than-average operation risk, which warrants a thorough preoperative assessment, particularly regarding the cardiac risk.

The most commonly used techniques in our experience are:
1 - extraperitoneal approach of the aorta with transection of the infrarenal aorta and endarterectomy to prepare the site for the proximal anastomosis;
2 - a bypass from the descending aorta.

An axillofemoral or bifemoral bypass procedure should be restricted to high-risk patients and those with critical ischemia due to occlusive lesions. The presence of an aortic crushing device is justified in all vascular surgical operation theatres. The use of this instrument should be applied only as an ultimate, last-resort solution.

REFERENCES

1 Doherty TM, Fitzpatrick L, Inoue D et al. Molecular, endocrine, and genetic mechanisms of arterial calcification. *Endocr Rev* 2004; 25: 629-672.

2 Doherty TM, Asotra K, Fitzpatrick L et al. Calcification in atherosclerosis: bone biology and chronic inflammation at the arterial crossroads. *Proc Natl Acad Sci USA* 2003; 100: 11201-11206.

3 Hak AE, Pols HA, van Hemert AM, et al. Progression of aortic calcification is associated with metacarpal bone loss during menopause: a population-based longitudinal study. *Arterioscler Thromb Vasc Biol* 2000; 20: 1926-1931.

4 Mundy G, Garrett R, Harris S et al. Stimulation of bone formation in vitro and in rodents by statins. *Science* 1999; 286: 1946-1949.

5 O'Rourke M. Arterial compliance and wave reflection. *Arch Mal Coeur Vaiss* 1991; 84: S45-48.

6 Fayad ZA, Fuster V. Clinical imaging of the high-risk or vulnerable atherosclerotic plaque. *Circ Res* 2001; 89: 305-316.

7 Sands MJ, Levitin A. Basics on magnetic resonance imaging. *Semin Vasc Surg* 2004; 17: 66-82.

8 Wilson PW, Kauppila LI, O'Donnell CJ et al. Abdominal aortic calcific deposits are an important predictor of vascular morbidity and mortality. *Circulation* 2001; 103: 1529-1534.

9 Walsh CR, Cupples LA, Levy D et al. Abdominal aortic calcific deposits are associated with increased risk for congestive heart failure: the Framingham Heart Study. *Am Heart J* 2002; 144: 733-739.

10 Hyde GL, Sullivan DM. Fogarty catheter tamponade of ruptured abdominal aortic aneurysms. *Surg Gynecol Obstet* 1982; 154: 197-199.

11 Crawford ES, Beckett WC, Greer MS. Juxtarenal infrarenal abdominal aortic aneurysm. Special diagnostic and therapeutic considerations. *Ann Surg* 1986; 203: 661-670.

12 Ricco JB, Dubreuil F. Aorte cœliaque. In: Branchereau A, Magnan PE, Rosset E (eds). *Voies d'abord des vaisseaux*. Paris, Arnette Blackwell publishing Inc, 1995: pp 167-176.

13 Mathieu JP, Hartung O, Branchereau A. Aorte sous-rénale. In: Branchereau A, Magnan PE, Rosset E (eds). *Voies d'abord des vaisseaux*. Paris, Arnette Blackwell publishing Inc, 1995: pp 177-196.

14 Sasajima T, Inaba M, Azuma N et al. Novel anastomotic method enables aortofemoral bypass for patients with porcelain aorta. *J Vasc Surg* 2002; 35: 1016-1019.

15 Branchereau A, Espinoza H, Rudondy P et al. Descending thoracic aorta as an inflow source for late occlusive failures following aortoiliac reconstruction. *Ann Vasc Surg* 1991; 5: 8-15.

16 Criado E, Keagy BA. Use of the descending thoracic aorta as an inflow source in aortoiliac reconstruction: indications and long-term results. *Ann Vasc Surg* 1994; 8: 38-47.

17 Branchereau A, Albertini JN, Amabile P. Small aorta syndrome or aortic hypoplasia: nosology and treatment. *G Ital Chir Vasc* 1996; 3: 25-33.

18 Kolvenbach R, Da Silva L, Schwierz E et al. Descending aorta-to-femoral artery bypass: preliminary experience with a thoracoscopic technique. *Surg Laparosc Endosc Percutan Tech* 2000; 10: 76-81.

19 Harrington ME, Harrington EB, Haimov M et al. Axillofemoral bypass: compromised bypass for compromised patients. *J Vasc Surg* 1994; 20: 195-201.

10

UNINTENTIONAL OCCLUSION OF THE RENAL ARTERY DURING EVAR

JEAN-PIERRE BECQUEMIN, PASCAL DESGRANGES
ERIC ALLAIRE, HISHAM KOBEITER

Unintentional occlusion of the renal artery during endovascular aneurysm repair (EVAR) is a relatively rare event. In the September 2004 report from the EUROSTAR database (which included 5686 patients), 1116 side branches were blocked. Among them, 767 were blocked intentionally, 228 inadvertently and 121 were not specified. However, in the vast majority of cases, the coverage concerned the hypogastric artery. Renal arteries were covered in only 192 cases, including 126 accessory renal arteries and 66 main renal arteries. Thus, the estimated frequency of occlusion of the renal artery is 1.1%. However, on the EUROSTAR case report form it was not specified whether the renal artery was definitively covered or if it was blocked and subsequently reopened by appropriate methods. Therefore, the real percentage might be a little bit higher. In our own series of 456 stent-grafts placed between 1995 and 2001, five patients (1%) were found to have stent-graft coverage of one or two renal arteries.

In this chapter, we address our personal experience of these cases and present suggestions on how to prevent the occurrence of this event and some tips and tricks for dealing with the problem once it has occurred.

Case reports

CASE 1

A 78-year-old man presented with an aneurysm of 5 centimeters in diameter. His medical history includes myocardial infarction and mild hyperten-sion. The CT scan showed the infrarenal neck to be 1.5 centimeter long and a Vanguard® prosthe-sis was then placed inside. The postoperative course was uneventful. At the two-year follow-up, the Duplex scan showed no endoleak and the correctly functioning graft. However, a tight stenosis of the left renal artery was detected. Renal artery angioplasty was considered and this was performed by means of an introducer sheath via the arm and catheterization of the left renal artery with a 0.035 Terumo guide wire. Following this, a 5 millimeter x 2 centimeter balloon was pushed on the wire. The balloon could not be advanced into the renal artery, probably as a result of a strut of the graft's proximal bare stent crossing the renal artery ostium. After several attempts, the renal artery occluded. The patient was taken to the operating room. A graft was attached from the left external iliac artery to the left renal artery through a retroperitoneal approach. Three years afterwards, the stent-graft is still in place and the renal bypass is patent.

CASE 2

This woman was 75 years old and suffered from congestive heart failure. She presented in an emergent condition with a painful 7-centimeter aneurysm. She was considered inoperable due to poor cardiac function. The neck was short and angulated on the CT scan, but a stent-graft repair was attempted anyway. Unfortunately, the graft migrated upward during the procedure, leading to the coverage of both renal arteries. A right renal artery repair was performed with a bypass from the right external iliac artery to the right renal artery. The intervention was straightforward. She had a normal renal function on the first postoperative days. She died on the fourth postoperative day from a massive myocardial infarction.

CASE 3

A 76-year-old man was referred to us for repair of an aortic false aneurysm. Ten years earlier he had been operated on for lower limb ischemia. A bifurcated aortobifemoral graft was inserted with an end-to-side proximal anastomosis. The duplex scan and CT scan showed a large 5-centimeter aneurysm at the level of the aortic anastomosis and dilatation of the aortic bifurcation. The distance between the renal arteries and the aneurysm was more than 2 centimeters. However, the neck was conically shaped. The patient refused an open repair and a stent-graft repair was undertaken. Under local anesthesia, an aortouniiliac Cook graft was correctly deployed. However, when it came to catching the capsule which contained the first row of bare stents and hooks, the pusher could not go through the graft. After several attempts the pusher went up but we realized that the entire graft had moved upward

covering the renal and superior mesenteric arteries. The patient was then given general anesthesia, draped for an open procedure and a left thoracolaparotomy was performed. A 6 millimeter graft was attached from the distal thoracic aorta to the left renal artery. The aorta was then clamped and the stent-graft removed. A tube graft was placed from the celiac aorta to the body of the previous graft. The celiac artery and superior mesenteric artery were attached to the graft using the Crawford technique. Then we observed that the right renal artery could not be repaired due to severe atheromatous disease at the ostium. We dissected the main trunk free, divided the artery, and performed an end-to-end anastomosis with a 6 millimeter graft which was then reattached to the left renal bypass. After surgery, renal function never recovered and, because of renal failure, the patient became dialysis dependant.

CASE 4

We observed a distal migration of the main body of the graft at the two-year follow-up in a 78-year-old man who had a 6 centimeter large aneurysm treated with an AneurX® device. We attempted to place a proximal aortic cuff and a Cook device was chosen. The cuff was partially deployed and an angiogram was performed to check proper positioning of the cuff. We then realized that the cuff, if fully deployed, would cover both renal arteries. We placed two 0.035 wires from the left arm into both renal arteries and were able to place two 4-centimeter long self-expandable stents into the renal arteries. The aortic part of the stent was long enough to remain in the aorta above the cuff. The cuff was then fully deployed. However technically demanding, the procedure was successful, with aneurysm exclusion and patent renal arteries.

CASE 5

An 81-year-old woman was brought to the hospital by the mobile emergency unit. She had been found at home in shock and complained of excruciating back pain. On arrival, CT scanning showed a large aneurysm with retroperitoneal hematoma. She was taken to the operating room and an on-table angiogram was performed. This showed that an endovascular treatment was feasible. A Cook stent-graft was placed but completion angiography depicted that both renal arteries were covered by the graft. A right renal bypass was performed but the patient died a few hours later.

Anatomical, functional and clinical consequences of renal artery coverage

In almost all cases, coverage of a major renal artery will lead to renal infarction, the extent of which depends on the presence of patent polar arteries. The incidence of renal infarction varies greatly among series. In the experience of Bockler et al. [1], 19% of patients had renal infarction, mainly associated with endograft with suprarenal fixation. Contrary to this, Kim et al. [2] reported no renal infarction in a series of 114 patients, despite the fact that the polar renal arteries were covered in 11 cases. In our personal experience, which includes more than 300 suprarenal fixations, the incidence of renal infarction was rather low (1.3%).

The functional and clinical consequences are benign in the majority of cases. Most cases of renal artery coverage remain unnoticed.

Renal infarction is detected only by means of accurate image assessment of the kidneys on post-implantation CT scan [3]. A rise of blood pressure as a sign of renal impairment has almost never been mentioned in the literature.

Serum creatinin increase during follow-up of patients with stent-grafts has been underlined by several groups, including our own. At one year, between 5% and 10% of patients have a decline of the glomerular filtration index [4,5]. This mechanism is not fully understood and is probably not unique. It may include micro and macro emboli into the renal arteries, the use of contrast medium for the subsequent CT-scan evaluation and, occasionally, administration of nephrotoxic drugs, such as antibiotics or inhibitors of conversion enzymes.

In the worst case scenario, however, dialysis can be the ultimate outcome. It may happen when both renal arteries are occluded or when a single patent renal artery is blocked and the rescue measures have failed. We encountered one such case (0.2%) in our series.

Onset and mechanisms of renal artery coverage

Inadvertent coverage of the renal artery can occur at any time during or after the stent-graft (Figure) placement. Unintentional covering during deployment can be explained by clumsiness during external sheath retrieval (Fig. C), mishandling of the graft and poor visualization of the ostium of the renal arteries. Once the graft has been properly placed, modelling of the first row of stents may displace the graft and subsequently cover a renal artery. Micro and macro emboli into the renal arteries may occur when the neck contains thrombus. Thrombus can be dislodged at any time of the procedure and may happen during wire placement, graft positioning, deployment and even after a straightforward procedure. Also, unstable atheromatous plaques can be crushed and displaced, thereby upwards obstructing the renal arteries' ostium.

Renal artery blockage can also occur during follow-up. Although infrequent, upward migration can lead to the coverage of the renal artery by the covered part of the stent-graft. The true incidence is unknown since, to our knowledge, it has never been reported. The role of the bare stent placed across the renal arteries has been extensively evaluated. The impact of different stent designs on renal function was minimal in animal experiments [6,7]. Healing the stent struts generally leaves enough space for uninterrupted blood flow. The size of the struts is not large enough to represent a real danger in humans. Atherosclerotic renal artery stenosis may develop months or years after stent-graft placement. Subsequently, renal artery angioplasty may become difficult when the balloon cannot enter the lumen of the renal artery, precluding endovascular attempts (Case 1).

Predisposing factors

DIFFICULT NECKS

The risk of renal artery loss is obviously increased when the aortic necks are not optimal. Short necks require great attention and precision in all maneuvers. A stent-graft placed too distally may leave a type I proximal endoleak. A stent-graft placed too proximally endangers the renal arteries. Angulated necks are a classical contraindication for stent grafting. However, in some high-risk patients there is no alternative if aneurysm repair is necessary. The risk is determined by the different level of renal artery ostia arising from the aorta and also by the fact that it may be difficult to anticipate where the stent will land when deployed. The angle of the aorta

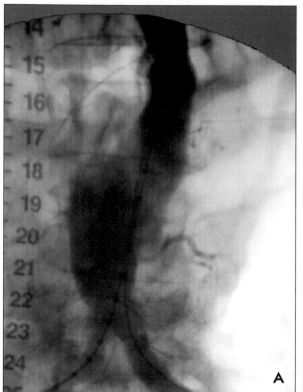

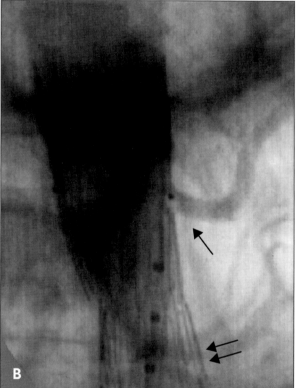

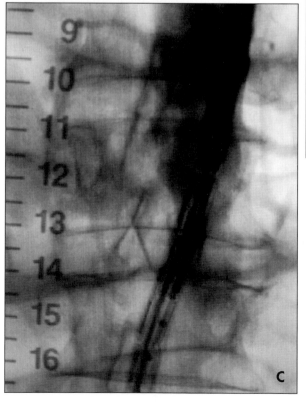

FIGURE   A - Arteriography before deployment.   B - Partially deployed stent-graft *(double arrow)* and adequate position with respect to the left renal artery *(arrow)*.   C - Following proximal deployment, arteriography shows occlusion of both renal arteries.

can be directed in the anterior-posterior plane but also in the lateral axis. Combined angles make it even more complex. It becomes even more demanding if both the angle between the renal artery segment of the aorta and the neck and the angle between the neck and the aneurysm itself are abnormal. Thrombus is an evident source of material migration into the visceral arteries. Avoiding endovascular manipulation in the neck is of prime importance when an endovascular option is chosen. Bulging necks also comprise technical difficulties because the level of apposition cannot be entirely controlled. In general, the grafts migrate upwards because of the pressure exercised by the distal aortic ring on the stent itself.

RENAL ARTERY ANATOMY

Renal arteries arise from the aorta at the same level in the majority of cases. However, asymmetry is not infrequent. In order to calculate the neck length, the level of the lowest renal artery must be taken into account. Polar arteries may be overlooked on CT scan and, therefore, can be covered unintentionally. Pre-existent renal artery stenosis may also favor renal artery occlusion. Ostial stenosis is rightly considered as an aortic disease and expansion of the stent-graft in the aorta may dislodge plaques and occlude the renal artery. A horseshoe kidney must also be recognized before graft deployment in order to avoid a catastrophic outcome.

STENT-GRAFT

So far, the rate of renal artery coverage does not appear to be associated with the type of graft. Suprarenal fixation has been proved to be safe and infrarenal fixation does not appear to be an issue [8-10].

In contrast, the technique of stent-graft deployment is a key point. With the Cook graft, the proximal deployment is always controlled. Once in a proper position, the first covered row is deployed by removing the outer sheath. A new angiogram is then performed to assess the lack of migration. If needed, the graft may be repositioned proximally or distally. During the following steps, the bare stents carrying the hooks are freed. At this stage, the risk of renal artery covering is low in normal anatomical conditions. However, deployment may be hazardous in patients with unfavorable morphology. With the AneurX® or Talent® devices, the sequential steps are similar, but the stent-grafts can-

not be pushed upwards in case the graft is placed too distally. That is the reason why the company advises starting deployment above the renal arteries and gently descending the whole system until the desired level is reached.

There is no repositioning possible with the Gore device. One has to be sure that the positioning is correct before pulling the thread which detaches the sheath in which the graft is wrapped.

IMAGING

Good quality imaging is essential. Modern equipment with recent generation C-arms is generally sufficient in the majority of cases. However, with intensive practice, the quality of images deteriorates within a period of three to four years. Poor assessment and software breakdown during procedures may be the cause of catastrophic events. Handling and manipulation of the equipment is also fundamental. There might be a discrepancy in competence during day and night working hours. This can be very unfortunate because many challenging cases, including ruptured aneurysms, appear outside working hours where competent technicians are not available.

What to do in case of inadvertent renal artery occlusion?

The first requisite is to understand the exact mechanism of the occlusion, which is not always easy. It is worthwhile spending time reviewing the video of the whole procedure carefully. By comparing the predeployment video and the final positioning with depiction of the metallic frame of the graft, the mechanism of occlusion might be understood. Rescue techniques can be undertaken based on the presumed mechanism, the anatomical condition and the duration of kidney warm ischemia.

ENDOVASCULAR MANEUVERS

In cases where the renal artery is covered and the endograft is not fully deployed, gentle traction with the sheath can solve the problem. With an aortic cuff it is much more difficult as the graft is very short (generally two rows of covered stent). An alternative valuable option is the placement of self-expandable bare stents in the renal arteries. We have used this technique successfully in Case 3.

When the graft is still attached to the delivery system, the first step is to exercise a gentle traction on the graft in an attempt to slip it down. A few millimeters may be gained, but hooks will not allow further movement.

If the graft is still free, a balloon can be placed in the bifurcation of the graft, inflated and used to pull the whole system downward. The balloon must not be too large because it might open the stent-graft and prevent repositioning. Another option is to place a wire over the graft bifurcation from one groin to the other. It can be done with the crossover technique, using a pigtail catheter, a 0.035 Terumo wire and a snare catheter to catch the proximal tip of the Terumo wire. This technique is obviously not feasible with an aortouniiliac graft.

Stent-graft perforation is another option. By placing a guiding catheter in the graft at the presumed location of the renal artery and pushing a stiff wire against the fabric of the graft, a perforation can be accomplished into the renal artery. A 5-millimeter cutting balloon can be used to enlarge the hole in the fabric and a balloon expandable stent (EV 3) can be placed distally in the renal artery and proximally into the lumen of the graft. A compliant balloon is then used to flare up the aortic part of the stent which fixates the fabric to the aortic wall. These maneuvers are rather similar to the techniques used for fenestrated grafts [11].

If renal artery occlusion is not caused by graft coverage, the first step is to catheterize the renal artery. Since it is generally obstructed by fresh thrombus, the maneuver is relatively easy. In these cases, the preferred access is via the brachial artery. Once the wire is in place, thromboaspiration can be performed. If not successful, local thrombolysis may be attempted and a stent may be placed in cases of residual stenosis.

OPEN REPAIR

Open repair is the second choice. However, it might be used as first attempt if the conditions are not favorable for endovascular repair. When the time elapsed between occlusion and reopening of the artery is too long, it is more appropriate to go directly for surgical repair. Renal artery bypass is probably the least invasive surgical option.

The condition for this limited surgical repair is that the aneurysm is excluded by the stent-graft. The trunk of the renal artery (right or left) is dissected free via a retroperitoneal approach. The fastest way is to suture the proximal end of the

renal bypass distal to the limb of the stent-graft on the external iliac artery. Splenorenal or hepaticorenal bypasses are other options but they are more time-consuming.

Surgical conversion has to be chosen when the stent-graft is not properly deployed in the aneurysm. A left retroperitoneal incision will allow renal artery repair first, followed by removal of the stent-graft and classic repair of the aneurysm. Occasionally, one can simply remove the upper part of the graft by cutting the main shaft and then suture the remaining distal stent-graft body directly on to the infrarenal aorta. This technique prevents extensive surgery and will limit blood loss.

How to prevent renal artery coverage?

It is obvious that the best treatment of renal artery coverage is its prevention. It is also evident that unfavorable anatomical conditions increase the risk of inadvertent accidents. These risk factors determine the decision whether an endovascular treatment should be chosen. Along that line it could be considered that high-risk patients with a poor morphology are left untreated, especially as surgical conversion is a serious threat. Experience, sound judgement, and evaluation of the risk benefit ratio should all be integrated in order to make the proper choice in the patient's best interest.

Careful planning may avoid disenchantment. In patients with a short or difficult neck, it may be preferable to perform renal artery translocation first. This enables the surgeon to gain a few centimeters necessary to place the stent-graft safely. In difficult necks, we place wires preemptively in the renal arteries. Because the location of the renal artery is known throughout, there is no need to repeat the contrast medium injection and, if problems occur, the rescue techniques can be performed instantaneously without the burden of trying to catheterize the target renal artery where the ostium has been lost.

Conclusion

Unintentional occlusion of the renal artery is a rare but unfortunate event during EVAR. Patient selection, proper planning and a careful procedure will avoid the majority of these events. However, physicians involved in EVAR must be well aware of all available rescue techniques which can be ap-plied in such occasions. Although relatively sophis-ticated, they might save kidneys and life when prop-erly performed.

REFERENCES

1 Bockler D, Krauss M, Mannsmann U et al. Incidence of renal infarctions after endovascular AAA repair: relationship to infra-renal vs. suprarenal fixation. *J Endovasc Ther* 2003; 10: 1054-1060.

2 Kim B, Donayre CE, Hansen CJ et al. Endovascular abdominal aortic aneurysm repair using the AneuRx stent-graft: impact of excluding accessory renal arteries. *Ann Vasc Surg* 2004; 18: 32-37.

3 Kramer SC, Seifarth H, Pamler R et al. Renal infarction follo-wing endovascular aortic aneurysm repair: incidence and clinical consequences. *J Endovasc Ther* 2002; 9: 98-102.

4 Mehta M, Cayne N, Veith FJ et al. Relationship of proximal fixation to renal dysfunction in patients undergoing endo-vascular aneurysm repair. *J Cardiovasc Surg* 2004; 45: 367-374.

5 Walker SR, Yusuf SW, Wenham PW, Hopkinson BR. Renal complications following endovascular repair of abdominal aortic aneurysms. *J Endovasc Surg* 1998; 5: 318-322.

6 Desgranges P, Hutin E, Kedzia C et al. Aortic stents covering the renal arteries ostia: an animal study. *J Vasc Interv Radiol* 1997; 8: 77-82.

7 Desgranges P, Kobeiter H, Coumbaras M et al. Placement of a fenestrated Palmaz stent across the renal arteries. Feasibility and outcome in an animal study. *Eur J Vasc Endovasc Surg* 2000; 19: 406-412.

8 Lau LL, Hakaim AG, Oldenburg WA et al. Effect of suprarenal vs. infrarenal aortic endograft fixation on renal function and renal artery patency: a comparative study with intermediate follow-up. *J Vasc Surg* 2003; 37: 1162-1168.

9 Marin ML, Parsons RE, Hollier LH et al. Impact of transrenal aortic endograft placement on endovascular graft repair of abdo-minal aortic aneurysms. *J Vasc Surg* 1998; 28: 638-646.

10 Surowiec SM, Davies MG, Fegley AJ et al. Relationship of proximal fixation to postoperative renal dysfunction in patients with normal serum creatinine concentration. *J Vasc Surg* 2004; 39: 804-810.

11 Verhoeven EL, Prins TR, Tielliu IF et al. Treatment of short-necked infrarenal aortic aneurysms with fenestrated stent-grafts: short-term results. *Eur J Vasc Endovasc Surg* 2004; 27: 477-483.

11

HOW TO DEAL WITH URETERAL INJURIES DURING AND AFTER AORTIC RECONSTRUCTION?

PIERRE BONNET, RAYMOND LIMET

Iatrogenic injuries of the ureter are encountered after various types of surgery. Brandes et al. [1] recently published a review on the diagnosis and treatment of all ureteric lesions on the basis of the literature, grouped according to the level of evidence. This chapter focuses on the lesions observed particularly in vascular surgery. These lesions are related to aneurysmatic and obstructive aortoiliac disease and its treatment. These complications are rarely dreaded by vascular surgeons. Twenty years ago, a ureteral lesion always required nephrectomy [2]. Later it was demonstrated that a ureteral perforation without urinary infection could be repaired without jeopardizing the vascular prosthesis [3]. On the basis of the literature and a personal series, we propose a diagnostic and therapeutic strategy led by the type and mechanism of the lesion, the acute or chronic character of the process, and the remaining function of the affected kidney. This approach is based on anatomic considerations and the progress of endo-urology.

Clinical picture

Iatrogenic ureteral lesions occur mainly after urologic surgery, less frequently after abdominopelvic surgery (general and gynecological surgery), and rarely after vascular surgery. Vascular surgery is regarded to be responsible for iatrogenic ureteral lesions in 0.8%-6.1% [4,5]; it accounts for the lesions of the middle third of the ureter, as opposed to pelvic (rectal, urologic and, especially, gynecologic) surgery, which causes lesions in the lower third of the ureter in particular. In addition to these iatrogenic lesions, aortic pathology may also be responsible for ureteral lesions, before any therapeutic action, which are directly related to the aortic pathology per se.

In a period of 14 years, 2297 patients were treated in our center with surgery for obstructive or aneurysmatic aortic pathology. We observed 41 patients with a ureteric lesion related to this pathology or its treatment who showed various clinical pictures.

DETECTION OF A HYDRONEPHROSIS DURING PREOPERATIVE ANALYSIS OF AN ABDOMINAL AORTIC ANEURYSM (AAA)

In this case, the eventually bilateral hydronephrosis often illustrates the inflammatory character of the aneurysm. These obstructions, discovered during the diagnostic procedure, occurred in 20% of the inflammatory aortic aneurysms and in 0.2% of the non-inflammatory ones. Our almost systematic application of preoperative CT scanning for aneurysms operated without rupture allows for the diagnosis of this complication. Ureteral obstruction may also be found during the surgical procedure or follow-up (within three months). Hydronephrosis due to ureteral compression may be mild and transient. The frequency varies between 0.1% and 20% [6,7]. Some hydronephroses may resolve spontaneously in the three-month postoperative period [8,9]. Others persist beyond that period, with the risk of a compromised function of the kidney involved. In cases of pronounced ureteral obstruction, the stasis will become symptomatic (lumbar pain) and may impair kidney function, particularly in case of bilateral obstruction.

DETECTION OF A URETERAL INJURY WITHIN THREE MONTHS AFTER SURGERY

In cases of ureteral injury, urine will appear in the operation field or in the postoperative drainage fluid. The lesion may not always be detected during surgery and may result in a symptomatic retroperitoneal urinoma (pain, subsequent passage disturbances, biological inflammatory response or superinfection).

DETECTION OF A URETERAL OBSTRUCTION MORE THAN THREE MONTHS AFTER SURGERY

In these cases, the discovery is by chance or as the result of an investigation for renal insufficiency. These chronic, progressive obstructions are seldom painful and are the result of stenoses from a periprosthetic inflammation. The duration of the obstruction and its bilateral occurrence explain the possible consequences for total renal function. Other obstructions diagnosed beyond three months postoperatively may show an acute or semi-acute progression. They betray the development of a recent progressive retroperitoneal complication such as an infection, a false aneurysm, or the growth of an aneurysm of an iliac artery with retrograde perfusion (*see below*).

Mechanisms of ureteral injuries

The obstructions comprise stenoses by external compression (compression by the aneurysm) and stenoses through ureteral involvement. These lesions are induced by fibrosing inflammatory responses due to the aortic disease (mycotic aneurysm) or due to a foreign body (vascular prosthesis). The external compression is provoked by the size of the aneurysm and, in some cases, by the pre-ureteral localization of the limb of the arterial prosthesis (Fig. 1).

Ureteral lesions are secondary to direct injury after the dissection, or ischemic events such as the use of electric bistouries or extensive dissection of the ureter (Figs. 1C and D). All these lesions can be explained by the close relation between the ureters, the aorta, and the iliac arteries in the retroperitoneal space, as shown in Fig. 2. The ureteral wall is supplied by an arterial network, in 80% of the cases fed by a single longitudinal artery, running between the adventitial and muscular layer of the ureter [10]. This longitudinal artery itself is supplied by branches of the aorta along the ureteral tract: renal, gonadic, iliac, hypogastric, uterine, vesical and obturator arteries, as well as infraperitoneal branches. These vessels reach the ureter at the external side of its upper part and the internal side of the lower part (Fig. 3). The middle part of the ureter receives a lesser vascularization than the superior and inferior parts. Dissection of this part of the ureter towards the iliac vessels changes its arterial supply. The majority of ureteral lesions involve the iliac ureter. Lesions of the lumbar ureter can be expected in case of extensive retroperitoneal fibrosis (mycotic aneurysm), false aneurysm of the proximal anastomosis, or direct peroperative injury. In our vascular context, lesions of the pelvic ureter (lower third) are rare and were never encountered in our series.

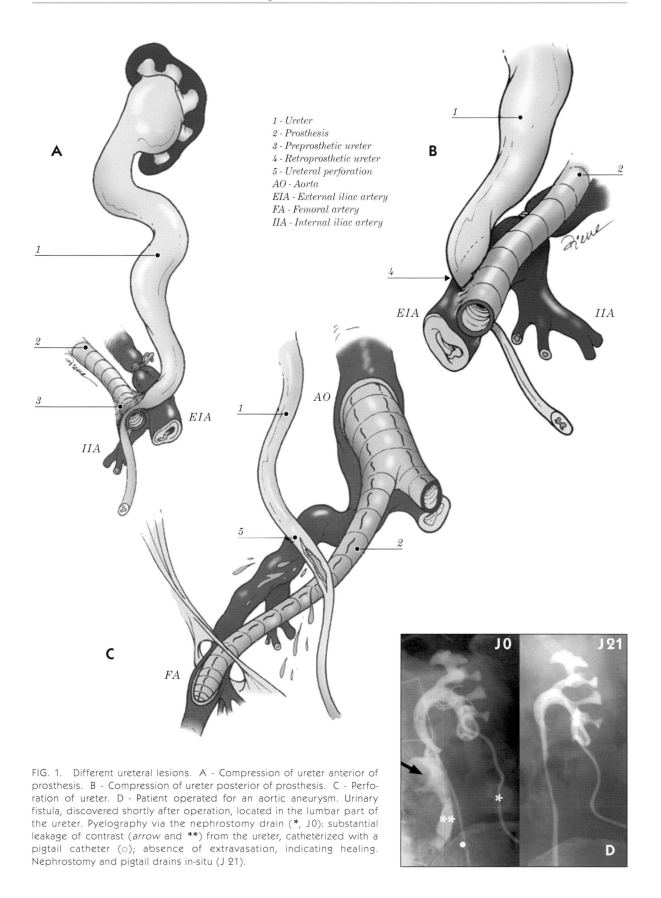

1 - Ureter
2 - Prosthesis
3 - Preprosthetic ureter
4 - Retroprosthetic ureter
5 - Ureteral perforation
AO - Aorta
EIA - External iliac artery
FA - Femoral artery
IIA - Internal iliac artery

FIG. 1. Different ureteral lesions. A - Compression of ureter anterior of prosthesis. B - Compression of ureter posterior of prosthesis. C - Perforation of ureter. D - Patient operated for an aortic aneurysm. Urinary fistula, discovered shortly after operation, located in the lumbar part of the ureter. Pyelography via the nephrostomy drain (*, J0): substantial leakage of contrast (*arrow* and **) from the ureter, catheterized with a pigtail catheter (○); absence of extravasation, indicating healing. Nephrostomy and pigtail drains in-situ (J 21).

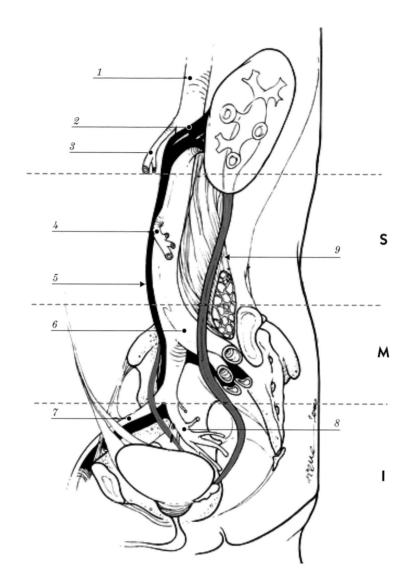

1 - Aorta
2 - Left renal vein
3 - Superior mesenteric artery
4 - Inferior mesenteric artery
5 - Inferior caval vein
6 - Common iliac artery
7 - External iliac artery
8 - Internal iliac artery
9 - Psoas muscle

FIG. 2   Left-lateral view, showing the anatomical relations of the three parts of the ureter *(in grey)*: S superior third, M middle third, I inferior third.

11
120

Predisposing factors for ureteral lesions

In our series we have identified four risk factors.
1 - Mycotic aortic aneurysms due to accompanying severe retroperitoneal fibrosis frequently results in ureteral obstruction, already present when being investigated.
2 - Previous surgery in that anatomic area increases the risk of a ureteral lesion in case of a reintervention.

3 - Infection of the vascular prosthesis increases the risk of ureteral involvement.
4 - A vascular prosthetic leg erroneously placed in front of the ureter augments the risk of ureteral compression.

Diagnosis

When a ureteral problem is suspected, its localization and etiology should be assessed. The total

ORIGIN OF THE
URETERAL VESSELS

1 - Renal artery
2 - Gonadic artery
3 - Common iliac artery
4 - Superior vesical artery
5 - Inferior vesical artery
  (uterine or prostatic artery)
6 - Deferent artery

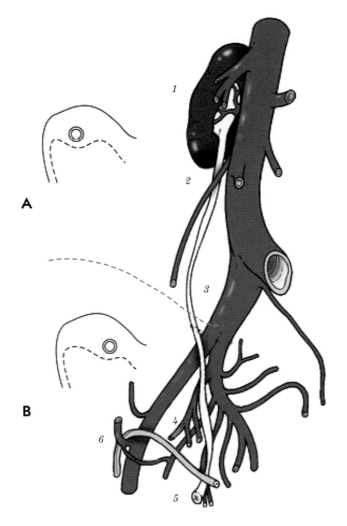

FIG. 3 Ureteral vascularization. A - Arteries approach the upper part of the ureter from its medial side. B - Arteries approach the lower part of the ureter from its lateral side.

and separate (left and right) renal functions need to be investigated. Hydronephrosis can be detected readily by abdominal ultrasound. CT scanning localizes the level of the obstruction. It allows appreciation of the function of the obstructed kidney (quality of contrast enhancement and emptying time of the renal cavities). In addition, a CT scan gives information as to the exact nature of the obstruction: periprosthetic inflammation (contrast absorbing), abscess, false aneurysm or retroprosthetic ureter. In case of renal insufficiency, magnetic resonance imaging using gadolinium offers a complete image of the urinary tract without a deleterious effect on renal function.

Urine loss is suspected from the appearance of urine during the procedure or in the postoperative drainage fluid. The ureate and creatinine concentration in this fluid differentiates between lymphorrhea and a urinary fistula. Intraoperatively, an intravenous injection of methylene blue typically colors the release of urine. This requires an adequate diuresis, which may sometimes be absent in case of hemodynamic disturbances during the procedure. Visualization in the surgical field of a ureteral drain placed preventively proves a ureteral perforation. A ureteral stenosis or injury is detected preferably by means of direct contrast imaging of the urinary tract, either via a retrograde (retrograde ureteropyelography via endoscopy) or antegrade (through a nephrostomy drain) route. Renal scintigraphy evaluates the total and separate function of the right and left kidneys. If the function of one kidney is less than 30% of the total function, a conservative approach should be weighed against nephrectomy. Combined with a furosemide test, the emptying curves from scintigraphy enable discernment between clear obstructions and simple delays in urinary passage.

Treatment

Minor obstructions due to a transient inflammatory response during the postoperative period may require only surveillance or may benefit from corticosteroids. This treatment may be combined with external or internal drainage of the urinary tract *(see below)*. Antibiotics are prescribed in case of an intraluminal foreign body (pigtail catheter, nephrostomy drain). The use of quinolones is generally accepted for this indication. Conventional surgery offers a large spectrum of reconstruction techniques (Fig. 4). For sutures in the urinary tract, slowly resorbable sutures are applied (to avoid stone formation on the foreign body), using 4 x 0 for the ureter by means of interrupted stitches to prevent stenoses. The ureteral segments to be stitched should be sufficiently mobilized to avoid tension at the suture site, which should be protected by adequate drainage (pigtail catheter). Open surgery allows for closure or partial resection of the ureter end-to-end anastomosis. If a substantial part of the ureter is lost, various techniques have been described to reconstruct the ureter. Mobilization of the upper angle of the bladder anastomosed with the upper stump of the ureter is mainly reserved to lesions limited to the lower part of the ureter; this is rarely possible when the lumbar or iliac part of the ureter is involved. The lower ureter may also be replaced by a tunneled vesical flap (Boari flap) which can bridge a larger defect. This technique too is not suited for the middle part of the ureter. Creation of an end-to-side uretero-ureteral anastomosis requires crossing the median line to reach the contralateral ureter. The aortic pathology and arterial prosthesis usually complicate this crossover. Moreover, in case of problems after this type of anastomosis, the two reno-ureteral units may be compromised. The ureter may partially or completely be replaced by an intestinal transplant onto the

small intestines. Autotransplantation of a kidney has also been described to overcome a substantial defect of the ureter. The latter two techniques are more aggressive and often not very suitable for vascular patients, particularly directly after a vascular intervention complicated by a urinary fistula.

Endoscopic treatment of stenoses or lesions of the ureter has been known for more than 60 years [11]. These treatments have benefited from the progress in medical imaging techniques (ultrasound-guided puncture) and miniaturization of endoscopes and drains. The endoscopic approach is the treatment of choice in the majority of ureteral injuries [12,13]. The common principle of all these treatments is drainage of the urinary tracts, while modelling the traumatized ureter (stenosis, perforation) during the healing process. Stenoses may be dilated or incised endoscopically during ureteroscopy. It has been shown experimentally that the ureteral wall can recover under these circumstances, with partial regeneration of the smooth muscle layers [14,15]. Ultrasound-guided percutaneous drainage of the urinary tract is performed under local anesthesia, at the patient's bedside if possible. This minimally invasive procedure is especially indicated for patients with a complication shortly after the operation. Ureteral pigtail catheters are placed via retrograde ureteroscopy. The pigtail-curved proximal and distal ends (double-J) of the catheter ensure maintenance of the correct position in the urinary tract. These multiperforated catheters enable drainage of the kidney as well as adaptation and remodelling of the ureter. In our experience, we have regularly chosen for double drainage using nephrostomy and pigtail drainage to treat urinary fistulas. In these cases the pigtail catheter ensures adaptation of the ureter and the nephrostomy drain ensures the urinary drainage, which may be insufficient when a single internal drainage is applied, especially in bedridden patients (Fig. 5). Nephrostomy allows for regular monitoring of the healing process (antegrade pyelography).

Percutaneous preoperative drainage of the hydronephrosis can improve kidney function before a vascular surgical procedure. Furthermore, preoperative placement of pigtail catheters is frequently performed in order to facilitate recognition of the ureter during surgery (reintervention, curation of the mycotic aortic aneurysm). This maneuver did not always seem effective to us, because the ureter and ureteral catheter could not be palpated due to the extensive perivascular fibrosis occurring in

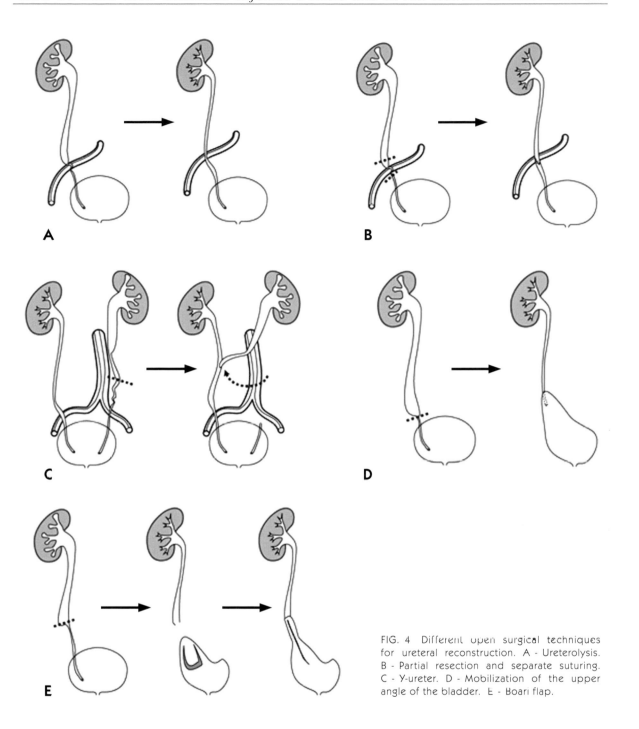

FIG. 4 Different open surgical techniques for ureteral reconstruction. A - Ureterolysis. B - Partial resection and separate suturing. C - Y-ureter. D - Mobilization of the upper angle of the bladder. E - Boari flap.

these cases. At present, this prophylactic drainage is indicated when an important pelvic mass is present but, except for these circumstances, it does not seem to improve identification of the ureter in other surgical procedures, such as rectal or gynecological surgery. In contrast, this drain facilitates preoperative identification of a possible trauma [1].

Therapeutic choices and results

The success of the techniques mentioned above varies with the clinical presentation and the type of found lesion. On the basis of our personal experience, we suggest an individual strategy for each of the situations described in the spectrum of

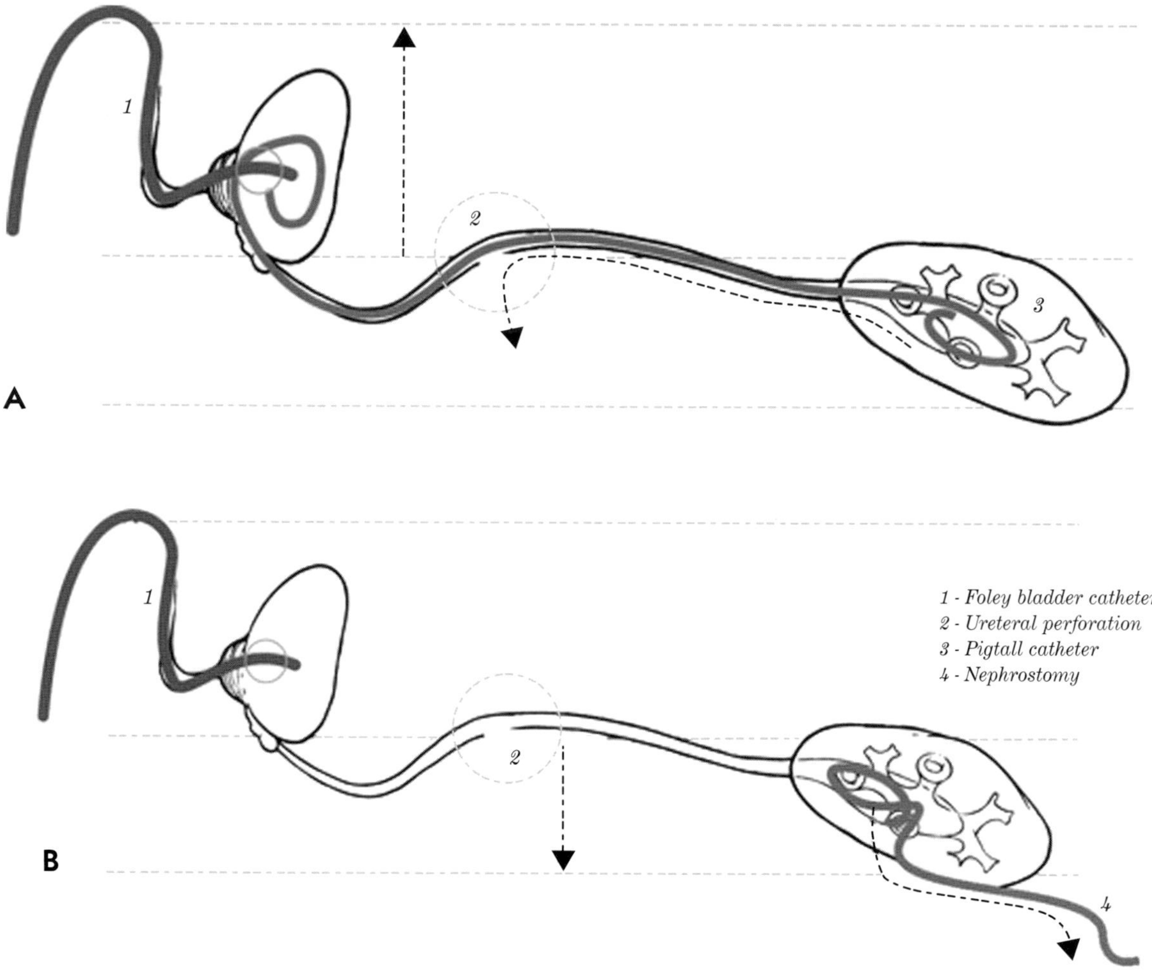

1 - Foley bladder catheter
2 - Ureteral perforation
3 - Pigtail catheter
4 - Nephrostomy

FIG. 5   Ureteral perforation (2), drained in a bedridden patient. A - The perforation is located low and sustains the fistula. B - Drainage by means of a nephrostomy, which is preferable, being lower than the opening in the ureter.

possibilities. This policy may vary from center to center, depending on the diagnostic and therapeutic facilities available. A lesion eligible for sole endoscopic treatment, according to our criteria, may benefit from classical surgical treatment rather than from poorly mastered endoscopic attempts if these techniques are not routine in that medical center.

HYDRONEPHROSIS DETECTED DURING EVALUATION OF AN AAA

CT scanning most often detects a mycotic aneurysm. Renal function should be assessed selectively by means of scintigraphy. Ideally, internal drainage using a pigtail catheter is performed before surgery in order to preserve renal function. Drainage by means of nephrostomy may be necessary if the placement of the drains appears impossible. Adding ureterolysis to the treatment of the aneurysm is debatable when a large obstacle is present. Still, treatment of a mycotic aneurysm most often terminates the active retroperitoneal process of fibrosis. Temporary internal drainage may be adequate. The duration of this drainage depends on the CT scan surveillance, showing regression of the fibrosis postoperatively. As long as no indication is present for a surgical intervention to treat the AAA, pigtail drainage is continued during the treatment with corticosteroids to counteract the inflammatory process. In our series, this treatment has protected 88% of the ureterorenal lesions, without having to perform an eventual nephrectomy. Functional loss of ureterorenal units (in 12% of the cases) probably represents irreversibility when the diagnosis is made. Absence of scintigraphic activity of a kidney, of which the cortex has become atrophic according to ultrasound and CT scanning, indicates irreversible loss of renal function. In this case, drainage is not necessary, except in case of superinfection or pain. Removal of the non-functional kidney then may be indicated during AAA surgery.

Isolated Ureteral Obstruction Discovered during or within Three Months of Surgery

A mild hydronephrosis detected by postoperative ultrasound requires surveillance and sometimes corticosteroids. In other cases, it is wise to perform a topographical and functional screening (scintigraphy, CT scan). If the kidney appears non-functional and beyond repair, no treatment is indicated. Nephrectomy may be indicated in case of complications (hypertension, superinfection, pain). Conservative treatment is indicated when the kidney is still functional. In case of a short ureteral stenosis (less than two centimeters) and if the prosthesis is placed correctly, endoscopic treatment may be performed successfully by placing a pigtail catheter or nephrostomy. When this treatment fails, surgical ureterolysis or partial resection of the ureter is indicated. If the stenosis is longer (more than two centimeters) or if the prosthesis is placed in front of the ureter, chances of success of endoscopy are small and surgery is preferable. In these cases, however, an endoscopic procedure may be indicated (pigtail or nephrostomy) to postpone a surgical intervention. Thus, an intervention can be planned after the directly postoperative phase, in which access to the ureter and realization of an ureterolysis can be achieved. When the prosthesis is poorly positioned, the intervention consists of uncrossing the ureter and prosthesis by means of an end-to-end anastomosis, either of the ureter or the vascular prosthesis, depending on the situation during operation. The success rate of these treatments is on the order of 64% in our series. We have never been led to do an autotransplantation or replacement of the ureter with an intestinal transplant. These interventions were considered too risky for such patients and when reconstruction was impossible, a nephrectomy was performed.

Ureteral Lesions (with or without Obstruction) Discovered during or within Three Months of Surgery

When a ureteral fistula is diagnosed preoperatively, the ureteral wall should be repaired and an internal drainage (pigtail) should be placed. If the fistula is diagnosed after surgery, a retrograde ureteropyelography should be added to the standard investigation (ultrasound, CT scan) and performed via a pigtail catheter placed endoscopically. In our series, all fistulas discovered directly postoperatively were treated successfully by means of endoscopic placement of a pigtail catheter, with or without nephrostomy (Fig. 1). Only one out of seven cases required additional ureterolysis because of a persistent ureteral stenosis after desiccation of the ureteral fistula. The recommended duration of pigtail drainage after endopyelotomy or ureteral incision is about a week [16]. We suggest a drainage period of three weeks to obtain adequate healing. In our series, two cases of uretero-arterial fistula were observed in patients having a pigtail catheter for more than six months. These sometimes comprised serious complications, as described earlier [17-19]. One patient developed a fistula between the ureter and an aneurysm of the common iliac artery with retrograde perfusion. The other one had a fistula between the retroprosthetic ureter and the prosthesis. Prolonged periods of pigtail drainage should be avoided whenever possible.

Ureteral Obstruction Discovered more than Three Months after Surgery

In these chronic lesions, silent destruction of the kidney function is most frequently seen. The remaining renal function should be assessed before any therapeutic intervention is undertaken. If the kidney is non-functional, but without complications (hypertension, superinfection, pain), abstention is preferred over any maneuver that may infect the poorly drained urinary tract. Nephrectomy is suggested in case of complications. When the remaining kidney function is to be preserved, the obstructing lesions should be treated surgically. The success rate of endoscopic procedures for this indication reached a mere 12.5% in our experience. If the obstruction is secondary to a subacute recent retroperitoneal fibrosis (development of a false aneurysm at the site of a suture, occurrence of a prosthetic infection), the treatment should be causal in the first place. In these cases, an adjuvant endoscopic procedure may still be indicated.

Prevention

Knowledge of the retroperitoneal anatomy and relations of the ureter will reduce the risk of ureteral devascularization. The proximal part of the ureter is to be approached from its lateral side and the distal part from the medial side to preserve its vascularization.

If the risk of a ureteral lesion appears high, for example when a mycotic AAA is present, prophylactic drainage may be considered. In our experience, this approach does not yield the expected benefits. In case of ureteral lesions, our personal series shows that the smaller the delay between the lesion and the treatment, the better the treatment effect is. Therefore, everything possible should be done to avoid delay in the diagnosis. Ultrasonography is a noninvasive investigation that may easily detect a hydronephrosis. This investigation should be recommended in the follow-up of patients treated surgically for obstructive or aneurysmatic aortoiliac pathology.

Reinterventions in which the risk of ureteral injury is increased deserve specific attention. Here, the preoperative localization of the ureters by means of pigtail catheters is an adjuvant method used by many centers.

Conclusion

In our experience, no ureteral lesion has led to mortality, but often to considerable morbidity, with prolonging of hospitalization, need for reinterventions and impairment of kidney function. Whichever lesions and therapies applied, the prognosis is improved by an early diagnosis. When a ureteral lesion occurs, a thorough investigation should be conducted including assessment of the involved kidney's function. Treatment should take into account the moment at which the lesion occurs, differentiating between preoperative, perioperative and postoperative lesions. Therapeutic options are chosen according to a simple algorithm (Figure 6). Single

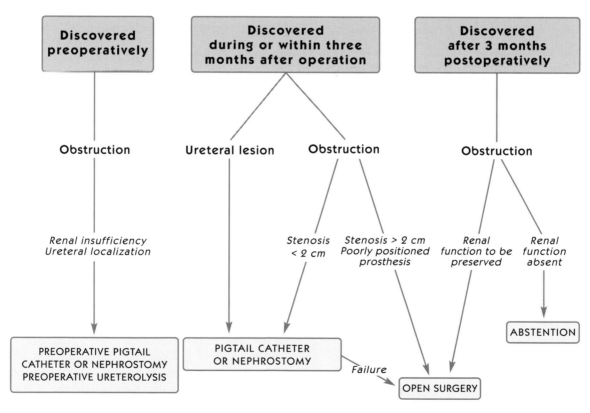

FIG. 6 Proposed algorithm to manage ureteral lesions.

endoscopic treatment appears particularly suitable for urinary fistulas, but it is less effective for pre-operative and perioperative obstructive lesions. In the remaining cases, open surgery is often necessary after temporary endoscopic urinary drainage.

A comprehensive knowledge of the predisposing factors for ureteral lesions, the ureteral anatomy and vascularization should reduce the frequency of iatrogenic injury to the ureter.

REFERENCES

1 Brandes S, Coburn M, Armenakas N, McAninch J. Diagnosis and management of ureteric injury: an evidence-based analysis. *BJU Int* 2004; 94: 277-289.

2 Schapira HE, Li R, Gribetz M et al. Ureteral injuries during vascular surgery. *J Urol* 1981; 125: 293-297.

3 Spirnak JP, Hampel N, Resnick MI. Ureteral injuries complicating vascular surgery: is repair indicated? *J Urol* 1989; 141: 13-14.

4 Wright DJ, Ernst CB, Evans JR et al. Ureteral complications and aortoiliac reconstruction. *J Vasc Surg* 1990; 11:29-35.

5 St Lezin MA, Stoller ML. Surgical ureteral injuries. *Urology* 1991; 38: 497-506.

6 Dalsing MC, Bihrle R, Lalka SG et al. Vascular surgery-associated ureteral injury: zebras do exist. *Ann Vasc Surg* 1993; 7: 180-186.

7 Schoeneich G, Perabo F, Heimbach D et al. Hydronephrosis after aorto bifemoral graft surgery: a marker for late graft complications. *Scand J Uro Nephrol* 1999; 33: 317-319.

8 Heard G, Hinde G. Hydronephrosis complicating aortic reconstruction. *Br J Surg* 1975; 62: 344-347.

9 Selzman AA, Spirnak JP. Iatrogenic ureteral injuries: a 20-year experience in treating 165 injuries. *J Urol* 1996; 155: 878-881.

10 Coburn M. Ureteral injuries from surgical trauma. In: Mcannish J, Carroll PR, Jordan JH (eds). *Traumatic and reconstructive urology.* Philadelphia, W.B. Saunders, 1996. pp 181-197.

11 Davis DM. Intubated ureterotomy: a new operation for ureteral and ureteropelvic stricture. *Surg Gyn Obst* 1943; 76: 513-523.

12 Cormio L, Battaglia M, Traficante A, Selvaggi FP. Endourological treatment of ureteric injuries. *Br J Urol* 1993; 72: 165-168.

13 Lask D, Abarbanel J, Luttwak Z et al. Changing trends in the management of iatrogenic ureteral injuries. *J Urol* 1995; 154: 1693-1695.

14 Begin LR, Selmy GI, Hassouna MM et al. Healing and muscular restoration of the ureteral wall following balloon-induced rupture: an experimental animal model with light microscopic and ultrastructural observations. *Exp Mol Pathol* 1993; 59: 58-70.

15 Galal H, Lazica A, Lampel A et al. Management of ureteral strictures by different modalities and effect of stents on upper tract drainage. *J Endourol* 1993; 7: 411-417.

16 Kerbl K, Chandhoke PS, Figenshau RS et al. Effect of stent duration on ureteral healing following endoureterotomy in an animal model. *J Urol* 1993; 150: 1302-1305.

17 Awakura Y, Yamamoto M, Fukuzawa S et al. A case of uretero-aortic fistula. *Hinyokika Kiyo* 1997; 43: 299-301.

18 Camps JI, Ortiz VN, Vargas J, Figueroa M. Uretero-arterial fistula: a case report and review of the literature. *Bol Asoc Med P R* 1998; 90: 82-84.

19 Van Damme H, Keppenne V, Sakalihasan N et al. Uretero-arterial fistula: two observations. *Acta Chir Belg* 1997; 97: 133-136.

12

RUPTURED MYCOTIC AORTIC ANEURYSM

ANDRÉ NEVELSTEEN, KIM DAENENS
INGE FOURNEAU, VALERIE COPPIN

Arterial infection represents a rare but dramatic and often lethal disease. Ambroise Paré described the first case of infected aneurysm in the mid-16th century when he reported the autopsy findings of a patient with a ruptured syphilitic aneurysm. In 1885 Sir William Osler introduced the term mycotic aneurysm to describe these infected aneurysms, which develop as a result of embolism from bacterial endocarditis. Since there was no apparent association with fungal disease, the term mycotic aneurysm has always been a source of discussion and confusion among vascular surgeons. Strictly speaking, the term mycotic aneurysms should be reserved for infected aneurysms resulting from bacterial endocarditis complicated by septic arterial emboli or an infected aneurysm of the sinus of Valsalva resulting from contiguous spread from an infected aortic valve. Nonetheless, the majority of the vascular surgeons nowadays keep to the commonly used definition of mycotic aneurysms to include all kind of infected aneurysms. In this chapter, we will focus on infected aneurysms of the thoracic and abdominal aorta, which is, after the common femoral artery, the most frequent anatomic location of this kind of disease. Aorto-enteric fistulas, postreconstruction septic anastomotic aneurysms and arterial graft infections are excluded.

Etiology of infected aneurysms

In the preantibiotic era, true mycotic aneurysms determined nearly 90% of all infected aneurysms. These aneurysms occurred -both in normal and abnormal arteries- as a result of septic emboli of cardiac origin, lodging in the lumen or vasa vasorum of the peripheral arteries. They were seen in virtually every artery: intracranially, in the great vessels, all over the aorta and in the visceral, extremity, pulmonary and also coronary arteries. The antimicrobial treatment of bacterial endocarditis and the reduction in rheumatic fever have fortunately caused a spectacular decrease in the incidence of these aneurysms. In most recent series, true mycotic aneurysms constitute less than 10% of all infected aneurysms [1].

At the other hand, there is no doubt that in recent decades the most frequent type of infected aneurysms is in fact the posttraumatic false aneurysm. This explains why the common femoral artery, used by drug addicts for repeated groin injections, has become the most common site for these lesions [2]. A second reason is without doubt the increasing frequency of arterial puncture, both in the femoral and brachial arteries, for monitoring of critically ill patients and also for imaging and endovascular treatment of arterial lesions.

Infected aortic aneurysms remain quite infrequent. They are reported at around 3% among all aortic aneurysms before 1960 and at around 1% in recent years. They occur all over the aorta, but nearly 50% will be seen at the infrarenal aorta. The juxtarenal or pararenal aorta is involved in 25% of cases. Thoracic or thoracoabdominal aneurysms make up another 25% [3]. They usually appear as solitary lesions, but multiple aneurysms have been described. Infected aortic aneurysms may be primary (aortitis) or secondary (infection of pre-existing aneurysm). The mechanism of infection is bacterial seeding of the aortic wall either by: hematogenous spreading (systemic sepsis, pneumonia); lymphatic spreading (tuberculous aortitis); or direct extension from an adjacent infected focus (osteomyelitis).

The normal aortic intima and adventitia are both quite remarkably resistant to infection. Therefore, normal arteries can only be invaded by extremely virulent organisms. The resistance to infection is, however, dramatically increased when the intimal barrier is disrupted by atherosclerosis. Chronic immunosuppression is another significant risk factor. In some series, nearly half of the patients are chronically immunosuppressed either by diabetes, corticosteroid therapy or malignancy [3]. Fungi causing infected aneurysms have been reported in patients receiving immunosuppressive therapy for transplantation or in cases of HIV infection. Whatever the mechanism, infection will invariably lead to suppuration, localized perforation and false aneurysm formation. Ultimately, rupture will follow and this can be seen as early as one week after the onset of infection.

It has already been common knowledge for several years that around 10% of the asymptomatic atherosclerotic infrarenal aortic aneurysms become colonized by bacteria. Ernst et al. showed that the incidence of positive cultures increased to 38% among patients with a ruptured aneurysm [4]. The clinical relevance of these findings is not completely understood and it is estimated that the incidence of infection in pre-existing atherosclerotic aneurysms is around 3.5%. It is also known that infection results in further weakening of the arterial wall and that it is associated with a highly elevated risk of rupture.

Bacteriology of infected aneurysms

Because true mycotic aneurysms develop as a complication of endocarditis, the responsible organisms will be those causing endocarditis. Most frequently, these are *Streptococcus viridans* (22%), *Staphylococcus aureus* (20%), *Streptococcus faecalis* (14%) and *Staphylococcus epidermidis* (11%). In endocarditis following venous injections in narcotic addicts, *Staphylococcus aureus* is seen the most frequent (36%), followed by *Pseudomonas* (16%), polymicrobial species (15%), *Streptococcus faecalis* (13%) and *Streptococcus viridans* (11%) [1].

The most frequently encountered micro-organism in infected false aneurysm will be *Staphylococcus aureus* (65%) and nearly 50% of these are methicillin resistant. Another characteristic of the aneurysms caused by self-injection with non-sterile needles is the high frequency of multiple organism infections. Thirty three percent will have polymicrobial cultures, including *Staphylococcus aureus, Escherichia coli, Streptococcus faecalis, Pseudomonas aeruginosa* and various enterobacter organisms [2].

Streptococcus is certainly the most virulent organism towards non-traumatized arteries. For centuries, *Treponema pallidum* has been the leading cause of infected aneurysms, especially in the thoracic region. Nowadays, it has become the exception and the predominant micro-organisms associated with bacterial aortitis and aneurysm formation are *Salmonella, Staphylococcus aureus* and *Escherichia coli*. *Salmonella* has a special affinity for the diseased aorta and the most common species are *S. typhimurium* (30.5%), *S. enteritidis* (20.3%), *S. choleraesuis* (12.1%), group D *Salmonella* (10.1%) and group B and C *Salmonella* (3.7%) [5]. Apart from this, there is a wide variety of organisms mentioned anecdotally in the literature, including *Streptococcus* species, *Pseudo-*

monas species, *Staphylococcus epidermidis*, *Proteus* and *Serratia* species and also anaerobes, such as *Bacteroides fragilis*. The overall negative culture rate is also quite high (25%) and this may indicate, according to some reports, a deficiency in obtaining anaerobic cultures.

The most common organisms causing infection of a pre-existing aneurysm are *Staphylococcus* species, either *aureus* or *epidermidis*. Gram-negative organisms (35%) are indeed less common than Gram-positive organisms (59%). Gram-negative infections are, however, more virulent and have an even less attractive prognosis, both towards rupture (84% vs. 10% for gram-positive infection) and patient's survival (16% vs. 50% for gram-positive infection) [6].

Diagnosis

Rupture of an infected aneurysm carries a very poor prognosis. Moreover, the operative management in case of infection is quite different from that of "ordinary" aneurysms. Consequently, every effort should be made to confirm a timely diagnosis. Infected aneurysms are indeed more often symptomatic and might show quite characteristic findings on imaging studies. Diagnosis remains, however, difficult and infected aneurysms are prone to early rupture. This explains that in up to 50% of the cases diagnosis is made at a late stage in combination with fulminant sepsis and aneurysm rupture [7].

CLINICAL PRESENTATION

Apart from "true" mycotic aneurysms which will also be seen at young age, the typical patient is elderly, atherosclerotic and often immunosuppressed. The majority will be symptomatic but the symptoms are somewhat vague and non-specific. Those most frequently reported are: fever, lumbar pain, abdominal pain, chest pain and painful palpable abdominal mass, which are present in 50% to 90% of cases [7]. Leucocytosis or an elevated erythrocyte sedimentation rate is present in over half of the patients. Sepsis or fever e causa ignota in the presence of an aneurysm should alert the physician. Hemocultures may be helpful although they might be negative in as many as 40% of the patients. Coprocultures should be taken when *Salmonella* is suspected. In fact, as *Salmonella* bacteremia will lead to septic arteritis in over 20% of cases in patients over 60 years of age, this possibility should be explored in any patient with *Salmonella* sepsis [8].

IMAGING STUDIES

Plain radiology and ultrasound usually offer little information. Plain radiography can demonstrate absence of calcifications or invasion of the vertebral spine. Ultrasound may be used to rule out the presence of an aneurysm, but is certainly not sensitive for infection. Both angiography and CT scan offer more characteristic information in the light of operative reconstruction as well. Angiographic findings suggesting infected aneurysms are: saccular aneurysm on an otherwise normal-appearing artery, multilobular aneurysm formation and eccentric aneurysm with a narrow neck (Fig. 1). Intravenous contrast enhanced CT scans may confirm the atypical angiographic shape of the aneurysm. In addition, it is able to demonstrate a periaortic soft tissue mass, contained rupture, stranding and/or fluid in nearly 50% of the cases [9] (Fig. 2). In an early stage, a CT scan might demonstrate subtle periaortic edema, followed by rapid aneurysm progression and development on sequential studies. Periaortic gas or gas within the aneurysm thrombus is diagnostic for infection, but is seen quite rarely (Fig. 3). Circumstantial suggestive findings include vertebral body destruction, abscess formation and absence of calcification in the aortic wall.

12

131

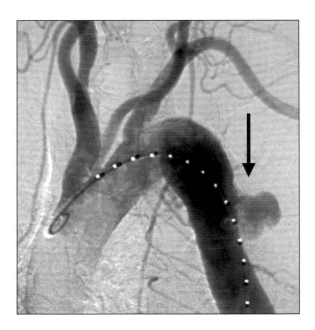

FIG. 1 Typical angiographic appearance of *Salmonella* aortitis (descending thoracic aorta). Patient refused operation and died one week later from rupture.

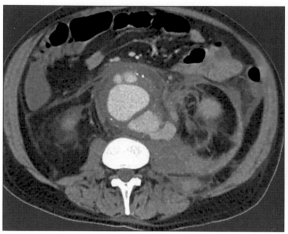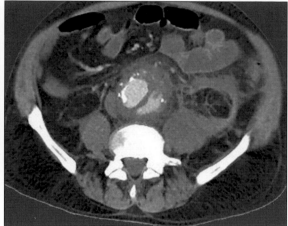

FIG. 2 Rupture of a pre-existing atherosclerotic infrarenal aortic aneurysm surinfected with *Salmonella enteritidis* and successfully treated with aneurysm resection and in-situ reconstruction with rifampicin bonded dacron graft.

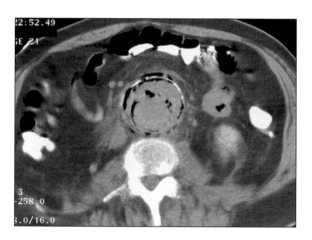

FIG. 3 Surinfection of pre-existing infrarenal aortic aneurysm with *Salmonella typhimurium*. Note, periaortic gas and gas formation within the aneurysm thrombus. Treatment consisted of aneurysm resection and in-situ reconstruction with dacron graft. Patient died after the operation.

The experience with MR imaging is still limited but it might have a similar diagnostic potential as CT scanning. Finally, nuclear medicine imaging will show increased radiotracer uptake in around 85% of the cases [9]. It cannot precisely show the site of increased uptakes, but correlation with CT findings allows better localization and therefore it might facilitate or confirm the diagnosis.

Surgical treatment

It has been known for years that there is no place for conservative medical treatment: surgery offers the only definite solution for an infected aortic aneurysm. Aneurysm rupture is a surgical emergency but, taking into account the propensity of rupture, any infected aneurysm should be treated on a semi-urgent base. Preoperative care should be kept as brief as possible and every effort should be made to identify the responsible micro-organism. Preoperative sepsis has to be controlled and, if attempts to identify the responsible organisms remain unsuccessful, intravenous antibiotics, according to the "best guess" principle should be instituted. This means that both aerobic and anaerobic organisms should be covered. In immunosuppressed patients, it might be wise to consider antifungal therapy as well.

General principles that apply to surgical treatment of infected aneurysms are a combination of both traditional aneurysm surgery and surgery for infected prosthetic grafts. Hemorrhage is controlled by aortic clamping well above the aneurysm. Supraceliac clamping is preferred for infrarenal aneurysms. Autotransfusion systems should definitely be avoided. The diagnosis is confirmed by Gram's stains of the aneurysm wall and the thrombus. Several culture specimens should be taken for aerobic and anaerobic bacteria and also for fungi.

Infection is controlled by complete resection of the aneurysm back to the healthy non-infected arterial wall. Equally important is a wide debridement of all surrounding infected tissues and irrigation with antibiotics and/or povidone-iodine solution. In the meantime, the surgeon has to decide on the method of revascularization, which remains a major point of discussion.

EXTRA-ANATOMIC REVASCULARIZATION

As for infrarenal aortic graft infection, aortic transsection and extra-anatomic revascularization through uninfected tissue planes (usually axillobifemoral bypass) is still popular for infrarenal infected aneurysms. Here, the presumed healthy infrarenal aorta is transsected and closed with monofilament sutures, preferably in a double suture line. An omental pedicle is brought through the transverse mesocolon and positioned around the aortic stump and in the bed of the excised aneurysm. The importance of omentum in containment of infections is well-recognized. Its gratifying effect is supposedly due to increased blood supply to the infected area which, in turn, intensifies inflammatory cell infiltration and increases tissue concentrations of antibiotics. Moreover, omentum will also absorb necrotic tissue and, by eliminating dead spaces, it will reduce the possibility of regrowth of residual bacteria. In cases of pararenal infection, transsection of the aorta above the renal arteries in combination with renal revascularization by venous bypasses from the splenic, hepatic or mesenteric arteries has been reported. More distally, the iliac arteries are also closed by monofilament sutures. Here it is important to preserve at least one hypogastric artery, which is usually sufficient to maintain adequate pelvic circulation and to avoid ischemic colitis. In cases of extensive iliac involvement, autogenous reconstruction of one hypogastric artery might be considered.

The major advantage of this technique is that there is no graft left in a possibly infected field. In elective cases, the operation can be staged with the axillobifemoral bypasses being done first, followed by the aneurysm resection afterwards. According to some authors, such a staged treatment will also reduce the hemodynamic stress caused by aortic clamping during the aneurysm resection and, therefore, it might produce better immediate results. In urgent cases, however, it certainly results in prolonged ischemia of the lower limbs since the extra-anatomic bypass has to be performed after hemostasis and resection of the aneurysm. Moreover,

extra-anatomic reconstruction is cumbersome in case of thoracic involvement and virtually impossible with thoracoabdominal infection. Other well-known disadvantages of this technique include the risk of aortic stump rupture, reinfection of the extra-anatomic bypasses, pelvic (interval) ischemia and the poor long-term patency of axillofemoral bypasses.

IN-SITU RECONSTRUCTION

In-situ reconstruction for mycotic aneurysms was introduced two decades ago. Initially, it was exclusively used for situations where extra-anatomic reconstruction was impossible, such as thoracic and thoracoabdominal aortic infections. However, thanks to the gratifying results and also the experience with in-situ grafting in case of prosthetic graft infection, in-situ reconstruction for infected aneurysms gained a lot of interest over the years and it is actually the preferred method in many centers. It offers a more physiological solution, it is frequently easier to perform and it is certainly superior to extra-anatomic grafting in terms of long-term patency. The key to success here is also wide and extensive debridement of all infected tissues and resection of the aorta back to the healthy non-infected wall. After completion, the reconstruction should be carefully covered with non-infected viable tissues. Here also, a pedicled flap of greater omentum is preferred since it can also be used in the thoracic and thoracoabdominal position. Although its use in virulent infection remains debated, the discussion at present is no longer whether in-situ reconstruction represents a safe and durable option but rather which materials are preferred. A first option might be prosthetic grafts (Fig. 4). They have the advantage of immediate availability in emergency situations. In addition, they can be adapted to any anatomical situation. The infectability remains a matter of concern. The superiority of rifampicin-bonded grafts and silver-coated grafts has actually not been proved in vivo but, from a pragmatic point of view, it seems logical that these grafts are preferred rather than "ordinary" dacron. Arterial homografts are a second option (Fig. 5). They are indeed more resistant to infection than prosthetic grafts. As with prosthetic grafts, they can also be adapted to any anatomical situation. The availability in urgent situations might, depending on the center, create a logistical problem. There is wide experience with arterial homografts, especially in prosthetic graft infection, but their use in virulent

12

133

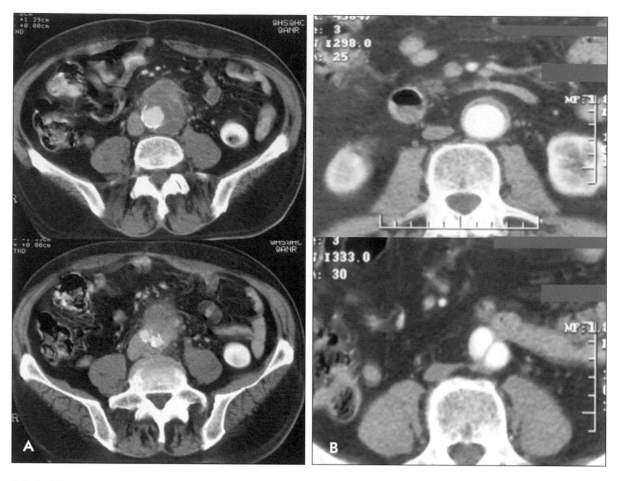

FIG. 4 Infrarenal aortitis (*Salmonella* group D). A - Preoperative CT scan. B - CT scan three years after aneurysm resection and in-situ reconstruction with rifampicin bonded dacron graft: normal graft healing, no reinfection.

infection is discouraged taking the risk of rupture into account. In addition, arterial homografts may pose problems of degeneration in the long term. Finally, it should be realized that, compared with other materials, homografts represent a very expensive solution.

The third option is autologous grafts (Fig. 6). In recent years, the femoral vein has been shown to be a very good, if not ideal, conduit in the aortic position. As an autogenous graft, it also offers the best resistance towards infection. Venous morbidity after resection of the femoral veins is minimal. Harvesting is, however, technically demanding and time-consuming, which might become problematic in urgent situations. The femoral vein can easily be adapted to the abdominal aorta. Favourable long-term results are well-documented, particularly in

cases of infrarenal aortic prosthetic graft infections, but its use as an interposition graft in the thoracic aorta is problematic. The limited amount of material might also be an additional disadvantage in complex reconstructions, but even then it can be used in combination with other techniques (Fig. 7). Finally, apart from its superior quality as an arterial conduit, it is also the cheapest material available.

Regardless of the surgical treatment, specific antibiotic therapy needs to be continued postoperatively. With regard to the length there is, once again, no consensus in the literature. The proposed duration varies between six weeks to one year. When the source of infection is unknown, some authors advise even life-long prophylactic antibiotic therapy, especially in case of *Salmonella* aortitis or if there is active infection during surgery. Since recurring or

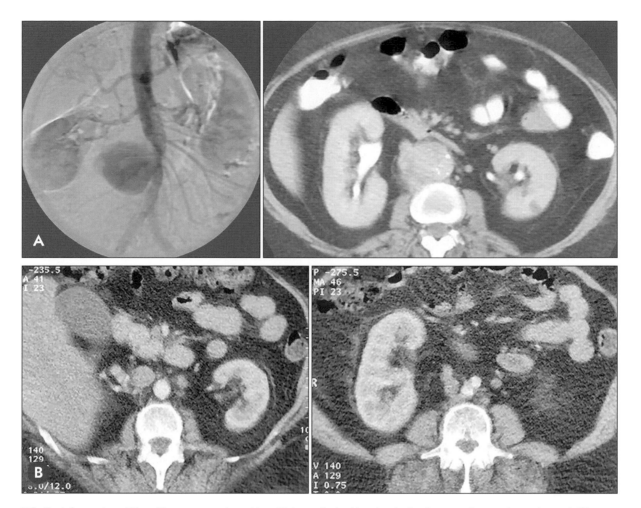

FIG. 5 Infrarenal aortitis with aneurysm formation *(Salmonella typhimurium)*. A - Preoperative angiography and CT scan. Treated by aneurysm resection and in-situ reconstruction with arterial homograft. B - CT scan after six years: calcified but well functioning arterial homograft, no reinfection.

persisting infection creates a major problem, serial imaging by CT scan and monitoring laboratory markers of inflammation are essential during follow-up. A CT scan prior to discharge provides a good starting base in this regard.

Personal experience

During the period 1990-2004, 32 patients were referred to the Department of Vascular Surgery because of a mycotic infected aortic aneurysm. One patient (male, 79 years old) presented with *Salmonella* aortitis located at the proximal descending thoracic aorta. He refused surgery and died one week after the diagnosis from rupture (Fig.1).

Thirty-one patients underwent surgical treatment. There were 27 men and 4 women with a mean age of 68.5 years (range 42-84 years). Thirteen patients (42%) showed at least one co-morbid condition associated with some degree of immunosuppression: chronic steroid use (n = 7), chronic renal failure (n = 4) or diabetes (n = 4). Another patient developed a fungal infection of a pre-existing infrarenal aortic aneurysm during multi-organ system failure after cardiac surgery.

Thirty patients were symptomatic. The mean duration of symptoms prior to surgical treatment was 53 days (range 1-224 days). The most common

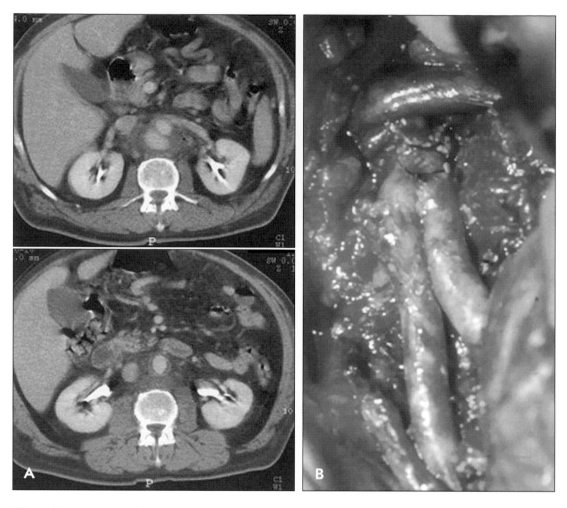

12
136

FIG. 6 Infrarenal aortitis (*Salmonella* group D). A - Preoperative CT scan. Treated by aneurysm resection and in-situ aorto-bi-iliac venous graft (femoral vein). B - Peroperative view: patient alive and well after four years.

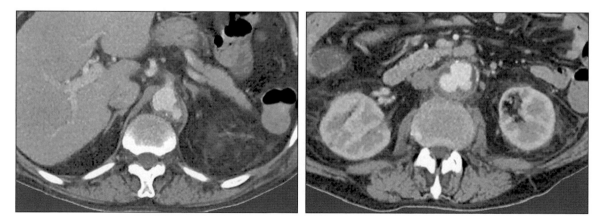

FIG. 7 *Escherichia coli* aortic infection starting at the level of the celiac trunk and extending distally to the aortic bifurcation. Treatment consisted of axillobifemoral bypass, followed the day afterwards by resection of the abdominal aneurysm, transsection of the aorta well above the celiac trunk and venous bypass (femoral vein) from the thoracic aorta to the visceral and renal arteries.

symptoms were: fever, n = 24; abdominal, back or thoracic pain, n = 21; and gastrointestinal symptoms (nausea, vomiting, diarrhoea, ileus), n = 8. Ten patients (32.5%) presented with hemodynamic instability due to aneurysm rupture.

Diagnosis, based on clinical presentation, imaging (CT scan and/or angiography) and blood cultures, was made preoperatively in 28 cases. Five patients (16%) presented with infection of a pre-existing aneurysm. The remaining 26 cases were due to aortitis. There were no patients with "true" mycotic aneurysms in these series. The location of the infection was: infrarenal, n = 23 (74%); para- or suprarenal, n = 7 (23%); and in the descending thoracic aorta, n = 1 (3%). Rupture was seen in 7 infrarenal aneurysms (30% of all infrarenal cases), in 2 suprarenal infections and also in the only patient with infection of the descending thoracic aorta.

The responsible organisms were identified in 30 cases, 2 or more micro-organisms were found in 3 patients (Table I). The majority of infections were due to *Salmonella* species (n = 13, 42%). These included *Salmonella* Group D (n = 9), *Salmonella typhimurium* (n = 2) and *Salmonella enteritidis* (n = 2). Three infections were due to *Escherichia coli* and *Streptococcus viridans* was noted in two patients.

The ten patients with ruptured aneurysms were taken immediately to the operating room. The majority (90%) of the remaining 21 cases were operated upon within one week after the diagnosis. One patient with *Salmonella* aortitis at the suprarenal level was diagnosed more than seven months and treated medically before he came to operation because of increasing pain and impending rupture. Overall, ligation of the aorta and extra-anatomic reconstruction was used in 5 patients; 25 underwent in-situ reconstruction with prosthetic polyester graft (n = 14), arterial homograft (n – 7) or femoral vein (n = 4). Finally, one patient presenting with both suprarenal and infrarenal aortitis *(Escherichia coli)* underwent combined extra-anatomic (axillobifemoral) grafting and in-situ visceral and renal revascularization (autologous femoral vein) (Fig.4). In-situ grafting was preferred in 8 (80%) out of the 10 patients with rupture as well as in 18 (86%) out of the 21 patients operated on "electively".

The patient with thoracic infection underwent in-situ prosthetic reconstruction. Six of the seven patients with para- or suprarenal involvement underwent in-situ grafting (polyester graft (n = 1), arterial homograft (n = 4), autologous femoral vein (n = 1)) in combination with renal (n = 6) and visceral revascularization (n = 2). As mentioned above, one patient underwent combined in-situ and extra-anatomic reconstruction. Aortic ligation and extra-anatomic revascularization was used on 5 occasions (22%) in patients with infrarenal aortic infections. The majority (78%) was handled by in-situ reconstruction (dacron prosthetic graft (n = 12), arterial homograft (n = 3), autologous femoral vein (n = 3)). The operation was completed in all patients by complete resection of the infected aorta, extensive debridement of all infected tissues and coverage of the reconstruction with viable tissue (omentum).

Eight patients (26%) died after the operation. The operative mortality increased from 19% after "elective" operation to 40% in patients with ruptured aneurysms. Apart from one patient with a ruptured suprarenal aneurysm, all deaths occurred

Table I	BACTERIOLOGY OF INFECTED AORTIC ANEURYSM (N = 31) (PERSONAL SERIES)	
Organism	*Number*	
Salmonella species	13	
Staphylococcus aureus	5*	
Escherichia coli	3	
Streptococcus viridans	2	
Bacteroides fragilis	1	
Campylobacter jejuni	1	
Pseudodiphteria	1	
Staphylococcus epidermidis	1	
Pseudomonas aeruginosa	1	
Acinetobacter species	1	
Klebsiella ozaenae	1	
Listeria monocytogenes	1	
Enterobacter species	1	
Candida	1	
No growth	1	

*MRSA, N = 1

in the group of infrarenal infections (Table II). *Salmonella* infection was associated with a poor prognosis and the overall mortality rate after in-situ reconstruction was 24% vs. 40% after extra-anatomic grafting. Causes of death included uncontrollable sepsis (n=3), respiratory insufficiency (n=2), multiple-organ system failure (n = 1), bowel ischemia (n = 1) and reinfection after in-situ prosthetic graft reconstruction (n = 1). Fifteen patients (71%) had significant postoperative complications: these included congestive heart failure (n = 2), renal insufficiency (n =6 of which 1 permanent dialysis), respiratory insufficiency (n = 6) and prolonged ileus (n = 5). Two patients presented postoperatively unilateral limb ischemia that was handled by thrombo-embolectomy. Wound complications occurred in seven patients. One patient developed ischemic colitis after aortic ligation and axillobifemoral grafting and underwent a hemicolectomy. Finally, two patients showed early reinfection after in-situ grafting. The first had an infrarenal dacron graft that was replaced by an autologous femoral vein graft. The second patient had reinfection after in-situ homograft reconstruction of a pararenal infection. He was handled by ligation of the aorta just below the superior mesenteric artery and axillobifemoral grafting. Both patients recovered (with permanent renal failure in the second). Antibiotic therapy was prolonged for 6 to 12 weeks

Table II OPERATIVE MORTALITY IN RELATION TO DIFFERENT RISK FACTORS (PERSONAL SERIES)

	Number	%
Clinical presentation (N = 31)		
Elective	4/21	19
Rupture	4/10	40
Location of infection (N = 31)		
Thoracic	0/1	0
Para/suprarenal	1/7	14
Infrarenal	7/23	30
Type of reconstruction (N = 31)		
Extra-anatomic	2/5	40
In-situ	6/25	24
Combined	0/1	0
Type of in-situ reconstruction (N = 26) *		
Prosthetic graft	3/14	21
Arterial homograft	2/7	28
Autologous femoral vein	1/5	20
Infrarenal infection (elective reconstruction – N = 16)		
Extra-anatomic	1/3	33
In-situ	2/13	15
Type of micro-organism (N = 30)		
Salmonella species	5/13	38
Non *Salmonella* species	2/17	12

*One patient with combined extra-anatomic and in-situ reconstruction

in all surviving patients. No patient in these series received life-long antibiotic therapy.

The mean follow-up period in the 23 surviving patients was 40 months (range 2 to 103 months). Follow-up consisted of clinical examination, laboratory blood markers and yearly duplex ultrasound and/or CT scan. Eight patients (35%) died during this period. Seven deaths occurred unrelated to the primary operation (cardiac (n = 4), pulmonary (n = 2), stroke (n = 1)). One patient with extra-anatomic reconstruction developed infection 14 months postoperatively. The axillofemoral graft was replaced by a thoracic aortofemoral graft but the patient died ultimately from sepsis and hemorrhage from suture dehiscence. Apart from this, morbidity during follow-up was minimal. There were no incidences of late infection or graft related complications in the in-situ group (n = 18). One patient in the extra-anatomic group developed graft failure one year postoperatively. He underwent a thoracic aorto-femoral dacron graft and survived for another seven years.

Literature data

It is clear that a mycotic aneurysm remains a catastrophic event. The results of surgery depend on several factors. The type of aneurysm, the location, the mode of presentation, the micro-organism responsible and the type of treatment are all equally important. In addition, patients with infected aortic aneurysms are usually in a poor general condition and several of them are immunosuppressed.

The overall mortality rate in the literature varies between 10% and 60% (Table III). Oderich et al. defined, in a series of 43 patients, 5 independent variables associated with operative mortality: extensive periaortic infection; female sex; *Staphylococcus aureus* infection; aneurysm rupture; and suprarenal location [7]. The negative effect of rupture on survival is clear from our own experience where the mortality rate of 19% increased to 40% in case of rupture. In the series of Müller et al. (n = 33), the operative mortality for rupture was 63% vs. 0% for

First author [ref.]	Year	Number of patients	Global	Infrarenal aneurysm %	Suprarenal aneurysm %	Intact aneurysm %	Ruptured aneurysm %
				Mortality rates			
Reddy [10]	1991	13*	31	20	67	11	75
Fichelle [11]	1993	25	20	20	-	NS	NS
Pasic [12]	1993	12	25	NS	NS	NS	NS
Moneta [13]	1998	17	18	0	43	NS	NS
Ihya [14]	2001	9	44	44	-	NS	NS
Müller [15]	2001	33	36	50	38	0	63
Oderich [7]	2001	43	21	9	40	18	44
Fillmore [16]	2003	10	40	0	67	40	-
Kyriakides [17]	2004	15	27	12	43	33	17
Hsu [18]	2004	35	11	NS	NS	0	37
Present series		31	26	30	12	19	40

Table III MORTALITY RATES AFTER SURGERY FOR INFECTED AORTIC ANEURYSMS (SELECTED PUBLICATIONS)

* Including three iliac aneurysms
NS: not significant

intact aneurysms [15]. The importance of the responsible organism was also stressed in the report of Hsu et al., who identified non-*Salmonella* infection and advanced age as risk factors for operative death [18]. Avoiding extensive infection and aneurysm rupture by early diagnosis is critical with regard to operative survival. However, the symptoms are usually non-specific and patients typically undergo an extensive investigation before operation is considered. This explains why, in contemporary series, the incidence of aneurysm rupture is still around 50%-70%.

With regard to the operative technique, in-situ reconstruction has been historically preferred, mostly for technical reasons in case of thoracic or thoracoabdominal infection. In a review through the period 1966-1999, Cinà et al. identified 73 cases of thoracoabdominal aortic infection reported in the literature [19]. Detailed surgical information was available for 40 patients. In-situ reconstruction was preferred in 85% of the patients with a mortality rate of 17%. The most commonly used materials were dacron, followed by polytetrafluorethylene (PTFE) and arterial homografts. Extra-anatomic bypass was used in 6 patients and only 2 survived the operation.

The method of surgical reconstruction in infrarenal aortic infection remains debated. According to the classic doctrine, extra-anatomic reconstruction is the treatment of choice for primary aortic sepsis. The theoretical advantage is revascularization through a plane remote from the infection, but even recent series report a high incidence of complications, going up to a 20% aortic stump rupture, a 20%-30% amputation rate and a 20% risk of reinfection [13,20]. As is true for prosthetic infections, there is an increasingly number of encouraging reports on in-situ reconstruction for mycotic aneurysms. As shown in Table IV, the operative results of in-situ reconstruction compete favourably with those of extra-anatomic recontruction. Admittedly, these are certainly not randomised studies. On the contrary, the operative method has usually been determined by the circumstances and the "clinical feeling" of the surgeon, which also means that these results need to be interpreted with some caution. Nevertheless, most authors will actually agree that in-situ reconstruction is an appropriate choice for most patients with aortic infection, especially in emergency situations and cases without extensive pus formation. Dacron grafts are used

Table IV MORTALITY RATES IN RELATION TO TYPE OF RECONSTRUCTION (SELECTED PUBLICATIONS)

First author [ref.]	Year	Number of patients	*Mortality* In-situ reconstruction %	(N death/N case)	Extra-anatomic reconstruction %	(N death/N case)
Reddy [10]	1991	12 •	28	(2/7)	40	(2/5)
Fichelle [11]	1993	25 •	14	(3/21)	50	(2/4)
Pasic [12]	1993	12 *	33	(2/6)	17	(1/6)
Müller [15]	2001	14 •	40	(2/5)	33	(3/9)
Oderich [7]	2001	41 *	20	(7/35)	17	(1/6)
Kyriakides [17]	2004	8 •	0	(0/6)	50	(1/2)
Hsu [18]	2004	35 *	11	(4/35)		-
Present series		30 *	24	(6/25)	40	(2/5)
Total		**177**	**19**	**(26/140)**	**32**	**(12/37)**

* Mixed infrarenal and suprarenal
• Infrarenal location

most frequently. Reinfection might create a problem and, in fact, in our own series we observed two cases of early reinfection (14%). It might be hoped that the results can still be improved by rifampicin-soaked and silver-coated grafts [21]. Encouraging results have also been reported with arterial homografts [22]. Others question these results because of the incidence of rupture in virulent infections and the propensity of late degeneration of arterial homografts. The incidence of early homograft related morbidity, consisting of persisting infection with perianastomotic haemorrhage, graft limb occlusion and pseudoaneurysm was 25% in the *United States Cryopreserved Aortic Allograft Registry* [23]. In a multicentric study, reported by Verhelst et al., the incidence of homograft rupture was 41% in case of virulent infection [24]. Experience with the autologous femoral vein, one of the better options in prosthetic infection [25], is still limited in cases of mycotic aneurysm. Apart from our 4 personal cases, there have been 8 others reported in the literature including one patient with a ruptured infected aortic aneurysm [16,26-28]. All these patients' recovery was uneventful, confirming once again the infection resistance of autogenous grafts.

Taken into account the mortality of open surgery and the technical difficulties, it should be no surprise that endovascular stent-grafts have been proposed in some centers as an alternative. There are at least ten papers documenting endovascular treatment of mycotic aneurysms (thoracic and abdominal) with an in-hospital mortality ranging from 0% to 40% [29]. The philosophy is clear: reduction of mortality and morbidity. A major disadvantage, however, is the inability to resect the infected aneurysm and to debride the infected area, which remains one of the key points in open surgery. Although some papers mention a follow-up of more than one year, the results are still premature. It is, therefore, too early to judge whether this therapy offers a definite solution or whether it might just serve as a temporary protection allowing a definite operation to be performed in more appropriate conditions in some patients.

REFERENCES

1 Maggilligan DJ, Quinn EL. Active infective endocarditis. In: Maggiligan DJ, Quinn EL (eds) *Endocarditis: medical and surgical management.* New York, Marcel Dekker, 1986: pp 207-214.

2 Reddy DJ, Smith RF, Elliott JP et al. Infected femoral artery false aneurysms in drug addicts: evolution of selective vascular reconstruction. *J Vasc Surg* 1986; 3: 718-724.

3 Miller DV, Oderich GS, Aubry MC et al. Surgical pathology of infected aneurysms of the descending thoracic and abdominal aorta: clinicopathologic correlations in 29 cases (1976 to 1999). *Hum Pathol* 2004: 35: 1112-1120.

4 Ernst CB, Campbell HC Jr, Daugherty ME et al. Incidence and significance of intra-operative bacterial cultures during abdominal aortic aneurysmectomy. *Ann Surg* 1977; 185: 626-633.

5 Veraldi GF, de Manzoni G, Laterza E et al. Extra intestinal infection by group C Salmonella: a case report and review of the literature. *Hepatogastroenterology* 2001; 48: 471-474.

6 Jarrett F, Darling RC, Mundth ED, Austen WG. Experience with infected aneurysms of the abdominal aorta. *Arch Surg* 1975; 110: 1281-1286.

7 Oderich GS, Panneton JM, Bower TC et al. Infected aortic aneurysms: aggressive presentation, complicated early outcome, but durable results. *J Vasc Surg* 2001; 34: 900-908.

8 Fernandez Guerrero ML, Aguado JM, Arribas A et al. The spectrum of cardiovascular infections due to salmonella enterica: a review of clinical features and factors determining outcome. *Medicine* 2004; 83: 123-138.

9 Macedo TA, Stanson AW, Oderich GS et al. Infected aortic aneurysms: imaging findings. *Radiology* 2004; 231: 250-257.

10 Reddy DJ, Shepard AD, Evans JR et al. Management of infected aortoiliac aneurysms. *Arch Surg* 1991; 126: 873-878.

11 Fichelle JM, Tabet G, Cormier P et al. Infected infrarenal aortic aneurysms: when is in-situ reconstruction safe? *J Vasc Surg* 1993; 17: 635-645.

12 Pasic M, Carrel T, Tönz M et al. Mycotic aneurysm of the abdominal aorta: extra-anatomic versus in-situ reconstruction. *Cardiovasc Surg* 1993; 1: 48-52.

13 Moneta GL, Taylor LM, Yeager RA et al. Surgical treatment of infected abdominal aortic aneurysms. *Am J Surg* 1998; 175: 396-399.

14 Ihya A, Chiba Y, Kimura T et al. Surgical outcome of infectious aneurysms of the abdominal aorta with and without SIRS. *Cardiovasc Surg* 2001; 9: 436-440.

15 Müller BT, Wegener OR, Grabitz K et al. Mycotic aneurysms of the thoracic and abdominal aorta and iliac arteries: experience with anatomic and extra-anatomic repair in 33 cases. *J Vasc Surg* 2001; 33: 106-113.

16 Fillmore AJ, Valentine RJ. Surgical mortality in patients with infected aortic aneurysms. *J am Coll Surg* 2003; 196: 435-441.

17 Kyriakides C, Kan Y, Kerle M et al. 11-year experience with anatomical and extra-anatomical repair of mycotic aortic aneurysms. *Eur J Vasc Endovasc Surg* 2004; 27: 585-589.

18 Hsu RB, Chen RJ, Wang SS Chu SH. Infected aortic aneurysms: clinical outcome and risk factor analysis. *J Vasc Surg* 2004; 40: 30-35.

19 Cinà CS, Arena GO, Fiture AO et al. Ruptured mycotic thoraco-abdominal aortic aneurysms: a report of three cases and a systematic review. *J Vasc Surg* 2001; 33: 861-867.

20 Taylor RM, Deitz DM, McConnell DB et al. Treatment of infected abdominal aneurysms by extra-anatomic bypass, aneurysm excision and drainage. *Am J Surg* 1988; 155: 655-658.

21 Batt M, Magne JL, Alric P et al. In-situ revascularisation with silver coated polyester grafts to treat aortic infection: early and midterm results. *J Vasc Surg* 2003; 38: 983-989.

22 Vogt PR, Brunner-La Rocca HP, Carrel T et al. Cryopreserved arterial allografts in the treatment of major vascular infection: a comparison with conventional surgical techniques. *J Thorac Cardiovasc Surg* 1998; 116: 965-972.

23 Noel AA, Gloviczki P, Cherry KJ et al. Abdominal aortic reconstruction in infected fields: early results of the United States Cryopreserved Aortic Allograft Registry. *J Vasc Surg* 2002; 35: 847-852.

24 Verhelst R, Lacroix V, Vraux H et al. Use of cryopreserved arterial homografts for management of infected prosthetic grafts: a multicentric study. *Ann Vasc Surg* 2000; 14: 602-607.

25 Daenens K, Fourneau I, Nevelsteen A. Ten-year experience in autogenous reconstruction with the femoral vein in the treat-ment of aortofemoral prosthetic infection. *Eur J Vasc Endovasc Surg* 2003; 25: 240-245.

26 Thrush S, Watts A, Fraser SCA, Edmondson RA. Primary autologous superficial femoral vein reconstruction of an emergency infected ruptured aortic aneurysm. *Eur J Vasc Endovasc Surg* 2001; 22: 557-558.

27 Brown PM Jr, Kim VB, Lalikos JF et al. Autologous superficial femoral vein for aortic reconstruction in infected fields. *Ann Vasc Surg* 1999; 13:32-36.

28 Benjamin ME, Cohn EJ Jr, Purtill WA et al. Arterial reconstruction with deep leg veins for the treatment of mycotic aneurysms. *J Vasc Surg* 1999: 30: 1004-1015.

29 Smith JJ, Taylor PR. Endovascular treatment of mycotic aneurysms of the thoracic and abdominal aorta: the need for level I evidence. *Eur J Vasc Endovasc Surg* 2004; 27: 569-570.

12

13

DISTAL EMBOLIZATION DURING ANEURYSMAL SURGERY: FROM BLUE TOE SYNDROME TO FATAL STROKE

GEORGE HAMILTON

Atheroembolism is a well-recognized condition which may present as a primary syndrome arising from dislodgement and fragmentation of atheromatous plaques or from associated thrombotic material. Depending on the distribution of these emboli, the clinical presentation may be cerebrovascular, spinal, visceral, renal, and lower limb ischemia and sometimes a combination of these. Emboli can develop from atheromatous plaques and aneurysms involving virtually any artery in the arterial tree, but most commonly primary embolization arises from the infrarenal aorta to the popliteal arteries and embolization to the lower limbs is the most common presentation. Aneurysms, and in particular popliteal aneurysms, have been recognized for centuries as a source of embolization but overall the most important sources are atheromatous plaques which are inflamed, degenerative, irregular and ulcerated.

Vascular interventions ranging from simple catheterization for angiography to complex reconstructions, are complicated by a small but significant risk of secondary atheroembolism. Often the result of this embolization can prove to be devastating with major morbidity and fatal outcome is not uncommon. This chapter is focused on embolization following aneurysmal surgery (secondary atheroembolism) where the likeliest source of embolic material is from the laminated porridge-like thrombus contained within the aneurysm. Widespread atheromatous degeneration of the contiguous non-aneurysmal aorta and, of the iliac arteries in particular, is frequently present and these sites must also be considered as possible sources for embolism.

Pathophysiology

Emboli may be constituted of fragmented atheromatous material, or of thrombus which is either associated with plaque or from an aneurysmal sac. The emboli arising from atheromatous plaque are mainly in the 100-200 μm size range but there can be considerable variation in particle size as confirmed by studies of embolic material retrieved from protection devices during stent angioplasty for renal and carotid artery disease [1]. Emboli arising from thrombus may be large enough to occlude vessels of the caliber of the distal superficial femoral, popliteal or tibial arteries but may also be friable and, therefore, likely to fragment further into sizes similar to those of cholesterol emboli. The size of the embolic particles is obviously of great clinical importance; a large embolus will result in critical lower limb ischemia, for example, which can be treated by embolectomy, while a showering of multiple small emboli will result in widespread occlusion of end arteries and arterioles. The latter situation may result in widespread patchy ischemia and infarction of the end organ and will not be amenable to revascularization by embolectomy. Thrombolysis is a possible therapeutic option which might be successful if the preponderance of microemboli were of thrombotic origin. The success of thrombolysis, however, is related to the age of the thrombus and in these clinical situations the thrombus is likely to be mature and resistant to the action of the thrombolytic agent. Consequently proximal and distal thrombosis will take place upon the arterial occlusion with release of platelet activated factors and activation of a response leading to inflammation, vasoconstriction and further downstream ischemic damage to the end organ. These changes may respond to anticoagulation and treatment with vasoactive drugs such as prostacyclin analogues (iloprost) and other prostaglandins.

Clinical features

The clinical pictures will obviously depend on the anatomical site, distribution and extent of embolization. The lower limb is the most commonly reported site of involvement with typical findings ranging from an obviously critically ischemic leg with absence of pulses and pallor, to focal digital ischemia usually in the presence of normal pulses which is universally known as *blue toe syndrome*. The presence of *livedo reticularis* (patchy non-blanching cyanosis, Fig. 1) involving the trunk, buttocks and lower limbs is indicative of widespread microembolization. Cerebrovascular embolization may present as transient ischemic attack or full-blown stroke, or more subtly as diminished cognitive function. The kidney is commonly involved and renal embolization should be suspected when renal failure develops after surgery. The presence of abdominal pain and tenderness, prolonged paralytic ileus and septicemia should raise the suspicion of colonic embolization. In many cases the microembolization is subclinical but, where there is preexisting compromise to colonic blood flow, embolization secondary to an intervention for an intra-abdominal aneurysm may lead to clinically significant stage II or III colonic ischemia. The buttock muscles are a further site for embolic damage presenting as severe buttock pain, renal failure from rhabdomyolysis and septicemia resulting from gluteal compartment syndrome. Spinal ischemia is a rare complication of infrarenal aortic surgery but is more commonly seen after interventions on the descending thoracic and thoracoabdominal segments. The pathophysiology of this spinal damage is complex but microembolization undoubtedly plays an important role.

Diagnosis

The diagnosis is primarily based on a high index of clinical suspicion in a patient developing unexpected complications following aneurysmal surgery. The presence of the clinical features as described above is of vital diagnostic importance, especially renal failure, hypotension, abdominal symptoms and signs, *livedo reticularis* and lower limb ischemia. There are no specific investigations which will confirm the diagnosis other than perhaps the confirmation of major embolic occlusion by duplex scanning of an axial lower limb artery. Proteinuria and hematuria may be present with elevated C-reactive protein, leucocytosis, and possibly a transient eosinophilia, which all indicate an acute phase response. In contradistinction to primary syndromes of atheroembolism, diagnosis after aneurysmal surgery may be clinically more obvious.

Open aortic surgery

THE ASCENDING AORTA AND AORTIC ARCH

Postoperative stroke due to cerebroembolization from atheromatous plaques of the ascending aorta and the aortic arch may complicate this surgery, particularly in elderly patients with vascular disease and diabetes. Over the last fifteen years, since the introduction of transesophageal echocardiography and its intraoperative use, this complication has been increasingly documented [2]. Preoperative assessment of the ascending aorta and aortic arch by transesophageal echocardiography, contrast enhanced spiral CT scanning or magnetic resonance angiography in order to exclude the presence of atheromatous disease or aortic ulceration should form part of the routine assessment of these patients. Deep hypothermia with circulatory arrest has been shown to reduce the incidence of stroke, particularly with the use of retrograde perfusion of the brain via the great veins during circulatory arrest. This may be as a result of a flushing out of microemboli from the cerebral circulation. Complications arising from embolization of the other vascular beds are rare in this situation.

DESCENDING THORACIC AND THORACOABDOMINAL ANEURYSM

Paraplegia or paraparesis is a major complication of these interventions which has a complex pathophysiology relating primarily to aortic cross-clamping. However, it is very likely that microembolization resulting from dissection, ostial endarterectomy and anastomosis of the intercostal vessels contributes to this process. Renal failure is a further major complication which is primarily related to preoperative renal dysfunction. However, renal atheroembolism has been shown to be a frequent occurrence in any aortic intervention, being found in up to 25% of renal biopsies performed, even after diagnostic renal angiography. The need for endarterectomy in the presence of renal artery stenosis will increase this risk significantly. In most cases, the atheroembolism results in a subclinical insult to renal function. Colonic and visceral ischemia is a very rare complication of this form for aneurysmal surgery.

13

145

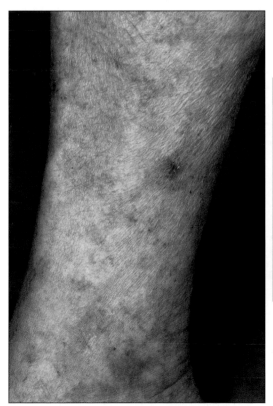

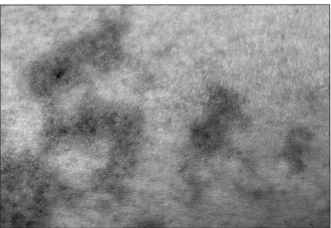

FIG. 1 This is the typical appearance of *livedo reticularis* of the leg resulting from atheroembolism; the close-up view shows the patchy non-blanching cyanosis.

JUXTARENAL AND INFRARENAL ANEURYSM

Embolization is most frequently reported after this most common form of aneurysm surgery. The embolization is mostly distal, primarily to the lower limb, with an estimated incidence of about 3% [3]. Perhaps less frequently appreciated is the incidence of proximal embolization that occurs above the clamp into the renal and upper visceral vessels.

Small bowel ischemia following infrarenal abdominal aortic surgery is very rare and is estimated to occur between 0.15% and 0.4%, out of which embolism accounted for a minority [4]. Renal failure complicating infrarenal abdominal aortic aneurysm surgery is reported to occur in 5%-10% of patients predominantly associated with preoperative renal dysfunction. It is impossible to quantify the contribution of atheroembolization to the development of renal failure in these patients. Proximal embolization to the kidneys and the viscera probably gives rise to subclinical renal damage but this, together with the other adverse factors associated with open aortic surgery, may predispose the significant renal failure seen in these patients.

In order to minimize the potential for distal embolization, many authors have long advocated initial clamping distal to the abdominal aortic aneurysm. Lipsitz et al. [5] reported a study in 1999 where a comparison of proximal and distal clamping was performed in dogs with fluoroscopic blood flow analysis in the infrarenal aorta being evaluated by injection of contrast and particles. This study showed that up to 90% of the particles placed in the aorta passed into the renal and mesenteric arteries when the initial clamps were placed distally. The probable mechanism for this phenomenon is pressure wave reflection from the occluded iliac artery orifices causing turbulent and retrograde flow (Fig. 2). In a clinical comparison of initial proximal or distal clamping of the aorta and iliac vessels, no difference was found in the number of emboli detected in the superficial femoral arteries using a transcranial doppler ultrasound system [6]. This clinical study provides evidence that there is no advantage to initial distal clamping of the iliac arteries but that this practice might actually increase the incidence of renal and visceral emboli-

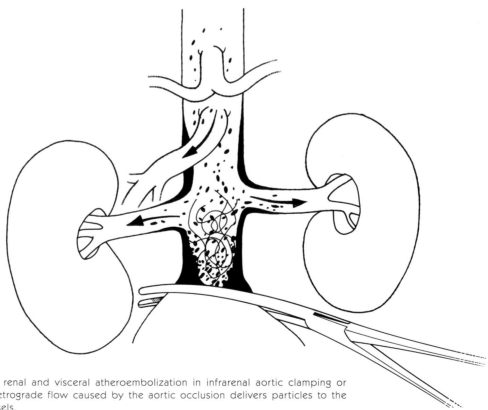

FIG. 2 Mechanism of renal and visceral atheroembolization in infrarenal aortic clamping or occlusion. Turbulent retrograde flow caused by the aortic occlusion delivers particles to the renal and visceral vessels.

zation due to the effects elegantly demonstrated by Lipsitz et al.

Clamping of the infrarenal aorta is also associated with a significant incidence of microembolization. In 1957, an autopsy series found atheromatous emboli to the kidneys in 77% patients following aortic surgery (both aneurysmal and occlusive disease - 22 cases) [7]. These emboli may arise from atheromatous fragmentation secondary to dissection but more probably from clamping of the infrarenal aorta. This process results in the release of atheroemboli which are taken up by the turbulent flow above the clamp and swept into the renal arteries. Obsessional assessment of the infra- and juxtarenal aortic neck, as is now common with endovascular repair of abdominal aortic aneurysms, is most important as it allows clamping of the aorta at the usually healthier diaphragmatic or supra-celiac level to minimize the potential for atheroembolism (Fig. 3).

FEMORAL AND POPLITEAL ANEURYSM

Aneurysms involving the femoral, superficial femoral and popliteal arteries are commonly associated with long standing spontaneous distal embolization resulting in silting up of the distal tibial circulation. Rough dissection of these vessels during repair can result in distal microembolization. Because of the high incidence of preexisting tibial atheroembolism, it is difficult to assess how frequently significant intraoperative embolization may complicate these interventions.

Endovascular aortic surgery

THORACIC AORTIC ANEURYSM

Endovascular repair of thoracic aortic disease is increasingly used with encouraging mid-term results for treatment of aneurysmal disease. This technique is much less invasive than open repair and several series report reduced morbidity and mortality in comparison. The approach offers several advantages in addition to the obvious avoidance of an extensive thoracic or thoracoabdominal incision. In particular, the avoidance of high aortic cross-clamping and the need for left-sided heart bypass are obvious benefits. It is difficult to assess from the data available what the incidence of atheroembolism complicating these interventions might be. In a recent assessment of the initial and one year outcome of endovascular treatment of thoracic aortic dissections by the EUROSTAR and the *United*

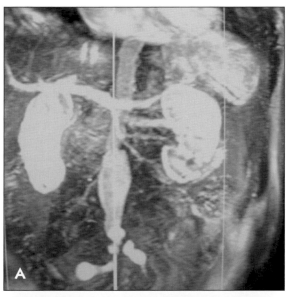

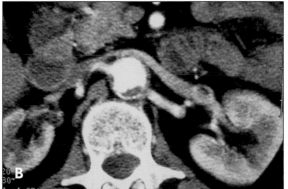

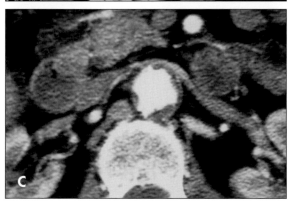

FIG. 3 This patient with aortic neck atheroma underwent open abdominal aortic aneurysm repair with infrarenal clamping of the aorta. He developed renal failure and hypertension from atheroembolism postperatively. Clamping at the non-diseased supraceliac aorta would have reduced the risk of this complication.

Kingdom Thoracic Endograft Registries, no cases of overt atheroembolism were reported in 443 patients undergoing these treatments [8]. The incidence of paraplegia and spinal cord ischemia was found to be consistently low after endovascular repair with rates of 0.8% for aortic dissection and 4% for patients with degenerative aneurysms. The authors reviewed the literature and found a range of risk for spinal complications of 0%-12%. This lower rate of spinal cord ischemia could be due to the avoidance of clamping of the aorta, the speed of the procedure and the avoidance of prolonged hypotension. The fact that multiple stents were frequently used covering several levels of intercostal arteries is a further important feature. The possibility that the endovascular approach might dramatically reduce the risk of atheroembolism is also present, but this must remain a speculative observation in the absence of direct clinical evidence.

INFRARENAL ABDOMINAL AORTIC ANEURYSM

Endovascular aneurysm repair (EVAR) has led to significantly diminished postoperative morbidity and mortality, a shorter in-hospital stay and a quicker recovery time. The hope that ischemic complications might similarly be reduced has not proved to be the case and is reported to occur in 3%-10% of patients [9]. Limb occlusion and internal iliac arterial embolization are the major factors which are implicated in these ischemic complications. Increasingly, however, atheroembolization is being recognized as a significant cause. In 2001, the *Montefiore Group* reported an analysis of their large experience of EVAR (278 procedures) with specific regard to development of overt colon ischemia [10]. They used a variety of devices and importantly all patients in whom postoperative colonic ischemia was suspected underwent colonoscopy. They reported a 2.9% incidence of colon ischemia (8 out of 278 patients after EVAR). Out of the 8 patients with colon ischemia, 4 patients had direct evidence of microembolization as seen on histological analysis, with a further 3 patients showing evidence of widespread ischemia involving the kidneys, small bowel and skin as a result. In 2004, Geraghty et al. [11] reported a similarly low incidence of ischemic colitis after EVAR (4 patients out of 233: 1.7%) with 3 of these patients needing colonic resection. Histological analysis of these specimens revealed atheroemboli in the colonic vasculature in all 3 (mortality was 66%). The *New York University School of Medicine* group reported that 4 out of 311 patients undergoing

EVAR had developed significant colon ischemia, with 3 requiring colectomy after which 2 patients died [9].

Embolization as a cause of bowel ischemia was investigated in a cohort of 702 patients with similar rates of colonic ischemia (1.4%) found in comparison to open aortic surgery. This study also found operative evidence of small bowel ischemia and infarction in 6 out of the 10 patients (0.8%) - a pattern which differs significantly from open repair [12]. The presumed mechanism for this atheroembolism is turbulence caused during the occlusive parts of graft deployment and aortic occlusion during balloon modeling and dilatation (Fig. 4). Similarly, paralytic ileus develops in about

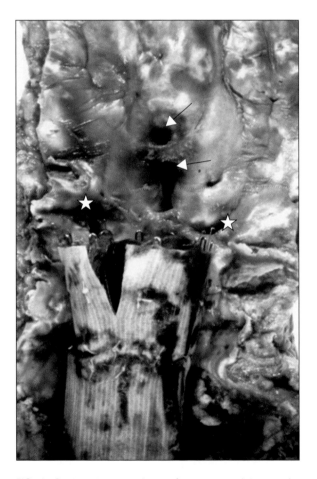

FIG. 4 Post-mortem specimen of a non-proprietary endovascular stent. This view of the anterior wall of the aorta at the infrarenal landing zone demonstrates the close proximity of the renal *(stars)* and superior mesenteric arteries and celiac axis *(arrowed)* and the potential for embolization from atheroma at the aortic neck.

4% of patients, which is similar to that seen after open aortic repair. It is difficult to explain this complication where the peritoneal cavity has not been opened, the bowel has not been handled and it is probable that microembolization into the mesenteric circulation is a contributing factor [13].

Postoperative renal failure complicating EVAR in patients with normal preoperative renal failure has been reported to occur in 6.2% of patients [14]. This incidence is similar to that typically seen after open aneurysm repair and is not related to contrast use. One possible reason is that it is the sicker cohort of patients which has been subjected to EVAR in comparison to those subjected to open repair. However, this is unlikely because it is well documented that EVAR minimizes hemodynamic upset and limits ischemic reperfusion injury [15]. Hopkinson's group from Nottingham found no difference in dose of contrast between patients who developed renal failure and those who did not, thus removing this potential cause. In the absence of any other good explanation, it is highly probable that atheroembolism plays a role in the development of postoperative renal failure. The possibility that transrenal fixation of aortic endografts might account for impaired renal function was recently investigated. A slight increase in serum creatinine concentration and decrease in creatinine clearance was found in the early period after aortic endografting but no difference was found between patients who had undergone endografting with transrenal fixation and those who had undergone infrarenal fixation [16]. This study identified a slight decline in renal function after EVAR suggesting that transrenal fixation was safe but providing further circumstantial evidence that atheroembolism may be an important factor affecting postoperative renal function.

An analysis of the EUROSTAR database of spinal cord ischemia after EVAR for infrarenal abdominal aortic aneurysms found an incidence of 0.21% (6 patients out of 2 862 consecutive EVAR procedures) [17]. This is a very low rate for this complication and in EVAR the two possible risk factors are interruption of the lumbar and pelvic circulation to the spine and embolization from the aorta. The most common cause of spontaneously occurring spinal cord ischemia is embolization from a diseased aorta and, although there is no direct clinical evidence, embolization must be implicated as a major factor in the etiology of this rare complication of EVAR.

Preprocedural embolization of the internal iliac arteries is being used increasingly in order to allow endovascular treatment of aneurysmal disease encroaching on the iliac bifurcation. Unilateral and bilateral internal iliac artery embolization has been implicated by several authors as an important cause of colonic, pelvic and spinal ischemic complications. Undoubtedly this procedure causes a significant incidence of buttock claudication and impotence. Gluteal compartment syndrome complicates 13%-36% of patients with unilateral and 25%-80% of patients with bilateral internal iliac artery embolization [18,19]. However, recent analysis of three large series of EVAR (821 procedures) found that preoperative internal iliac occlusion had not contributed significantly to the development of colonic ischemia. Each publication came to the conclusion that intraoperative microembolization was the major cause of postoperative ischemic colitis, even in the presence of internal iliac artery occlusion.

Lower limb ischemia after EVAR is most commonly due to graft limb occlusion with a mean incidence of this complication of 5.1% (range 0.6%-9.9% of early follow-up) [20]. Analysis of lower limb ischemia after 12 months in the EUROSTAR database found 18% of patients requiring a secondary intervention for treatment of limb occlusions [21]. With specific regard to lower limb embolization or *trash foot*, the reported incidence lies between 0.9%-2% [9].

It is clear from the above that EVAR carries a significant risk of atheroembolization, which is similar to that seen with open aortic surgery. This is due to several factors and the most important of which would include interventions on severely atheromatous aorta and iliac arteries, dislodgment of atheromatous plaques and aneurysmal sac thrombus as a result of guide wire and catheter manipulations and the passage of large diameter EVAR sheaths. Thompson et al. [22] reported an ultrasound-based comparison of the number of emboli thrown off into the superficial femoral artery during conventional and endovascular aneurysm repair, and found significantly more particulate and gaseous emboli detected during endovascular aneurysm repair. The authors concluded that manipulation of the devices within the aneurysm sac might not be the sole cause of embolization as no correlation could be found between the length of the procedure and the clinical experience of the operatives. The experimental study reported by Lipsitz et al. [5] comparing initial distal clamping and proximal clamping in open aneurysm repair perhaps provides an explanation in that distal clamping was found to cause reflected pressure waves with turbulent flow generated within the occluded iliac arteries in the aorta, thus increasing the potential for disruption of embolic material. In EVAR patients with difficult, tortuous or narrowed iliac arteries there is the potential for quite prolonged iliac occlusion and for the potential mechanism for embolization to take place (Fig. 5).

Treatment

The general principles of treatment similarly apply to embolization complicating both open and endovascular aneurysmal surgery. The principal mainstay of treatment is supportive, with resuscitation of the patient, treatment of any sepsis complicating colonic or buttock ischemia, for example, and renal support. The use of heparinization is controversial based on the observation that anticoagulation per se is a common cause of primary atheroembolic syndromes. In atheroembolism complicating aortic interventions, however, it is preferable to anticoagulate these patients fully with the specific aim of limiting propagated thrombosis at the site of embolic occlusions in the distal arterial trees. Treat-

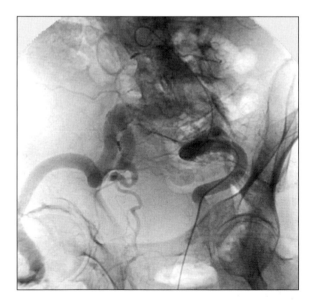

FIG. 5 Tortuous iliac arteries are a relative contraindication for endovascular aneurysm repair (EVAR). EVAR deployment through such iliac arteries would involve prolonged total iliac occlusion and increase the risk of proximal and distal embolization.

ment with systemic or directed thrombolysis is not appropriate in these cases because of recent surgical intervention and the probability of hemorrhage. The use of vasodilators such as iloprost or other prostaglandins may be of value although there is little objective clinical evidence to support their use. Corticosteroids have not been shown to be of value.

Where the clinical picture suggests colonic ischemia, contrast enhanced spiral CT scanning and colonoscopy are of value in diagnosis. If transmural colonic ischemia is clinically suspected, surgical exploration and colectomy must be undertaken although this is a very high-risk intervention in these elderly patients who frequently have multi-organ failure. In patients with *trash foot*, where the arterial pulses have disappeared, urgent duplex or digital subtraction angiography should be undertaken (if the degree of neurovascular compromise of the lower limb allows it). Urgent embolectomy, either by the femoral or popliteal approach, should be undertaken and, where there is poor or absent backbleeding, the use of intraoperative thrombolysis should be considered. Where there is no occlusion of a major arterial tree, *trash foot* should be treated conservatively. Sympathectomy may have a role to play in the treatment of severe atheroembolic foot and toe lesions where it may be particularly useful to control the pain, which is often quite severe. Gangrene of the toes and forefoot is best treated by auto-amputation in order to preserve the greatest amount of functioning tissue in the foot.

In the rare occasion when a patient has multiple episodes of microembolization following an aortic intervention, either conventional or endovascular, a potential source must be sought. Kinking or occlusion of an aortic limb is the most frequent cause but, in the absence of this complication, areas of potential embolization in the remainder of the aorta and the iliac arteries should be sought by contrast enhanced spiral CT scanning or duplex scanning. High dose statin therapy may be useful in these circumstances, although the evidence for stabilization and successful treatment of atheroembolism in these cases remains largely anecdotal.

How to avoid atheroembolism

In both open and endovascular repair, meticulous preoperative assessment of the anatomy and luminal structure of the clamping and attachment sites around the aneurysm is the key to avoiding atheroembolism. A hostile juxtarenal aortic neck with luminal atheroma or thrombus should be a contraindication to EVAR although fenestrated stent-grafts may have a role to play in the future. In open repair such necks must never be clamped directly since with suprarenal, or more usually supraceliac clamping, the risk of renal or visceral embolization is virtually abolished and suturing can be accomplished onto an endarterectomized or thrombectomized aortic neck. Similar attention to the anatomy of iliac clamping or landing zone sites will avoid atheroembolization into the pelvic and lower limb circulations. The need for the same assessment applies to thoracic or thoracoabdominal aneurysm work-up.

In order to minimize atheroembolism from turbulence above an occluded aorta, clamping should follow the sequence of proximal aorta first and distal iliac arteries secondly. In EVAR, aortic occlusion times should be kept to a minimum with prompt and direct proximal deployment, thus avoiding dragging down the stent. The configuration and size of the iliac arteries merits careful assessment with narrow or tortuous vessels increasing the likelihood of prolonged iliac occlusion and renal and visceral embolism (Fig. 5). Catheter and device manipulations must be kept to a minimum during deployment of the stent-graft.

measures are all that can be employed and the administration of vasodilators and vasoactive agents, such as prostaglandin analogues, are justified.

Table I	CLINICAL FEATURES OF ATHEROEMBOLISM
✔ Blue toe syndrome: digital ischemia and normal pulses	
✔ Livedo reticularis: patchy non-blanching cyanosis	
✔ Renal failure post intervention - *Hematuria and proteinuria*	

✔ Visceral ischemia
  - *Abdominal pain*
  - *Prolonged paralytic ileus*
  - *Peritonism*
  - *Metabolic acidosis*
  - *Septicemia*	

✔ Gluteal compartment syndrome	
✔ Stroke	
✔ Paraplegia/paraparesis	
✔ Elevated CRP	
✔ Leukocytosis	
✔ Transient eosinophilia	
✔ Shock	

How to deal with atheroembolism

It is important to maintain a high index of clinical suspicion for atheroembolism when immediate postoperative complications become apparent (Table I). Resuscitation, hydration to maintain good renal function and full anticoagulation are basic components of treatment in all cases. In severe cases, renal support will be required (Table II). In the lower limbs, treat major occlusions by embolectomy. Careful assessment of the abdomen for possible bowel ischemia is extremely important, with urgent colonoscopy and laparotomy performed in all cases where this diagnosis is made. Gluteal compartment syndrome is usually not clinically obvious and is another complication that must be excluded in the sick postoperative patient suspected of having suffered atheroembolism. In most cases, general supportive

Tableau II	MANAGEMENT OF ATHEROEMBOLISM
✔ Resuscitation and support	
✔ Heparinization	
✔ Treatment of septicemia	

✔ Lower limb
  - *Embolectomy if possible (macroembolism)*
  - *Prostaglandin therapy, sympathectomy (microembolism)*
  - *Auto-amputation*	

✔ Visceral
  - *Colonoscopy and contrast CT scan*
  - *Surgical exploration and resection*	

✔ Gluteal compartment syndrome: fasciotomy	
✔ Cerebrovascular and spinal: supportive treatment	
✔ Aggressive statin therapy	

Conclusion

There is considerable anecdotal evidence in the reported series implicating atheroembolism as a major complication of aneurysmal surgery. The reported incidence is low but it is probable that this is underestimated with atheroembolism being a frequent complication, albeit in subclinical forms. The evolving experience of EVAR documents clinical atheroembolism occurring at least as frequently as in open aneurysm repair.

Meticulous preoperative assessment of clamping and landing zones for atheroma and thrombus of the aorta is the key step in avoiding atheroembolism. Prevention of this complication is much simpler than treatment.

REFERENCES

1 Henry M, Klonaris C, Henry I et al. Protected renal stenting with PercuSurge GuideWire device: a pilot study. *J Endovasc Ther* 2001; 8: 227-237.

2 Davila-Roman VG, Barzilai B, Wareing TH et al. Intraoperative ultrasonographic evaluation of the ascending aorta in 100 consecutive patients undergoing cardiac surgery. *Circulation* 1991; 84: 47-53.

3 Johnston KW. Multicenter prospective study of non-ruptured abdominal aortic aneurysm. Part II. Variables predicting morbidity and mortality. *J Vasc Surg* 1989; 9: 437-447.

4 Brewster DC, Franklin DP, Cambria RP et al. Intestinal ischemia complicating abdominal aortic surgery. *Surgery* 1991; 109: 447-454.

5 Lipsitz EC, Veith FJ, Ohki T, Quintos RT. Should initial clamping for abdominal aortic aneurysm repair be proximal or distal to minimize embolisation? *Eur J Vasc Endovasc Surg* 1999; 17: 413-418.

6 Webster SE, Smith J, Thompson MM et al. Does the sequence of clamp application during open abdominal aortic aneurysm surgery influence distal embolisation? *Eur J Vasc Endovasc Surg* 2004; 27: 61-64.

7 Thurlbeck WM, Castleman B. Atheromatous emboli to the kidneys after aortic surgery. *N Engl J Med* 1957; 257: 442-447.

8 Leurs LJ, Bell R, Degrieck Y et al. Endovascular treatment of thoracic aortic diseases; combined experience from the EUROSTAR and the United Kingdom Thoracic Endograft Registries. *J Vasc Surg* 2004; 40: 670-679.

9 Maldonado TS, Rockman CB, Riles E et al. Ischemic complications after endovascular abdominal aortic aneurysm repair. *J Vasc Surg* 2004; 40: 703-709.

10 Dadian N, Ohki T, Veith FJ et al. Overt colon ischemia after endovascular aneurysm repair: the importance of microembolization as an etiology. *J Vasc Surg* 2001; 34: 986-996.

11 Geraghty PJ, Sanchez LA, Rubin BG et al. Overt ischemic colitis after endovascular repair of aorto-iliac aneurysms. *J Vasc Surg* 2004; 40: 413-418.

12 Zhang WW, Kulaylat MN, Anain PM et al. Embolization as a cause of bowel ischemia after endovascular abdominal aortic aneurysm repair. *J Vasc Surg* 2004; 40: 867-872.

13 Malinzak LE, Long GW, Bove PG et al. Gastrointestinal complications following infra-renal endovascular aneurysm repair. *Vasc Endovascular Surg* 2004; 38: 137-142.

14 Walker SR, Yusuf SW, Wenham PW, Hopkinson BR. Renal complications following endovascular repair of abdominal aortic aneurysms. *J Endovasc Surg* 1998; 5: 318-322.

15 Baxendale B. Anaesthetic implications. In: Hopkinson B, Yusuf WS, Whitaker S et al. (eds). *Endovascular surgery for abdominal aortic aneurysms.* W B Saunders, London, 1997; pp 289-297.

16 Cayne NS, Rhee SJ, Veith FJ et al. Does trans-renal fixation of aortic endografts impair renal function? *J Vasc Surg* 2003; 38: 639-644.

17 Berg P, Kaufmann D, van Marrewijk CJ, Buth J. Spinal cord ischaemia after stent-graft treatment for infra-renal abdominal Aortic aneurysms. Analysis of the EUROSTAR database. *Euro J Vasc Endovasc Surg* 2001; 22: 342-347.

18 Su WT, Stone DH, Lamparello PJ, Rockman CB. Gluteal compartment syndrome following elective unilateral internal iliac artery embolisation before endovascular abdominal aortic aneurysm repair. *J Vasc Surg* 2004; 39: 672-675.

19 Mehta M, Veith FJ, Darling RC et al. Effects of bilateral hypogastric Artery interruption during endovascular and open aorto-iliac repair. *J Vasc Surg* 2004; 40: 698-702.

20 Aljabri B, Obrand DI, Montreuil B et al. Early vascular complications after endovascular repair of aorto-iliac aneurysms. *Ann Vasc Surg* 2001; 15: 608-614.

21 Laheij RJ, Buth J, Harris PL et al. Need for secondary interventions after endovascular repair of abdominal aortic aneurysms; intermediate-term follow-up results of a european collaborative registry (EUROSTAR). *Br J Surg* 2000; 87: 1666-1673.

22 Thompson MM, Smith J, Naylor AR et al. Ultrasound-based quantification of emboli during conventional and endovascular aneurysm repair. *J Endovasc Surg* 1997; 4: 33-38.

14

TECHNICAL DIFFICULTIES OF TOTAL LAPAROSCOPIC AORTIC ANASTOMOSES

ISABELLE JAVERLIAT, MARC COGGIA
ISABELLE DI CENTA, OLIVIER GOËAU-BRISSONNIÈRE

During the last decade, minimal invasive techniques have been developed in vascular surgery in order to reduce the perioperative morbidity of infrarenal aortic surgery. Recently, aortic surgery entered the field of laparoscopic surgery [1]. Laparoscopic infrarenal aortic surgery contains three main technical problems: the exposure of the aorta; arterial clamping; and the performance of laparoscopic anastomoses. Laparoscopic aortic surgery has not gained widespread acceptance to date, probably because of the highly specific technical skills necessary to perform laparoscopic aortic anastomoses. However, contrary to general surgery, the most challenging problem of laparoscopic aortic surgery remains aortic clamping time, depending on the performance of the aortic anastomoses.

Recently, we have developed a technique of total laparoscopic aortoiliac surgery using a new and simplified technique for total laparoscopic aortic anastomoses and this allows performing the same sutures as in conventional aortic surgery [2]. In this chapter, we describe the principles of these total laparoscopic aortic anastomoses. We also reveal the different tricks used in difficult anastomoses, particularly in cases with a heavily calcified aorta.

Basic technique

As in open surgery, total laparoscopic aortic bypasses require a stable exposure of the aorta [2]. Before performing the proximal aortic anastomo-sis, it is important to prepare the aortic anastomotic site very carefully. As described by Creech, in cases of aortic aneurysm, the posterior wall of the proximal aneurysmal neck is transected. This transection of the posterior aortic wall facilitates the placement of the posterior sutures and allows wrapping of the anastomosis if necessary. Great care should be taken to avoid any injury to the lumbar arteries or a retroaortic left renal vein. One should not cut the aortic wall too close to the proximal aortic clamp. To avoid skewed cutting, the operating surgeon must hold the scissors in their left hand. These tips all simplify the aortic anastomosis.

Sutures are prepared for the aortic anastomosis before aortic clamping. Multiple 3/0 or 4/0 polypropylene sutures are knotted on teflon pledgets [2]. Two polypropylene sutures, 18 centimeters in length and knotted on 10 x 10 millimeter teflon pledgets, are needed to perform a total laparoscopic aortic anastomosis. A third and shorter stitch (10 centimeters in length) is also knotted on a 5 x 5 millimeter

teflon pledget to begin the aortic anastomosis. Several additional 10-centimeter-long sutures are also prepared for additional stitches. Our technique of aortic anastomosis is used both for end-to-end anastomoses and for end-to-side anastomoses. To perform an end-to-side aorto-prosthetic anastomosis (Fig. 1), the length of the aortotomy is adapted to the length of the prosthetic spatula. The anastomosis begins at the heal with a short polypropylene stitch, already knotted on a teflon pledget. The left side of the anastomosis is performed first. End-to-end anastomoses start on the left side of the aorta with a short polypropylene stitch, already knotted on a teflon pledget. The posterior wall of the anastomosis is performed first (Fig. 2).

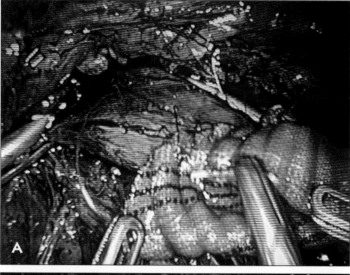

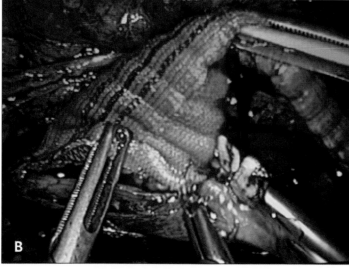

FIG. 1 Laparoscopic end-to-side anastomosis. A - The suture is started at the heel of the anastomosis, running at the left side first. B - Right site of the anastomosis. Note the two pledgets at the heel of the anastomosis.

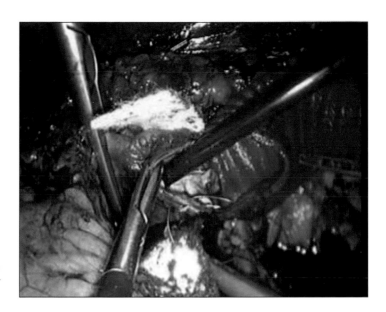

FIG. 2 End-to-end anastomosis between aorta and prosthesis with two running hemicircumferential sutures.

The proximal aortic anastomosis is performed with two hemi-circumferential running sutures. At the end of the anastomosis, both ends of the threads are tied together intracorporally. After unclamping, additional short stitches, blocked on 5 x 5 millimeter teflon pledgets, can be added if suture line bleeding is seen.

As in conventional surgery, the motion of the wrist ideally allows passing the needle cleanly through the aortic wall without tearing it. Moreover, the bites on the aortic wall must be 4-5 millimeter deep in order to prevent aortic tearing. This allows the running suture to spread after unclamping.

The stitches blocked on teflon pledgets avoid intracorporeal knots at the beginning of the suture. This is an important technical point in avoiding any suture material trauma and in reducing the time required to perform the anastomosis. Instead of using a single running suture, the use of two short sutures used separately avoids the obstructing the operative field. This is all the more significant as the surgical instruments' mobility is restricted in a small operative field. This technical point is a fundamental difference between laparoscopic and open aortic surgery.

It is important to underline that the use of this technique to create aortic anastomoses allows performing the same revascularizations as with conventional surgery. Laparoscopic anastomoses are stable and safe. The vascular prosthesis is the same as used in conventional surgery, with well known long-term reliability. Therefore, results similar to the excellent long-term results of gold standard open aortic surgery can be expected.

As in conventional surgery, the polypropylene sutures should never be held by grasping forceps. In our technique, the first assistant introduces the suction device through a left iliac fossa trocar to maintain the tension of the suture, through a system of triangulation with the surgeon's instruments.

For total laparoscopic iliac anastomoses, the technique used to perform an end-to-end anastomosis between the graft limb and the common iliac artery, or an end-to-side anastomosis between the graft limb and the external iliac artery, is the same as for aortic anastomoses. The suture length is less. Since iliac anastomoses are smaller, they can be carried out using little grasping forceps *(Karl Storz Endoskope, Tuttlingen, Germany)*. When performing an iliac anastomosis, the operating surgeon typically does not use the same operator trocars as used during the aortic anastomosis.

Total laparoscopic aortic anastomosis and a heavily calcified aorta

Infra- or juxtarenal circumferential aortic calcifications are not contraindications for total laparoscopic aortic anastomosis with our laparoscopic approaches of the abdominal aorta [2-4]. In these cases, suprarenal clamping is possible and simple. The control of the suprarenal aorta is performed via a mediovisceral rotation. After suprarenal aortic clamping, forceps endarterectomy of the infrarenal aorta can be performed, which facilitates aorto-prosthetic anastomosis. As in open surgery, the aortic wall can be weakened after endarterectomy. It is necessary to reinforce the aortic neck with a teflon cuff (Fig. 3) in order to avoid a tear of the aortic wall during suturing. This wrapping can be stabilized with three or four stitches prior to performing the aortic anastomosis. The anastomosis is then performed as previously described under supra- or infrarenal aortic clamping.

Closure of the aortic stump

When an end-to-end aorto-prosthetic anastomosis is performed, distal aorta closure can be achieved with 2-0 or 3-0 polypropylene double running sutures, always with the stitches blocked on teflon pledgets. As previously described, an aortic endarterectomy can be performed at this level in cases of severe calcifications of the aortic stump. In such a case, the suture can be buttressed with two teflon sheets to strengthen friable aortic tissue.

At the beginning of our experience, we used a mechanical stapler (Multifire endoGIA® *30, USSC, Autosuture Company, Elancourt, France)* to close the aortic stump in case of non-calcified aortas. Currently, we prefer to close the aortic stump with a double running suture. This stapling technique was described in conventional aortic surgery by Blumenberg et al. [5]. Hartung et al. [6] evaluated the efficacy of commercially available staplers to ligate major intra-abdominal arteries. They concluded that commercially available staplers can be used on moderately or non-calcified arteries and should be avoided for severely calcified arteries.

Sutureless vascular anastomoses and total laparoscopic aortic surgery

Since vascular anastomoses are considered as the more difficult technical problem in laparoscopic aortic surgery, several techniques have been described in order to facilitate laparoscopic sutures. Some authors have proposed mechanical devices [7-10] or gluing [11] in order to reduce operative time, but the use of these devices remains limited and controversial in clinical practice. Mechanical sutures have not gained widespread use in vascular surgery

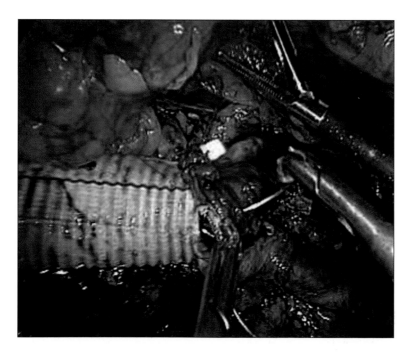

FIG. 3 End-to-end anastomosis with teflon reinforcement in case of endarterectomized calcified aorta.

contrary to the daily practice in pulmonary or gastrointestinal surgery. This is explained by the fact that vascular anastomoses are generally performed on non-healthy arteries.

Each device is associated with technique-related complications. Although mechanical anastomoses can be made more rapidly than classical sutures, the disadvantages of non-suture techniques include rigidity obstruction, large diameter and high cost of devices. Moreover, these sutures are not warranted and seem to be less effective than polypropylene sutures [12]. Garitey et al. [12] have shown that anastomoses made with clips or stents were ten to fifteen times weaker than those made with stitches. He observed that a continuous suture is far too resistant in relation to the aorta's own resistance. Our technique of laparoscopic aortic anastomosis is reliable, readily available and can be adapted to almost any tissue condition that may be encountered. As a consequence, suturing continues to be our standard approach.

Future for robotic-assisted laparoscopic aortic anastomoses?

The main technical difference between laparoscopic and conventional aortic anastomoses is that, in laparoscopic aortic surgery, there is a lack of direct manual contact with the tissue. Moreover, the operating surgeon does not view the laparoscopic field with direct binocular vision. To circumvent these problems, several authors [13-15] recently developed the use of robotic technology to simplify endoscopic surgical manipulations, by increasing the degrees of freedom of motion and through the use of facilitated hand-eye coordination. The Da Vinci® System *(Intuitive Surgical, Sunnyvale, CA, USA)* enhances visualization using a true three-dimensional view based on a double optical system. For Desgranges et al. [14], robotic surgery allows them to gain natural dexterity and precision. Contrary to manual laparoscopic anastomoses, robotically-assisted laparoscopic aortic anastomoses do not require prior training in laparoscopic surgery to obtain the required level for suturing [13,14]. Ruurda et al. [15] reported that, after only three cases, every surgeon was able to perform aortic anastomosis with robotic assistance in approximately 20 minutes.

A major disadvantage of robotic technology is the lack of sensory feedback which can break polypropylene running sutures. To avoid this problem, some surgeons use Gore-Tex® sutures which are less prone to breakage [14]. Robotic, as compared to conventional, laparoscopic aortic surgery has a prohibitive cost [14] and it is not widespread, which limits its use for training. Compared with robotic technology, our technique of laparoscopic aortic anastomoses is relatively inexpensive. Moreover, robotic technology is not always compatible with space limitations [14], with an external conflict between robotic arms altering the procedure. In addition, the setting-up is more time-consuming than a simple change of laparoscopic instruments (30 minutes vs. 30 seconds for Desgranges et al. [14]).

In our department, we do not have access to robotic technology to perform aortic surgery. However, we are studying the different possibilities of robotic technology use for aortic surgery in vitro (unpublished data). In fact, we think that robotic-wristed instruments are probably interesting and can be useful in performing difficult and small anastomoses, such as those in laparoscopic inferior mesenteric artery reimplantation [16] or laparoscopic renal revascularization. However, even if training is less important with this new technology, prior training in laparoscopic aortic suturing appears mandatory in case of robotic technical failure. The lack of easy availability for training and the high cost of robotic technology remains a serious drawback. Our simplified technique of total laparoscopic aortic sutures allows performing safe and stable anastomoses, as is the case in conventional surgery. We want to underline the importance of the laparo-training, which allows surgeons to obtain the required level of expertise to perform laparoscopic anastomoses, even in difficult cases.

14

157

REFERENCES

1 Dion YM, Gracia CR. A new technique for laparoscopic aortobifemoral grafting in occlusive aortoiliac disease. *J Vasc Surg* 1997; 26: 685-692.

2 Coggia M, Bourriez A, Javerliat I, Goëau-Brissonnière O. Totally laparoscopic aortobifemoral bypass: a new and simplified approach. *Eur J Vasc Endovasc Surg* 2002; 24: 274-275.

3 Coggia M, Di Centa I, Javerliat I et al. Total laparoscopic aortic surgery: transperitoneal left retrorenal approach. *Eur J Vasc Endovasc Surg* 2004; 28: 619-622.

4 Javerliat I, Coggia M, Di Centa I et al. Total videoscopic aortic surgery: left retroperitoneoscopic approach. *Submitted to Eur J Vasc Endovasc Surg,* 2004.

5 Blumenberg RM, Gelfand ML. Application of intestinal staplers to aortoiliac surgery. *Am J Surg* 1982; 144: 198-202.

6 Hartung O, Garibodi V, Garitey V et al. Are laparoscopic staplers effective for ligation of large intraabdominal arteries? *Eur J Vasc Endovasc Surg* 2004; 28: 281-286.

7 Richard T, Eloi R, Godet G et al. Anastomoses mécaniques en chirurgie vasculaire. In: Kieffer E (ed). *Le remplacement artériel: principes et applications.* Paris, AERCV, 1992: pp 303-312.

8 Tozzi P, Corno AF, Marty B, Von Segesser LK. Sutureless video-endoscopic thoracic aorta to iliac artery bypass: the easiest approach to occlusive aortoiliac diseases. *Eur J Vasc Endovasc Surg* 2004; 27: 498-500.

9 Ahn SS, Clem MF, Braithwaite BD et al. Laparoscopic aorto-femoral bypass. Initial experience in an animal model. *Ann Surg* 1995; 222: 677-683.

10 Zegdi R, Martinod E, Fabre O et al. Video-assisted replacement or bypass grafting of the descending thoracic aorta with a new sutureless vascular prosthesis: an experimental study. *J Vasc Surg* 1999; 30: 320-324.

11 Glock Y, Roux D, Leobon B et al. Experimental technique of aorto-prosthetic anastomoses by gluing (Bioglue®-Cryolife). In Juhan C, Alimi YS, (eds). *Laparoscopic aortoiliac surgery for occlusive disease and aneurysm.* Marseille, Angio-techniques 2000: pp 16-26.

12 Garitey V, Rieu R, Alimi YS. Prostheto-prosthetic and aorto-prosthetic anastomosis using stents, threads, clips and staples. In vitro comparative study. *J Mal Vasc* 2003; 28: 173-177.

13 Wisselink W, Cuesta MA, Gracia C, Rauwerda JA. Robot-assisted laparoscopic aortobifemoral bypass for aortoiliac occlusive disease: a report of two cases. *J Vasc Surg* 2002; 36: 1079-1082.

14 Desgranges P, Bourriez A, Javerliat I et al. Robotically assisted aorto-femoral bypass grafting: lessons learned from our initial experience. *Eur J Vasc Endovasc Surg* 2004; 27: 507-511.

15 Ruurda JP, Wisselink W, Cuesta MA et al. Robot-assisted versus standard videoscopic aortic replacement. A comparative study in pigs. *Eur J Vasc Endovasc Surg* 2004; 27: 501-506.

16 Javerliat I, Coggia M, Di Centa I et al. Total laparoscopic abdominal aortic aneurysm repair with reimplantation of the inferior mesenteric artery. *J Vasc Surg* 2004; 39: 1115-1117.

15

INADVERTENT COVERAGE OF SUPRA-AORTIC ARTERIES DURING ENDOGRAFTING OF THE THORACIC AORTA

PIERRE ALRIC, JEAN-PHILIPPE BERTHET
PASCAL BRANCHEREAU, REUBEN VEERAPEN
JÉRÔME ALBERTIN, CHARLES MARTY-ANE

Since the first endovascular treatment of an infrarenal abdominal aorta by Parodi et al. [1], endoluminal techniques have developed rapidly. In 1994, Dake et al. [2] showed the feasibility of treating descending thoracic aortic aneurysms by means of self-expandable covered endografts in 13 patients. Only 8% of their patients suffering from a thoracic aortic aneurysm were eligible for endovascular treatment. Ten years on, endovascular treatment of thoracic aneurysms has changed from homemade, experimental stent-grafts for anatomically favorable aneurysms to an established treatment using commercially manufactured devices in acute and chronic thoracic aortic diseases (such as aneurysms, dissections, traumatic ruptures, ulcerations and intramural hematomas) [3].

Initially, these techniques were mainly applied in patients with high surgical risks but indications for endovascular treatment progressively extended to patients eligible for conventional surgery.

The evident interest of these covered stents is to avoid a surgical procedure comprising: thoracotomy; double lumen tube intubation with a collapsed lung; extracorporeal circulation with systemic heparinization; and proximal clamping in patients with atherosclerotic comorbidities or associated lesions as a result of trauma.

The majority of recent studies shows reduced morbidity and mortality after endovascular treatment as compared to conventional surgery. However, specific complications of endovascular techniques have become apparent, including periprosthetic endoleaks, migration, kinking and prosthetic thrombosis.

Technical limitations

The main technical limitations for endovascular repair of thoracic aortic pathology are associated with problematic vascular access when inserting the graft, rapid availability of a customized prosthesis and the level and morphology of the lesion, requiring adequate necks for safe proximal and distal fixation [3,4]. Vascular access problems should be carefully assessed preoperatively by means of complete anatomic studies of the aorta and iliac arteries. If necessary, vascular access via the common iliac artery, infrarenal aorta, descending thoracic aorta (sometimes thoracoscopically guided [5]), ascending aorta [6] or common carotid artery [7] should be anticipated. Availability of endografts with variable lengths and diameters is increasingly common in vascular centers with thoracic endograft experience. Many of these centers do have a stock of endografts in order to treat urgent cases. As a matter of fact, delivery of a specific endograft nowadays takes less than 24 hours.

The main limiting factor of endoluminal treatment is actually the location and morphology of the lesion. Deployment of a thoracic endograft requires proximal and distal necks, with a neck of at least 15 millimeter length. The diameter of the graft has to be 10%-20% larger than the diameter of the aortic neck [3,4]. The proximity of a major side branch is also a limiting factor. The left subclavian artery (LSA), left common carotid artery (LCA) and brachiocephalic trunk (BCT) proximally and the celiac axis distally can be accidentally covered by the prosthesis. In treating diseases of the proximal descending thoracic aorta or the aortic arch, technical challenges concentrate on preserving the patency of the supra-aortic arteries, especially the LCA and BCT.

How to foresee the risk of covering a supra-aortic artery during thoracic aortic endografting

Increasing the length of the proximal aortic neck represents a key issue in the endovascular treatment of thoracic aortic pathologies in order to propose this treatment to a larger number of patients and to reduce the risk of failure due to type I endoleak or migration.

The decision to cover the ostium of the LSA intentionally in order to deploy the endograft just distal to the LCA remains subject to discussion. The potential risks of this technique are ischemia of the left arm, vertebrobasilar insufficiency (even stroke) and a type II endoleak by retrograde bleeding of the LSA. According to some authors [4,8,9], this technique should not be adopted after performing a left subclavian-carotid transposition or a left carotid-subclavian bypass and ligation proximal to the vertebral artery. Given the relative simplicity of this revascularization and the security for a normal cerebral perfusion, coverage of the LSA is only intentionally performed in emergency cases. According to other authors [3,10-12], coverage of the LSA is well-tolerated and revascularization only indicated if symptomatic ischemia occurs.

Among the reported vascular complications in the literature, inadvertent coverage of the LCA and, even worse, the BCT rarely occurs. However, this is surprising because of the frequency of covering the LSA and the short distance between the LSA and LCA. Orend et al. [13] only reported one unintentional coverage of the LCA in 74 patients undergoing endovascular treatment for type B aortic dissection. Pulling back the endograft failed and a carotid-carotid bypass was uneventful. Schumacher et al. [14] have treated 80 patients with various descending thoracic aortic diseases. Eight patients suffered from aortic arch lesions and in one of these patients the LCA was covered accidentally, requiring extra-anatomic revascularization. Kieffer et al. [15] describe a series of 113 aortic arch aneurysms of which 15 were treated by means of endovascular techniques; in one patient, maneuvering the graft proximally caused occlusion of the BCT, requiring conversion to sternotomy and circulatory arrest with profound hypothermia. Our experience comprises 53 covered stents in 45 patients: 23 thoracic aneurysms, of which 9 ruptures; 18 acute traumatic ruptures; and 4 complicated type B dissections. The ostium of the LCA was covered in only one patient (traumatic rupture) and careful traction by means of an inflated balloon could solve the problem. In general, it seems that this kind of complication is not reported often enough in the literature to define its prevalence.

Inadvertent coverage of the carotid artery should specifically be suspected and avoided in type B dissections and traumatic ruptures because the origin of the dissection or tear is most frequently located just distal to the ostium of the LSA. The topography of thoracic aneurysms is extremely variable and a large number originate at the distance of the supra-aortic vessels. In contrast, the aortic arch aneurysms represent the most difficult cases to treat because the aortic neck is very short, or even absent if the supra-aortic arteries originate directly from the aneurysm.

There are differences in material and basic concept in the thoracic endografts currently available in France. The common feature is the self-expandable nitinol structure. The Talent® device *(Medtronic)* consists of polyester and has a non-covered part to improve its proximal anchoring quality; the first row of the nitinol stent which forms the metallic cage of the endograft has large webs and is not covered with polyester, therefore allowing deployment over supra-aortic ostia without occluding these vessels [16]. Deployment is performed by progressively pulling back the sheath which contains the endograft. This maneuver allows the surgeon to position the covered part at the level of the carotid ostium and subsequently pull the partially deployed graft back under fluoroscopy until its ideal location is reached. The Endofit® device *(Endomed, Edwards)* is made of PTFE and deploys like the Talent® graft. The Zenith® prosthesis *(Cook)* consists of polyester but has a non-covered part at the distal site and hooks and barbs at both ends.

The principle of deployment is similar to the Talent® device but requires an additional maneuver to launch the proximal fixating hooks. The Excluder® *(Gore)* is completely covered with PTFE and has a different deployment system; rapid launching of the device is performed by pulling a PTFE deployment sleeve. This device deploys from the middle outwards to both ends. Accurate positioning requires a certain level of experience, especially in keeping the graft at the external curve of the aortic arch in order to avoid distal movement during its opening. Regardless of the endograft used, the launching seems to be less accurate with large diameter endografts; in fact, the parallax errors on positioning and alignment of the proximal radio-opaque markers are more obvious with phased deployment devices (Talent®, Endofit®, Zenith®) and the distal movement during deployment might not be noticed anymore with the Excluder®, especially in large aneurysms.

The risk of accidental coverage of the LCA or BCT is substantially increased if the aortic neck is short and the aortic arch is markedly angulated. Complete preoperative anatomic assessment is crucial.

CT angiography allows accurate measurement of the descending aortic diameter. Investigation of the aortic arch is more difficult, especially in measuring the length and diameter of the proximal neck, because of the inaccurate visualization of the supra-aortic ostia at the transversal slices. Measurement of the required length of the endograft and diameter of the aortic necks are, however, possible with the 3D reconstructions obtained by the latest generations of scanners. Arteriography remains complementary to CT scanning: it allows us to visualize the entire arch, its angulation and the exact anatomy of the supra-aortic arteries, including its variants (such as a LCA originating from the BCT, a left vertebral artery coming off the arch, and a retro-esophageal right subclavian artery). In addition, aortoiliac vascular access can be studied with regard to stenoses, calcifications, tortuosity, iliac diameter less than 7-8 millimeters and spasms. Using an endoluminal marker, accurate assessment can be performed of the length of the necks and the length of the aortic segment to be covered (Fig. 1). MRA is less frequently used but comprises the advantages of both the above-mentioned techniques, especially in patients suffering from renal failure. Pre- and intraoperative transesophageal echography has specific value, especially in endovascular treatment of aortic dissections and traumatic ruptures, as well as to detect endoleaks. It only offers moderate information about the proximal aortic necks because of the blind region caused by the trachea which is in front of the esophagus. In summary, combined CT scanning and arteriography are most commonly used as preoperative assessment of thoracic aortic pathology.

How to prevent accidental coverage of the BCT or LCA?

Accurate deployment of an endograft is crucial in patients with a short and/or angulated aortic neck. Several general principles have to be respected. A radio-transparent table is indispensable when performing these procedures. An angiography catheter should be introduced via the right brachial artery in order to perform angiography during positioning and deployment of the endograft and to depict the origin of the BCT. Intraoperative angiography should be performed in a left anterior oblique manner usually between 30 degrees and 60 degrees in order to visualize the origin of all supra-aortic arteries

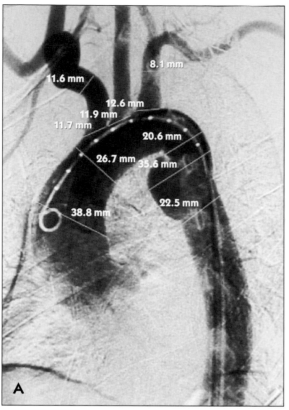

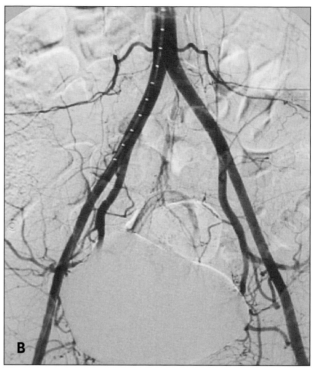

FIG. 1   A - Preoperative arteriographic assessment of the aortic arch.   B - Control of aortoiliac access.

perfectly, without superposition. In case of a short aortic neck between the LSA and LCA, a guide wire can be introduced via the right brachial artery and positioned in the LCA. If the endograft covers the ostium of the LCA following deployment, a stent can be placed to recanalize this carotid axis.

Several authors have addressed the importance of arterial hypotension, even short cardiac arrest, in order to increase the accuracy of deploying the endograft. Controlled hypotension with a systolic pressure between 60 and 70 mmHg can be obtained by administrating nicardipine or sodium nitroprusside [3,4]. Adenosine-induced transient cardiac asystole has been described by Dorros et al. [17] and Schumacher et al. [14]. Other techniques to reduce systolic flux temporarily have been reported [18], including: induction of ventricular fibrillation, controlled hypotension caused by balloon occlusion or simply by Valsalva maneuvers with hyperventilation, and prolonged inspiration to reduce arterial pressure and cardiac volume. The most appealing technique remains pharmacologically-controlled hypotension.

An aortic arch map has been proposed by Ishimaru in order to identify the different landing zones of the proximal endograft in thoracic aortic diseases (Fig. 2). In cases where the distance between the LCA and LSA (zone 2) is 15 millimeters or greater, a covered endograft can be deployed in this area, with or without a left carotid-subclavian transposition (Fig. 3) or carotid-subclavian bypass with ligation of the LSA proximal to the vertebral artery (Fig. 4). In cases where zone 2 is shorter than 15 millimeters, performing a reconstruction of the LCA prior to stent placement is recommended. Two different scenarios can be described.

First, if the distance between the BCT and LCA in zone 1 is greater than 15 millimeters, endovascular treatment can be performed after transposition of the LCA and LSA. This vascular reconstruction can be carried out according to several techniques, using prosthetic or venous grafts as follows:

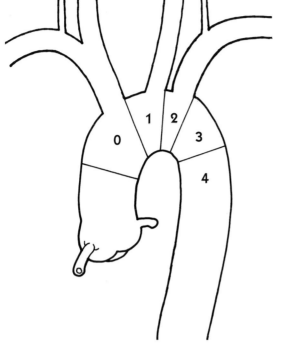

FIG. 2 Aortic arch map according to Ishimaru.

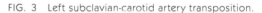

FIG. 3 Left subclavian-carotid artery transposition.

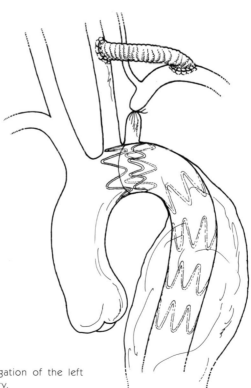

FIG. 4 Left subclavian-carotid bypass with ligation of the left subclavian artery proximal to the vertebral artery.

- retro-esophageal carotid-carotid bypass and transposition of the LSA [19-21] (Fig. 5);
- right carotid-left subclavian bypass and end-to-side reimplantation of the LCA (Fig. 6), which represents a simple variant of the previous technique;
- subclavian-subclavian bypass with side-to-side anastomosis of the LCA. In this variant, the right carotid artery (RCA) can not be used as a source for bypass;
- bypass from the BCT to the LCA and LSA [14]. In this case, the RCA and right subclavian artery (RSA) cannot serve as a donor site for bypass;
- bypass from the ascending aorta to the LCA and LSA [6], requiring partial or total median sternotomy. The RCA, RSA and BCT cannot be used as a donor arteries;
- extra-anatomic bypass from femoral or iliac artery to left subclavian artery and subclavian-carotid transposition (Fig. 7). This procedure can be applied in exceptional cases in which the RCA, RSA

and BCT cannot be used as inflow arteries or sternotomy is not feasible.

Deployment of the endograft should be performed with all precautions in order to avoid coverage of the brachiocephalic trunk. Endovascular treatment can be carried out during the same procedure of supra-aortic artery transposition or in a staged sequence in order to verify the neurologic status of the patient.

Secondly, if the distance between the BCT and LCA in zone 1 is less than 15 millimeters, the endograft will have to be deployed in zone 0, proximal to the ostium of the BCT. This can only be performed if the ascending aorta has a normal diameter and transposition of all supra-aortic arteries is feasible according to one of the following techniques:
- bypass from the ascending aorta to the BCT, LCA and LSA [14,15] (Fig. 8), requiring partial or total sternotomy, using a single sequential or bifurcated

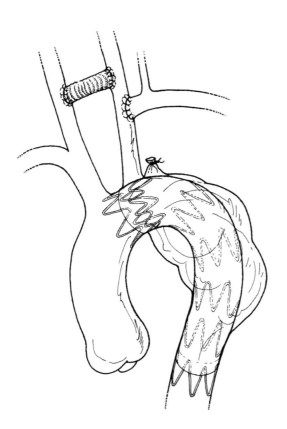

FIG. 5 Retroesophageal carotid-carotid bypass and left subclavian carotid transposition.

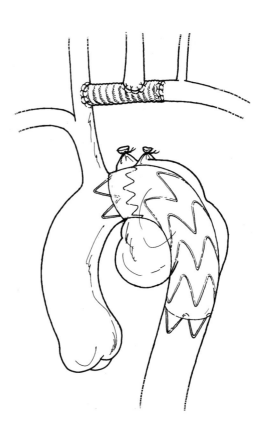

FIG. 6 Right carotid-left subclavian bypass with end-to-side reimplantation of the left carotid artery.

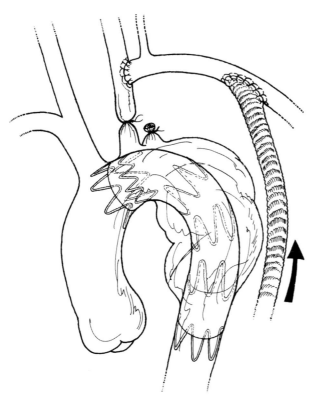

FIG. 7   Extra-anatomic bypass from the femoral or iliac artery
to the subclavian artery and subclavian-carotid transposition.

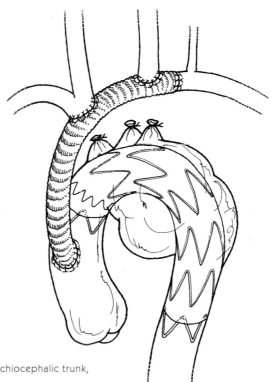

FIG. 8   Sequential bypass from the ascending aorta to the brachiocephalic trunk,
the left common carotid artery and the left subclavian artery.

graft. Metallic clips at the level of the proximal end-to-side anastomosis at the ascending aorta will allow accurate positioning of the proximal endoprosthesis;
- extra-anatomic bypass from femoral or iliac artery to right subclavian artery and carotid-carotid bypass (Fig. 9) in high-risk patients in whom sternotomy is not possible;
- non-manufactured and non-commercialized specific endografts as developed by Inoue et al. [22] in Japan and Chuter et al. [7] in the United States. Inoue's device comprises one or more side branches which revascularize one or several supra-aortic arteries during endovascular treatment of aortic arch aneurysms not requiring surgical repair. Chuter's endoprosthesis is a bifurcated endograft, positioned in the ascending aorta via the RCA following carotid-carotid bypass and left subclavian transposition. One of the two limbs of the bifurcated endograft serves as the inflow to the BCT and the other limb receives the arch-endograft inserted via the femoral access. Both devices are astute solutions but are relatively complex and infrequently applied at this moment.

What to do if inadvertent coverage of a carotid artery occurs

Despite complete preoperative anatomic assessment, revascularization of one or more supra-aortic arteries and cautious deployment of the endograft, inadvertent coverage of a carotid branch can still occur. It comprises a serious intraoperative complication which should immediately be detected and corrected. It is extremely important to eliminate other sources of occlusion of the BCT or LCA, especially occlusions due to thromboembolic causes or traumatic dissection which can occur as a result of intra-aortic manipulations. Intraoperative arteriography is the diagnostic modality of choice to detect the cause of arterial occlusion. Intraoperative duplex scanning of both carotid arteries can be performed if the diagnosis is still uncertain.

It is important to underline that the abstention of therapy has no place in inadvertent carotid artery

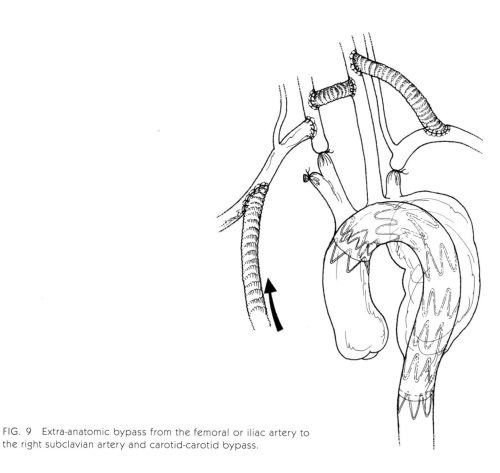

FIG. 9 Extra-anatomic bypass from the femoral or iliac artery to the right subclavian artery and carotid-carotid bypass.

covery, except in limited, partial coverage or preexisting homolateral occluded internal carotid arteries.

The therapeutic strategy should be graded as follows.

- Pulling back the endograft prudently should be attempted by means of an aortic balloon. In order to avoid complete fixation at the proximal aortic neck, the balloon should be inflated distal to this level. During this maneuver arteriography can confirm release of the carotid or BCT ostium and can inform the decision to continue or stop the retraction. This technique should not be used with a Zenith® device because the barbs can tear the interior aortic wall.

- In case retraction fails, introducing a guide wire between the endograft and the aortic wall to catheterize the covered carotid axis should be attempted, allowing stent placement at the ostium and subsequently revascularizing the artery. In case the BCT is inadvertently covered, it is relatively easy to deploy a stent at the ostium of the BCT, if the angiography catheter was introduced via the right brachial access and positioned in the ascending aorta at the moment of endograft deployment.

In LCA coverage, catheterization of the left carotid artery by antegrade access might be extremely difficult. Retrograde catheterization will be easier, either by percutaneous or open access of the LCA in the neck. Balloon-mounted stents are recommended because positioning is more accurate. In cases of extensive coverage of the BCT or LCA, Rousseau et al. [12] have considered perforating the endograft by means of a wire and deploying a transprosthetic stent. This technique, however, comprises difficulties due to the resistance of the prosthetic material and can cause endoleaks at the transfixated zone.

- If pulling back of the endograft or stent placement at the ostium fails, surgical repair of the covered artery should be considered during the same procedure. Revascularization of the LCA can be performed by using the RCA, RSA, BCT or ascending aorta as the inflow source for a bypass; revascularization of the RCA should be carried out by means of a bypass from the ascending aorta or femoral/iliac axis according to the techniques described previously.

- Complete failure of endovascular treatment with a periprosthetic leak and coverage of the BCT or LCA justifies surgical conversion with explantation of the endograft and subsequent conventional repair of the aortic pathology.

Conclusion

Inadvertent coverage of the BCT or LCA is a serious complication which can occur during deployment of an endoprosthesis for the treatment of aortic arch or proximal descending aortic pathologies. Preoperative morphologic assessment should allow the surgeon to detect short aortic necks and/or angulated aortic arches which predispose the patient to inadvertent coverage. Despite a lack of long-term results, transposition of the supra-aortic arteries seems to be an efficient strategy for extending the indications for endovascular treatment of aortic arch lesions and avoiding the complication of accidental coverage. Technical developments in the future should allow more accurate deployment of endografts and adaptation to variable anatomies in patients with different thoracic aortic pathology.

REFERENCES

1 Parodi JC, Palmaz JC, Barone HD. Transfemoral intraluminal graft implantation for abdominal aortic aneurysms. *Ann Vasc Surg* 1991; 5: 491-499.

2 Dake MD, Miller DC, Semba CP et al. Transluminal placement of endovascular stent-grafts for the treatment of descending thoracic aortic aneurysms. *N Engl J Med* 1994; 331: 1729-1734.

3 Dake MD. Endovascular stent-graft management of thoracic aortic diseases. *Eur J Radiol* 2001; 39: 42-49.

4 Alric P, Berthet JP, Branchereau P et al. Endovascular repair for acute rupture of the descending thoracic aorta. *J Endovasc Ther* 2002; 9: II 51-59.

5 Bernier PL, Turcotte R, Normand JP, Dagenais F. Video-assisted mini-thoracotomy for thoracic stent-graft implantation: a novel vascular access for endovascular repair. *J Endovasc Ther* 2004; 11: 180-182.

6 Buth J, Penn O, Tielbeek A, Mersman M. Combined approach to stent-graft treatment of an aortic arch aneurysm. *J Endovasc Surg* 1998; 5: 329-332.

7 Chuter TA, Schneider DB, Reilly LM et al. Modular branched stent graft for endovascular repair of aortic arch aneurysm and dissection. *J Vasc Surg* 2003; 38: 859-863.

8 Grabenwoger M, Fleck T, Czerny M et al. Endovascular stent graft placement in patients with acute thoracic aortic syndromes. *Eur J Cardiothorac Surg* 2003; 23: 788-793.

9 Saccani S, Nicolini F, Beghi C et al. Thoracic aortic stents: a combined solution for complex cases. *Eur J Vasc Endovasc Surg* 2002; 24: 423-427.

10 Hausegger KA, Oberwalder P, Tiesenhausen K et al. Intentional left subclavian artery occlusion by thoracic aortic stent-grafts without surgical transposition. *J Endovasc Ther* 2001; 8: 472-476.

11 Görich J, Asquan Y, Seifarth H et al. Initial experience with intentional stent-graft coverage of the subclavian artery during endovascular thoracic aortic repairs. *J Endovasc Ther* 2002; 9: II 39-43.

12 Rousseau H, Soula P, Perreault P et al. Delayed treatment of traumatic rupture of the thoracic aorta with endoluminal covered stent. *Circulation* 1999; 99: 498-504.

13 Orend KH, Scharrer-Pamler R, Kapfer X et al. Endovascular treatment in diseases of the descending thoracic aorta: 6-year results of a single center. *J Vasc Surg* 2003: 37: 91-99.

14 Schumacher H, Bockler D, Bardenheuer H et al. Endovascular aortic arch reconstruction with supra-aortic transposition for symptomatic contained rupture and dissection: early experience in 8 high-risk patients. *J Endovasc Ther* 2003; 10: 1066-1074.

15 Kieffer E, Koskas F, Cluzel P et al. Chirurgie de la crosse et des troncs supra-aortiques. In: Kieffer E (Ed). *Chirurgie des troncs supra-aortiques.* Paris, AERCV, 2003, pp 83-96.

16 Burks JA Jr, Faries PL, Gravereaux EC et al. Endovascular repair of thoracic aortic aneurysms: stent-graft fixation across the aortic arch vessels. *Ann Vasc Surg* 2002; 16:24-28.

17 Dorros G, Cohn JM. Adenosine-induced transient cardiac asystole enhances precise deployment of stent-grafts in the thoracic or abdominal aorta. *J Endovasc Surg* 1996; 3: 270-272.

18 Diethrich EB. A safe, simple alternative for pressure reduction during aortic endograft deployment. *J Endovasc Surg* 1996; 3: 275.

19 Kato N, Shimono T, Hirano T et al. Aortic arch aneurysms: treatment with extra-anatomical bypass and endovascular stent-grafting. *Cardiovasc Intervent Radiol* 2002; 25: 419-422.

20 Criado FJ, Barnatan MF, Rizk Y et al. Technical strategies to expand stent-graft applicability in the aortic arch and proximal descending thoracic aorta. *J Endovasc Ther* 2002; 9: II 32-38.

21 Criado FJ, Clark NS, Barnatan MF. Stent-graft repair in the aortic arch and descending thoracic aorta: a 4-year experience. *J Vasc Surg* 2002; 36: 1121-1128.

22 Inoue K, Hosokawa H, Iwase T et al. Aortic arch reconstruction by transluminally placed endovascular branched stent graft. *Circulation* 1999; 100: II 316-321.

16

ABNORMALITIES REQUIRING IMMEDIATE CORRECTION AFTER INTRAOPERATIVE CONTROL DURING CAROTID RECONSTRUCTION

PETER TAYLOR, SOUNDRIE PADAYACHEE

Randomized controlled trials have shown carotid endarterectomy to be highly effective in symptomatic patients with severe carotid stenosis. However, these trials also show that the operation carries a significant risk of stroke. Indeed, poor outcome following the operation may well invalidate the efficacy of surgical treatment particularly in patients who are asymptomatic. Perioperative stroke also has adverse consequences for the cost-effectiveness of carotid endarterectomy.

It is important therefore, for both clinical and economic reasons, that perioperative stroke is reduced to a minimum. Carotid thrombosis and embolism are both major contributing factors to early stroke and death and the majority are probably related to technical error. Internal carotid thrombosis is a disaster and associated with poor outcome. In a large series of 2250 operations, carotid thrombosis was associated with perioperative stroke in 41 patients of whom 49% died, and postoperative stroke in 18 patients of whom 22% died [1]. The most common cause of early restenosis is fibrointimal hyperplasia, which is likely to be related to a disruption of laminar flow caused by technical problems. Some series postulate that almost half of the cases of early restenosis are related to technical problems [2,3]. Quality control methods to identify technical errors are, therefore, important. Various techniques have been described in the literature including: simple palpation of the artery, angiography, angioscopy, continuous wave doppler, B-mode imaging and duplex scanning [4].

Historical perspective

The first report of intraoperative assessment for quality control of carotid endarterectomy was by Blaisdell et al. [5] in 1967. The technique used was completion arteriography which showed that the incidence of technical error was 26% (Fig. 1). The authors emphasized the superiority of angiography over clinical methods. However, angiography was associated with complications of its own, particularly adverse reactions to the contrast media. Continuous wave doppler was able to detect flow disturbance but was limited in its usefulness. Zierler et al. [6] in 1984 showed that duplex scanning had significant advantages in detecting intraoperative technical problems. Flanigan et al. [7] in 1986 reported a series of patients having intraoperative ultrasound and showed that 28% had technical errors. These were classified as intimal flaps, stenoses, kinks, residual plaques and intraluminal thrombi. However, not all of these required correction, and only 7% underwent re-exploration of the artery to correct the problem. However, the incidence of stroke in the group of patients who had undergone corrective surgery at 3.3% was found to be the same as those with normal ultrasound scans at 3.8%. They suggested that intimal flaps measuring more than 1 millimeter should be corrected if present in the internal carotid artery, but needed to be greater than 3 millimeters if they were present in the common or external carotid arteries. They also suggested that stenoses less than 30% could be left alone safely. This study highlights two of the major problems of techniques used for intraoperative quality control. The first is the lack of randomized controlled trials, as most surgeons consider it unethical to leave defects uncorrected in order to determine their immediate and late effect on outcome. The second is the empirical nature of the decision concerning which defects should be corrected, and which can be left untouched safely. There is no consensus concerning the objective criteria on which this decision should be based.

Techniques used for imaging

The educated surgeon's finger has been used for a number of years but is essentially useless for detecting intraoperative problems. All vascular surgeons are aware of the strong pulse associated with complete occlusion of a newly inserted vein graft. Unfortunately, palpation of the pulse gives no information about flow. Continuous wave doppler can show flow within the vessel, but cannot detect anatomical problems unless they are associated with significant stenosis. Angiography is still a useful technique particularly if the problem lies outside the operative field, i.e. proximally in the common carotid or innominate arteries or distally in the higher reaches of the internal carotid artery or in the intracranial arteries. Angiography is very limited in the detection of subtle lesions and offers gross anatomical rather than functional information. Angioscopy can detect problems before the restoration of flow, so that they can be corrected before they cause problems [4]. Angioscopy is excellent in detecting luminal thrombi and intimal flaps. Thrombi can be removed before restoration of flow, and large intimal flaps over 3 millimeters in size can be repaired. However, angioscopy gives

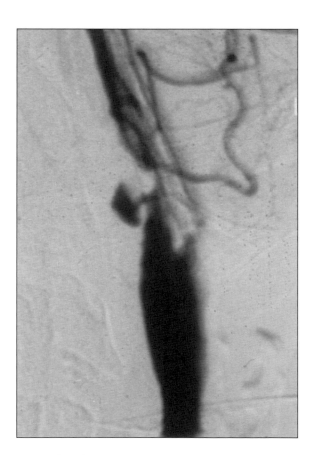

FIG. 1 Completion angiography showing kinking of the posterior wall.

no functional information about the blood flow in the endarterectomy site.

High resolution duplex imaging can provide both anatomical and hemodynamic information. The early duplex probes were large and unsuited to intraoperative imaging. More recently a small intra-operative transducer has become available which allows high resolution imaging of the full extent of the endarterectomy (Fig. 2). Small sub-millimeter defects can be seen easily with the high resolution probe. Duplex is able to detect a range of anatomical defects including intimal flaps and fronds, shelves, vessel kinks, clamp damage and thrombus formation. Hemodynamic information allied to anatomical data suggests which defects require correction. We currently consider these to be intimal flaps associated with severe stenosis (superior to 70%). The disadvantage of duplex is that flow has to be restored within the vessel lumen and, therefore, any adherent thrombus is likely to have embolized before it is detected. It is also operator dependent as are all ultrasound techniques.

Which abnormalities require immediate correction?

There are no objective criteria relating to defects detected on carotid completion imaging which stipulate the requirement for revision. However, certain empirical criteria have been suggested. It would seem sensible to revise a lesion causing a significant

degree of stenosis of the internal carotid artery. Defects in the internal carotid artery may cause more problems than those in the common carotid artery, simply because of the differential diameter of the vessels (Fig. 3). Unstable lesions loosely connected to the artery, which move with the blood

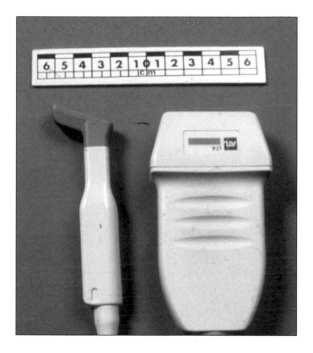

FIG. 2 Different ultrasound probes: probe for intraoperative use *(left)* and probe for transcutaneous application *(right)*.

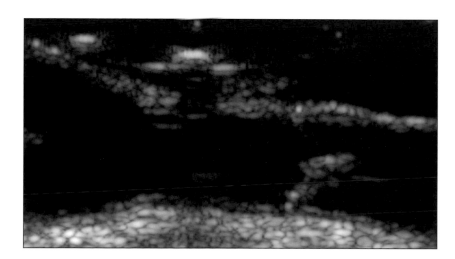

FIG. 3 Control duplex showing dissection of the common carotid artery due to shunt fixation by means of a tourniquet.

flow, may also be prone to break off and embolize into the cerebral circulation.

In an initial study of 100 patients undergoing standard carotid endarterectomy, duplex was performed prior to wound closure and repeated at six-eight weeks [8]. Stenoses were classified into non-significant, moderate or severe on duplex criteria. Intimal flaps, shelves, kinks, fronds and clamp damage were identified. The mortality for this series of patients was 2%, the stroke and death rate 3%, the transient ischemic attack rate 3% and the total neurological event rate was 5%. Primary patches were performed in six patients because of small vessels. Five moderate stenoses were found at the proximal endarterectomy site of which three resolved at six weeks. Adherent fronds were found in 83% of vessels and resolved in all but three cases at six weeks. There were 10 severe and 12 moderate stenoses at the distal endarterectomy site. Three of the severe stenoses were patched immediately as they were associated with an intimal flap. Of the remaining seven, one with vasospasm resolved with papaverine, and one disappeared with manipulation which extended the vessel. Of the remaining five, four were associated with vessel kinks. At six weeks, three remained severe, two had remodeled to moderate and five had no significant stenoses. Kinked vessels were detected in 20 vessels, 4 were associated with moderate and 4 with severe stenosis. At six weeks, one patient had died. Six stenoses detected intra-operatively persisted but one had remodeled to moderate. Two patients with kinks which were not associated with stenoses became moderately stenosed. Therefore 8 of the 19 kinked vessels showed a significant stenosis at 6 weeks.

This study was continued and followed out to one year [9] and 244 patients were studied prospectively. The stroke rate for this group was 0.8% and the stroke and death rate was 1.6%. There were 52 residual stenoses (18%), nine of which were re-explored for a more than 70% stenosis with an intimal flap. Nine (3.7%) further severe stenoses were not associated with a flap and were left. There were no carotid thromboses. There was an increased incidence of recurrent stenosis at one year in vessels with residual stenoses, and in vessels containing a residual anatomical defect. There was no significant difference in recurrent stenosis with respect to the type of closure (primary or patch) or the seniority

of the surgeon. However, recurrent stenosis was significantly increased in females. Over 70% of the recurrent stenoses were localized to the origin of the internal carotid artery. The late stroke rate was 0.9% and was not related to recurrent stenosis or symptoms. The etiology of recurrent stenosis is multifactorial and does not relate only to residual stenosis at completion of the endarterectomy.

One further advantage of duplex is that it can give feedback to trainees being taught the technique of carotid endarterectomy. Any technical error can be detected, shown to the trainee and corrected immediately [10]. The main advantage of duplex scanning intra-operatively is the detection of significant severe stenoses associated with anatomical defects such as intimal flaps which may cause carotid thrombosis and subsequent stroke and even death. If all 9 patients, detected by duplex to be in this category, had progressed to stroke then the stroke rate in the latter series would have increased from 0.8% to 4.5%.

Several series have shown that not all abnormalities require correction. The table shows that defects may be present in 11% to 42% of operations, but the percent corrected is much lower ranging from 3% to 18% [11]. Currently, we limit re-exploration and correction of defects to those at the distal end of the endarterectomy in the internal carotid which are associated with severe carotid stenoses. This means that intimal flaps causing at least a 70% stenosis are corrected (Fig. 4). We also have a low threshold for repairing kinks which are associated with 70% stenoses of the internal carotid artery, but some of these can remodel (Fig. 5). Rarely, the duplex shows residual atheroma to be the cause of the stenosis (Fig. 6). Corrective surgery usually involves patching a vessel, or taking the arteriotomy higher in the case of residual atheroma, which may then require a patch. Large flaps should be removed, and rarely, tacking sutures are used to correct intimal problems. Tacking sutures can be associated with significant restenosis, and the artery should probably be patched if they are used. The Fluoro-passiv® thin wall carotid patch *(Vascutek Terumo, Renfrewshire, UK)* is ultrasound friendly, allowing immediate interrogation of the artery. However, other patches do not allow the transmission of ultrasound waves for a few days and so are not useful for intra-operative duplex imaging.

First author [ref.]	Technique	Detected lesions		Corrected lesions	
		Number	%	Number	%
Flanigan [7]	B-mode	43/155	28	11/155	7
Schwartz [12]	Duplex	17/84	22	8/84	11
Baker [13]	Duplex	62/316	20	9/316	3
Papanicolaou [14]	Duplex	10/78	11	10/78	11
Dorffner [15]	Duplex	19/50	38	9/50	18
Walker [16]	Duplex	21/50	42	3/50	6
Padayachee [8]	Duplex	27/100	27	3/100	3
Seelig [3]	Duplex	14/102	14	14/102	14
Padayachee [9]	Duplex	54/244	18	9/244	4
Gaunt [7]	Angioscopy	12/100	12	12/100	12
Branchereau [17]	Angioscopy	26/103	25	5/103	5
Raithel [18]	Angioscopy	63/196	32	12/196	6
Donaldson [19]	Angiography	71/410	17	66/410	16
Zanetti [20]	Angiography and angioscopy	112/1305	9	48/1305	4

Table INCIDENCE OF INTRAOPERATIVE LESIONS, AND THOSE CORRECTED

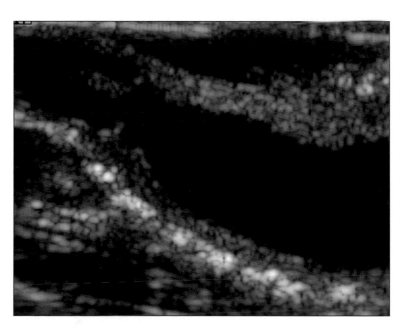

FIG. 4 Duplex image of distal flap causing severe stenosis.

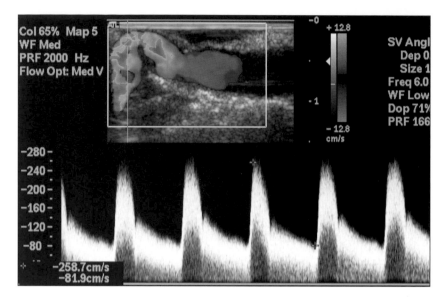

FIG. 5 Duplex showing distal kinking and severe stenosis.

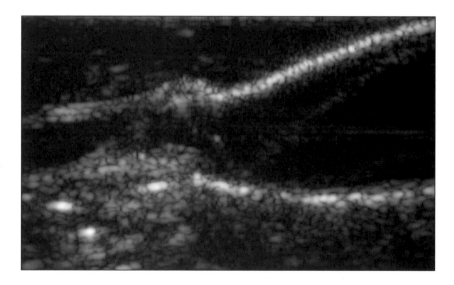

FIG. 6 Control duplex showing a residual plaque just distal to the patch closure.

Do different techniques of carotid endarterectomy affect the incidence of technical error?

It is possible to conjecture that obligatory patching following standard surgical endarterectomy will reduce technical error to a minimum. However, this has been shown not to be the case. Seelig et al. [3] demonstrated that in patients having carotid patch angioplasty closure, completion duplex imaging demonstrated technical defects requiring immediate correction in 14% of operations. The EVEREST trial of standard vs. eversion endarterectomy reported the results of completion studies, the method being left to the individual centers [20]. Angiography was performed in 77% of the patients having completion studies, angioscopy in 22% and duplex scanning in only 1%. Revisions were performed in 4% of the patients. There was a significant association between the incidence of revised defects in either the common or internal carotid arteries and perioperative ipsilateral stroke. All five of the patients who had an ipsilateral stroke associated with a revised defect had an eversion endarterectomy, and four of them were women. However, the overall incidence of stroke in this study was very low at 1.2%. Interestingly, there were 48 patients who had no completion imaging and they had an incidence of ipsilateral stroke of 4% and carotid occlusion of 2%. There was no significant difference between angiography and angioscopy in detecting defects, although angioscopy showed a higher number of defects requiring revision. This study is at variance with our own experience and that of others, which shows that revision of technical problems reduces the rate of stroke to that of arteries without defects [7-9]. It is possible that duplex is a more sensitive method to detect intraoperative defects than either angiography or angioscopy, and this may also be true of revision procedures. Another reason for this finding may be the difficulty in repairing such defects after eversion endarterectomy.

A combination of techniques may give the best results

We have had recently four patients who were found to have low flow in the internal carotid artery on intraoperative completion duplex imaging (Fig. 7). None of the patients had any detectable lesion on duplex scanning which was responsible for the low flow state. However, one patient died of a massive stroke which was caused by thrombosis of the intracerebral arteries. One patient had a silent occlusion of the internal carotid artery in the immediate perioperative period, and two asymptomatic patients were subsequently shown to have tandem stenoses of the distal internal carotid artery immediately beneath the skull base, outside the range of intraoperative duplex. The finding of low flow in the internal carotid artery on intraoperative imaging is therefore highly significant, and should be an indication for immediate on-table angiography to try to identify the cause in the distal vasculature.

Angioscopy and duplex scanning are not mutually exclusive, in fact they may well be complementary in their ability to detect problems during carotid

16
175

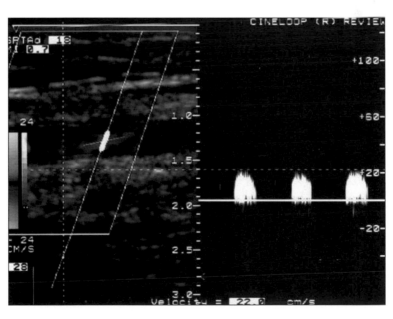

FIG. 7 Control duplex showing a low carotid flow with absent diastolic flux, illustrating high peripheral resistance.

endarterectomy. Angioscopy can be used to detect intraluminal thrombi and intimal flaps before the suture line is completed and flow restored. Duplex scanning can be used after flow is restored to the vessel, to ensure that the operation is anatomically and functionally perfect. In the event of poor flow in the internal carotid artery, angiography can then be used to identify any high lesion which may then be treated with endoluminal techniques such as catheter aspiration of embolized atheromatous debris or balloon angioplasty of tandem stenoses. Catheter directed thrombolysis is another technique which may have a role to lyse thrombus in distal cerebral vessels.

Conclusion

Intraoperative completion studies have been adopted widely and have helped to reduce the overall stroke and death rate associated with carotid en-

darterectomy, although direct evidence for their independent effect is lacking. The techniques discussed in this chapter form an essential part of the quality control to exclude technical error which remains an important cause of stroke and death. Angioscopy and high resolution duplex imaging are probably additive in their detection of defects, and selective angiography may also be useful when low flow is detected in the internal carotid artery. It is very difficult to prove that these techniques are cost-effective, and given the multiple causes of operation-related strokes, it is also difficult to show clinical effectiveness [11]. However, centers which have adopted them have shown a significant decrease in perioperative stroke and death rates. Randomized controlled trials would be very difficult to perform to prove their effectiveness, given the difficult ethical problems involved in not correcting technical defects to see if they cause carotid thrombosis, stroke and death. Objective criteria to establish those lesions which require revision have yet to be defined.

REFERENCES

1 Radak D, Popovic AD, Radicevic S et al. Immediate reoperation for perioperative stroke after 2250 carotid endarterectomies: differences between intraoperative and early postoperative stroke. *J Vasc Surg* 1999; 30: 245-251.

2 Moore WS, Kempczinski RF, Nelson JJ, Toole JF. Recurrent carotid stenosis: Results of the asymptomatic carotid atherosclerosis study. *Stroke* 1998; 29: 2018-2025.

3 Seelig MH, Oldenburg WA, Chowla A, Atkinson EJ. Use of intraoperative duplex ultrasonography and routine patch angioplasty in patients undergoing carotid endarterectomy. *Mayo Clin Proc* 1999; 74: 870-876.

4 Gaunt ME, Smith JL, Ratliff DA et al. A comparison of quality control methods applied to carotid endarterectomy. *Eur J Vasc Endovasc Surg* 1996; 11: 4-11.

5 Blaisdell FW, Lim RJ, Hall AD. Technical result of carotid endarterectomy: arteriographic assessment. *Am J Surg* 1967; 114: 239-246.

6 Zierler RE, Bandyk DF, Thiele BL. Intraoperative assessment of carotid endarterectomy. *J Vasc Surg* 1984; 1: 73-83.

7 Flanigan DP, Douglas DJ, Machi J et al. Intraoperative ultrasonic imaging of the carotid artery during carotid endarterectomy. *Surgery* 1986; 100: 893-899.

8 Padayachee TS, Brooks MD, Modaresi KB et al. Intraoperative high resolution duplex imaging during carotid endarterectomy: which abnormalities require surgical correction? *Eur J Vasc Endovasc Surg* 1998; 15: 387-393.

9 Padayachee TS, Arnold JA, Thomas N et al. Correlation of intra-operative duplex findings during carotid endarterectomy with neurological events and recurrent stenosis at one year. *Eur J Vasc Endovasc Surg* 2002; 24: 435-439.

10 Padayachee TS, McGuinness CL, Modaresi KB et al. Value of intraoperative duplex imaging during supervised carotid endarterectomy. *Br J Surg* 2001; 88: 389-392.

11 Flanigan DP, Naylor AR. Is there any evidence that perioperative monitoring and quality control assessment alter clinical outcome? In: Naylor AR and Mackey WC (Eds). *Carotid artery surgery: a problem-based approach.* London, WB Saunders 2000: pp 298-312.

12 Schwartz RA, Peterson GJ, Noland KA et al. Intraoperative duplex scanning after carotid artery reconstruction: a valuable tool. *J Vasc Surg* 1988; 7: 620-624.

13 Baker WH, Koustas G, Burke K et al. Intraoperative duplex scanning and late carotid artery stenosis. *J Vasc Surg* 1994; 19: 829-832.

14 Papanicolaou G, Toms C, Yellin AE, Weaver FA. Relationship between intraoperative color-flow duplex findings and early restenosis after carotid endarterectomy: a preliminary report. *J Vasc Surg* 1996; 24: 588-595.

15 Dorffner R, Metz VM, Tratting S et al. Intraoperative and early postoperative colour Doppler sonography after carotid artery reconstruction: follow-up of technical defects. *Neuroradiology* 1997; 39: 117-121.

16 Walker RA, Fox AD, Magee TR, Horrocks M. Intraoperative duplex scanning as a mean of quality control during carotid endarterectomy. *Eur J Vasc Endovasc Surg* 1996; 11: 364-367.

17 Branchereau A, Ede B, Magnan PE, Rosset E. Value of angioscopy for intraoperative assessment of carotid endarterectomy. *Ann Vasc Surg* 1995; 9 Suppl: S67-75.

18 Raithel D. Intraoperative angioscopy after carotid endarterectomy. *J Mal Vasc* 1993; 18: 258-261.

19 Donaldson MC, Ivarsson BL, Mannick JA, Whittemore AD. Impact of completion angiography on operative conduct and results of carotid endarterectomy. *Ann Surg* 1993; 217: 682-687.

20 Zannetti S, Cao P, De Rango P et al. Intraoperative assessment of technical perfection in carotid endarterectomy: a prospective analysis of 1305 completion procedures. Collaborators of the EVEREST study group. Eversion versus standard carotid endarterectomy. *Eur J Vasc Endovasc Surg* 1999; 18: 52-58.

17

UNEXPECTED SITUATIONS AFTER CAROTID PTA

PAOLA DE RANGO, FABIO VERZINI
AGOSTINO MASELLI, LYDIA ROMANO
LUCIA NORGIOLINI, PIERGIORGIO CAO

It is now nearly 20 years since angioplasty and stenting were first performed to treat carotid artery stenosis and, during these two decades, the technology for carotid artery stenting (CAS) has evolved rapidly. Several studies based on multicenter registries report morbidity and mortality rates comparable to carotid endarterectomy (CEA) [1-3].

Despite all advances, the use of CAS remains controversial. CAS is considered to be an ideal procedure for patients who do not have a surgical option and for those at higher risk of complications following CEA. The SAPPHIRE (Stenting and Angioplasty with Protection in Patients at High Risk for Endarterectomy) *trial is the first published randomized trial comparing CEA and CAS [4]. It included 334 patients with carotid artery stenosis at high risk for comorbidities. The authors observed a 30-day composite end-point rate including death, stroke and myocardial infarction of 5.8% in the CAS group compared to 12.6% in the CEA group; the same end-point rate at one year was 12% vs. 20%. The major difference between the two treatment groups was related to the incidence of perioperative myocardial infarction in the CEA group, whereas there were no significant differences in major and minor stroke or death.*

The more controversial area regarding CAS relates to treatment of "all comers" (patients who would normally undergo CEA for preventing stroke from carotid stenosis). CAS has not yet achieved the status of standard care for all such patients because of persisting doubts concerning safety of the procedure and the paucity or absence of data on long-term clinical efficacy.

Equipment and technical approaches for CAS have reached a high level of maturity with an excellent safety profile but they are still evolving and progressing, and the ideal technology has not been reached yet. In this respect, the use of Cerebral Protection Devices (CPDs) has played a crucial role in lowering the risks of stroke resulting from embolization of thrombus or atheromatous debris [5-9]. However, the use of protection devices will probably not reduce the rate of major complications to zero, because embolism is not always a predictable event and a variety of other complications may occur.

Predicting complications

When a neurological complication occurs during the procedure, the patient has to be promptly evaluated for signs of a true neurological event as opposed to a drug reaction. Patient evaluation includes a review of the level of consciousness, motor and sensory functions and speech, together with morphological evaluation of cerebral vessels. Angiograms of the cerebral circulation in anteroposterior and lateral views should be carefully compared to pre-treatment studies.

The timing of the event is a crucial point. Both the catheterization and the interventional phases of CAS carry the risk of neurological complications. In this regard, patient selection is a major point. Embolic complications during CAS may be reduced by excluding patients with unfavorable anatomy or high-risk lesions, such as a severely diseased and tortuous aortic arch, severe proximal common carotid artery (CCA) lesions or evidence of mobile thrombus at the carotid bifurcation.

Mathur et al. performed a multivariate analysis to individualize predictive factors of brain embolism and found three factors: elderly patients (older than 80 years), severe (more than 90%) stenosis and double long plaque [10]. Furthermore, symptomatic stenoses are generally known to predispose to a higher risk of periprocedural stroke due to a higher frequency of fracture of the plaque [11].

The possibility to predict the plaque at higher risk of mobilization with ultrasonographic criteria has been recently explored [12].

Some authors suggested criteria to identify the type and frequencies of cerebral embolism by transcranial doppler (TCD) monitoring during CAS, similarly to those used with CEA. The possibility of differentiating gaseous emboli or other artefacts (contrast or fluid injection, patient movement) from particulate embolic material has been speculated upon. However, to date there are no standardized criteria or clinical evidence to define risk of plaque by ultrasonography or TCD signals of embolism during CAS [13-14].

Avoiding complications: tips and tricks

All morphological and clinical predictors of risk should prepare the way for accurate planning of the procedure and a choice of appropriate pharmacological and technical measures to reduce the incidence of complications during CAS. Detailed strategies should be planned before starting the procedure and the choice of material should be adapted to the individual patient's vessel morphology.

During CAS it is possible to identify three technical phases that should be performed one at a time, as an unsuccessful attempt may increase the risk of complications. These three phases can be summarized as follows.

1 - CATHETERIZATION PHASE

Placement of the guiding sheath in the CCA in a safe and expeditious manner is the key to successful carotid angioplasty. Recognizing and appropriately responding to difficult access situations constitutes a great and important part of the learning curve.

The first step is to perform standard diagnostic angiography to evaluate the anatomy of the aortic arch, the origin and morphology of the main supraaortic vessels and the carotid artery that need treatment, as well as the intracranial circulation. Once the diagnostic study is completed, a 5-8 Fr guiding catheter or a shuttle sheath with smooth profile is introduced over a 0.035" diameter, 260 millimeter long guide wire positioned below the carotid bulb. The shuttle sheath is advanced over the guide wire into the common carotid artery and positioned below the carotid bifurcation. Sometimes it may be necessary to locate the guide wire in the external carotid artery branch to have a more stable positioning (in case of narrow aortic arch or vessel tortuosity) and to facilitate the progression of the shuttle sheath. Care must be taken in choosing the appropriate sheath conformation (straight, multipurpose, etc.) in order to have a gentle advancement of the sheath through the aortic arch and a smooth cannulation of the CCA up to the target position. A forceful advancement of the catheter or sheath may result in dislodgment of atherosclerotic debris from the aortic wall with massive embolization or disastrous dissection or, at least, in the expulsion of the entire system out of the carotid artery. If the carotid artery is tortuous, when placing the shuttle sheath in the CCA, existing tortuous loops can be exaggerated and the tortuosity displaced cephalad. These disappear once the sheath is withdrawn but can complicate the stenting procedure altering the flow profile of the artery at the end of the procedure.

2 - CROSSING THE STENOSIS PHASE

Appropriate technical planning and proper choice of CPD, stent, and pre- and postdilation balloons are crucial. Different CPDs have been introduced, such as distal balloon occlusion and flow reversal devices and filters, with the latter being the mostly common used. Most of CPDs available in Europe are listed in Table I.

Table I	COMMON TYPES OF CEREBRAL PROTECTION DEVICES	
Type	*Manufacturer*	
Filters		
Accunet	Guidant	
AngioGuard	Cordis Endovascular	
FilterWire EX (EPI)	Boston Scientific	
Interceptor	Medtronic Vascular	
Emboshield	Abbott Vascular Devices	
Rubicon	Rubicon Medical	
Sci-Pro	Scion Cardio-Vascular	
Spider	ev3	
TRAP	ev3	
Occlusion Balloons		
GuardWire	Medtronic Vascular	
TriActiv	Kensey Nash	
Retrograde Flow Devices		
MoMa	Invatec	
PAES	ArteriA	

In the flow reversal devices, the protection is conferred by the combination of the inflated common carotid and external carotid occlusion balloon determining a flow reversal in the ICA so that any emboli generated during the procedure will travel away from the distal cerebral bed. Protection is activated prior to crossing the stenosis in the ICA, conferring protection during all stages of carotid manipulation, and is particularly useful in cases of tortuous anatomy. On the other hand, as flow reversal is the crucial part of the protection mechanism, stenosis of the origin of the external carotid artery should be avoided. The system requires an average occlusion time of 7-12 min, even in the hands of experienced operators, and it is not the proper option in the presence of isolated hemisphere (contralateral carotid occlusion and transhemispheric collateral circulation not well developed).

The filter CPDs can maintain flow while affording embolic protection, but they need to cross the lesion and to be located properly. Filters are developed on a 0.014" fixed-wire system, and present a crossing profile of smaller than 3 French range. Sometimes it may be difficult to negotiate the system through a severe stenosis with a very friable and irregular plaque, or when the origin of the internal carotid artery is markedly eccentric and the artery is severely tortuous distally. Infrequently, another 0.014" guide wire may be placed first into the distal ICA (the so-called *buddy-wire*) to straighten the origin of the ICA, in order to facilitate the crossing of the stenosis by the CPD system. The CPD has to be placed sufficiently cephalad to the stenosis. If the protection filter is placed too close to the stenosis, there will not be an adequate chance to accommodate the tip of the stent delivery system and satisfactory coverage of the lesion with the stent will not be possible.

Proper filter location and stability during the procedure is crucial to ensure correct protection. Release of the filter in a curved segment of the vessel should be avoided and extreme care should be taken to minimize the up and down movement of the distal protection device during the procedure, to reduce the chance of spasm or filter and cerebral vessel damage. Currently most of the commercially available filters are using monorail systems. Not only are exchanges with monorail systems faster compared to the over-the-wire systems, but the entire system is also much more stable, as the operator has control over both the wire carrying the distal protection device and the balloon or the stent. The risk of neurological complications using CPD varies from less than 1% to 4.8%. On the other hand, there are other experiences showing a similar low risk of neurological complications in CAS performed without CPD. In a series of 528 CAS without protection, Roubin et al. reported a major stroke/death and minor stroke rate of 4.8% [2]. Criado et al., found only 1 major stroke (0.7%) and 2 minor strokes (1.4%) in a series of 135 patients treated with CAS without protection [15]. Wholey et al., using a multicenter international registry of over 8000 CAS (only 15% of these with cerebral protection), demonstrated a stroke and death rate of 4.2% without cerebral protection and 1.7% with protection [16]. Similarly, a meta-analysis performed by Kastrup et al. does support the use of cerebral protection devices, showing a reduction in neurologic events from 5.5% to 1.8%. Despite the lack of conclusive evidence, the use of such devices has become widespread as CAS evolves [7].

3 - INTERVENTIONAL PHASE

If the stenosis is preocclusive, a gradual step-up protected predilatation is planned to facilitate the exact location of the stent and the smooth retrieval through the stent of the delivery system. The first predilatation is performed with a 2 millimeter balloon, followed by a second predilatation using a 4 millimeter balloon. Rarely, and usually in heavily calcified lesions, if the stent does not pass through the stenosis easily after predilatation, a 5 millimeter balloon may be needed for additional predilatation. In all other cases, primary stenting with postdilatation is advisable.

Stent design. Balloon-expandable stents are not used any longer because of the risk of deformation and crushing. The nitinol stents are less rigid, conform well to the curve of the vessel and do not straighten the ICA as much as steel stents. Furthermore, since there is no foreshortening with nitinol stents, they can be placed more precisely using the distal and proximal markers. The drawback is that nitinol stents present an *open-cells* structure. The geometry of the stent presents a zig-zag open cell configuration (e.g. Smart Precise, Protégé) allowing a better alignment on the contour of complex lesions, but less ability to trap debris coming from plaque fragmentation. Moreover, in the case of severe tortuosity of the treated segment, the strut of the stent can protrude inside the lumen making progression of the retrieval catheter of the filter difficult. On the other hand, stents with *closed cell* stent

geometry, made of stainless steel, can better stabilize the plaque but are more rigid and can displace cranially a tortuosity present in the treated segment leading to a severe kinking of the native artery at the end of the stent. Finally, the operator has to compensate during deployment for the tendency of these stents to jump distally if released too fast in case of severely calcified plaque.

The choice of proper size and length of stents reduces the risks of deployment. The internal diameter of the ICA ranges from 5-7 millimeters, and the diameter of CCA ranges from 7-10 millimeters. When the stent is placed across the bifurcation it must cling to different arteries of different diameter. Some commercially available stents present a tapered shape that accommodates the difference of diameter between the internal and common carotid arteries.

Accurate preprocedural measurements of arteries must address the type and proper size of stents and filters to avoid over- or undersizing problems.

Balloon size and use. As the balloons can be inflated to a range of sizes, they should be accurately matched to the size of the distal vessel to avoid overdilation and reduce the risk of plaque fragmentation and dissection. In any event, small linear dissections do not compromise flow and usually do not require additional stents. The following measures are recommended to minimize the embolic load:

a) using balloons that are no larger than 5.5 millimeters in diameter;

b) inflating to nominal, not very high pressures;

c) accepting a 10%-20% residual stenosis (this will not cause hemodynamic problems and self-expanding stents have a tendency for late, progressive expansion);

d) restricting to a single postdilatation effort, gradual deflation of the balloon.

DRUG MANAGEMENT

Appropriate pharmacological agents before, during, and after CAS are strongly recommended to reduce cerebral risks.

1) Antiplatelet drugs. The standard protocol on antiplatelet drugs requires aspirin (325 mg) daily and clopidogrel (75 mg daily) preferably for three days before the procedure and for one month after. In a recent retrospective analysis on 204 CAS, Tan et al. found that, of the overall 18 neurological complications detected, 55.6% occurred after the first day of the procedure and suggested a role for the aortic arch or the heart as potential sources of late embolism, discouraging performing CAS as an outpatient procedure [17]. In this regard, the use of appropriate full antiaggregation could be useful. On the other hand, a number of studies have pointed to the risk of cerebral hemorrhage during CAS. The lack of an exaggerated antiplatelet antiaggregation could allow the surgeon to avoid this devastating complication.

2) Heparin. Immediately after sheath placement into the femoral artery, the patients should receive anticoagulation with intravenous heparin: 5000 units of heparin are usually administered as excessive doses may increase the risk of catastrophic brain hemorrhage.

3) Atropin. The use of atropin during the procedure is routine to prevent vagal reaction because the manipulation of the carotid artery, as well as stent or balloon insertion, can activate important baroreflex stimulation, with significant bradycardia.

4) Vasopressor and antihypertensive medications. Some degree of hemodynamic changes, such as hypotension, hypertension or bradycardia, occurs in up to 68% of patients during and/or after CAS [18].

CAS patients who experience hemodynamic instability may have serious clinical consequences. The greater the change in blood pressure, the greater the risk of cerebral hyper- or hypoperfusion with a consequent increase of hemorrhagic or ischemic infarction. It is not unusual to encounter spasm in the segment of the ICA that contains the CPD at the end of the procedure, especially in the case of excessive oversizing of the filter diameter compared to the diameter of the native vessel. A small dose of intra-arterial nitro-glycerine may infrequently be needed, but most of the times pulling back the shuttle sheath to the carotid origin aids in relieving the spasm, relaxes the artery, and helps the operator to get a better idea of the status of the stented vessel.

5) Fibrinolysis. When intraprocedural complications lead to carotid occlusion associated with major stroke, administration of intra-arterial thrombolysis associated with heparinization has been suggested [19]. Both urokinase and rtPA have been used for intraprocedural thrombolysis, although the efficacy and the best dosage are not evidence-based. With these actions, hemorrhage risks are inevitably high.

RISK FROM CONVERSION

Risks, timing, and need for conversion to open surgery after CAS failure are seldom analyzed in the literature, if at all. Similarly, the intention-to-treat principle, including all conversion-related complications, is rarely, if ever, applied to reports dealing with CAS procedures. Although the rates of failure are generally low, the opportunity to convert to open surgery or medical treatment a patient planned to undergo CAS for severe comorbidities remains a challenging issue.

Personal experience

From May 2001 to August 2004, 982 procedures were performed on 904 patients with carotid stenosis at our institution. In 281 patients, 309 procedures were performed by CAS (28 patients underwent staged bilateral CAS), which represents 31% of the overall procedures employed for treatment of carotid artery disease. During the same period 673 CEAs were performed on 623 patients. Patient data were collected in a prospective database.

The mean age of the CAS patients was 71.3 + 7.8 years (range 50-86 years) and 30% were female (85 out of 281). The primary criteria for intervention were symptomatic ICA stenosis in 22% (69 out of 309) of the cases or asymptomatic severe ICA stenosis in 78% (240 out of 309). Patients were selected for CAS vs. CEA, based on severity of comorbidities, unfavorable anatomy that may increase the risk for surgery (including a high bifurcation in severely obese patients), restenosis or a hostile neck.

Procedural technical success was achieved in 292 of 309 CASs (94.5%) with a less 30% residual stenosis.

INTRAPROCEDURAL UNEXPECTED PROBLEMS

Some technical problems accompanied the standard CAS. One patient had an asymptomatic intraprocedural occlusion of the stent immediately after stent deployment, which was completely solved by intra-arterial urokinase infusion with no neurological sequelae. Flow-limiting vessel spasm occurred in five procedures and all resolved spontaneously or with intra-arterial administration of nitrates. Clinical signs of intolerance of carotid occlusion appeared in seven CAS patients during balloon inflation, all promptly recovering with balloon deflation. No carotid dissection or stent entrapment requiring surgical intervention occurred.

COMPLICATIONS AND DEATHS

In-hospital and 30-day major stroke/death rate was 3.6% (11 out of 309).

Details of all events are summarized in Table II. The complication rate of our single center series appeared higher than many published reports on CAS from the most experienced centers. However, it should be emphasized that most patients in this series are classified at higher risk both for comorbidities and anatomical findings, the intention-to-treat principle is applied, and the complication rate is comparable to reports dealing with higher risk group patients, as in the SAPPHIRE study.

The following are some examples of devastating and unexpected events of CAS in our experience.

Case 1. One fatal stroke due to massive cerebral hemorrhage occurred four hours after the procedure in a 79-year-old patient with preocclusive carotid stenosis. Neurologic symptoms appeared immediately during catheterization of the aortic arch and common carotid artery (motor deficit of the upper contralateral limb) but progressively improved until the end of this phase of CAS. Due to the small size of ICA a TRAP-ev3 filter was chosen. However, during balloon inflating/deflating maneuvers, it was not possible to maintain filter stability and the TRAP displaced distally requiring repeated attempts to retrieve it because of partial entrapment into the distal internal carotid artery wall. The procedure was completed and the patient was neurologically intact. However, four hours after the procedure, further neurological deterioration occurred. An immediate CT scan revealed massive hemorrhagic infarction (Fig. 1). There was no clinical improvement and the patient remained unresponsive in the stroke unit and died the following day.

Case 2. One fatal vertebrobasilar ischemic stroke occurred during crossing of the lesion (Phase 2) in a symptomatic patient with a long preocclusive carotid lesion associated with tortuosity of vessels, high carotid bifurcation (above C2) and absence of anterior cerebral artery. During the crossing of the lesion with FilterWire EX® (EPI) the guiding catheter was pulled out from the right common carotid into the aortic arch and the patient suddenly experienced confusion, global neurological impairment and loss of consciousness. Filtered particles were detected in the filter at the end of the procedure. Accurate stent deployment and intracranial carotid patency were shown in the final angiographic examination. However, the occlusion of the basilar artery was evident. The patient failed to

Table II	PERIOPERATIVE COMPLICATIONS IN 309 CAS ON 281 PATIENTS		
		N	%
Neurological complications			
Major stroke /death		11	3.6
Major stroke		10	3.2
Minor stroke		12	3.9
TIA		16	5
Non neurological complications			
Myocardial infarction		3	0.9
Peripheral neurological complication		1	0.3
Access complication		8	2.6

TIA: transient ischemic attack

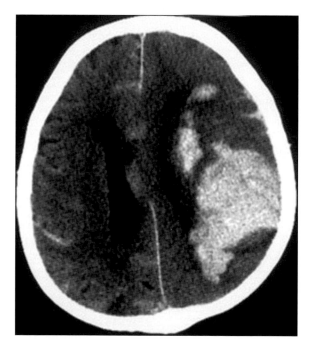

FIG. 1 Massive cerebral hemorrhage four hours after carotid artery stenting (CAS).

improve and at the end of the procedure he progressively worsened and remained unresponsive. He died on postprocedural day 2.

Case 3. An unexpected disaster occurred in a 61-year-old female patient with acute stroke. The patient presented with left hemiplegia of 24 hours duration due to a preocclusive long stenosis of the right carotid artery. A preprocedural cerebral CT scan showed right parietal infarction. Due to the evolution of clinical symptoms and high carotid bifurcation in a hostile neck, urgent carotid repair by CAS was undertaken. Severe diffuse calcification of the intracranial ICA during preprocedural angiography was observed. Cannulation of the right carotid vessels and filter placement FilterWire EX® (EPI) were straightforward. Due to the subocclusive stenosis of the ICA, staged predilatation with 3, 4 and 5 millimeter balloons was needed before placement of a carotid Wallstent®. During the postdeployment dilatation of the stent, the patient became uncounscious. When the filter was retrieved, a large tear in the FilterWire EX (EPI) was evident (Fig. 2). Due to the patency of the ICA and intracerebral arteries seen on the final angiographic examination,

thrombolytic therapy was not administered. Two hours later, her condition deteriorated and a CT scan, performed on day 1, showed a new massive right cerebral infarction.

Conclusion

Today CAS represents an alternative to surgery, potentially of value for some subgroups of patients affected by carotid stenosis. In our experience, cerebral embolic risk of the procedure is higher during phase 1 (catheterization phase) and phase 3 (stent deployment and ballooning phase), and is much less after the first 24 hours following the procedure.

Accurate selection of cases, excellent technique, appropriate antiplatelet therapy and "knowing when to quit" are essential criteria to ensure success and reduce the risk of the procedure.

Further broadening of clinical indications may be justified only if ongoing randomized trials give a final answer to questions about the safety and late efficacy of CAS.

17

183

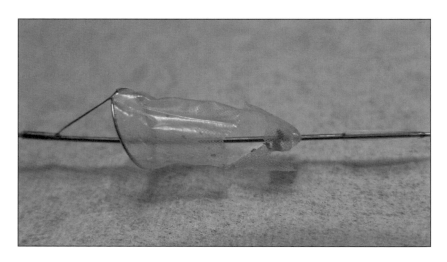

FIG. 2   Tear in the FilterWire EX® (EPI) during CAS for acute stroke in a patient with intracranial carotid calcification.

REFERENCES

1   Reimers B, Schluter M, Castriota F et al. Routine use of cerebral portection during carotid artery stenting: results of a multicenter registry of 753 patients. *Am J Med* 2004; 116: 217-222.

2   Roubin GS, New G, Iyer SS et al. Immediate and late clinical outcomes of carotid artery stenting in patients with symptomatic and asymptomatic carotid artery stenosis: a 5-year prospective analysis. *Circulation* 2001; 103: 532-537.

3   Wholey MH, Al-Mubarek N. Updated review of the global carotid artery stent registry. *Catheter Cardiovasc Interv* 2003; 60: 259-266.

4 Yadav JS, Wholey MH, Kuntz RE et al. Protected carotid-artery stenting versus endarterectomy in high-risk patients. *N Engl J Med* 2004; 351: 1493-1501.

5 Reimers B, Corvaja N, Moshiri S et al. Cerebral protection with filter devices during carotid artery stenting. *Circulation* 2001; 104; 12-15.

6 Muller-Hulsbeck S, Jahnke T, Liess C et al. In vitro comparison of four cerebral protection filters for preventing human plaque embolization during carotid interventions. *J Endovasc Ther* 2002; 9: 793-802.

7 Kastrup A, Groschel K, Krapf H et al. Early outcome of carotid angioplasty and stenting with and without cerebral protection devices. A systematic review of the literature. *Stroke* 2003; 34: 813-819.

8 Kasirajan K, Schneider PA, Kent KC. Filter devices for cerebral protection during carotid angioplasty and stenting. *J Endovasc Ther* 2003; 10: 1039-1045.

9 Powell RJ, Schermerhorn M, Nolan B et al. Early results of carotid stent placement for treatment of extracranial carotid bifurcation occlusive disease. *J Vasc Surg* 2004; 39: 1193-1199.

10 Mathur A, Roubin G, Iyer S et al. Predictors of stroke complicating carotid artery stenting. *Circulation* 1998; 97: 1239-1245.

11 Qureshi AI, Luft AR, Janardhan V et al. Identification of patients at risk for periprocedural neurological deficits associated with carotid angioplasty and stenting. *Stroke* 2000. 31: 376-382.

12 Biasi GM, Froio A, Diethrich EB et al. Carotid plaque echolucency increases the risks of stroke in carotid stenting. The Imaging in Carotid Angioplasty and Risk of Stroke (ICAROS) study. *Circulation* 2004; 110: 756-762.

13 Tegos TJ, Sabetai MM, Nicolaides AN et al. Correlates of embolic events detected by means of transcranial Doppler in patients with carotid atheroma. *J Vasc Surg* 2001; 33: 131-138.

14 Henry M, Henry I, Klonaris C et al. Benefits of cerebral protection during carotid stenting with the PercuSurge GuardWire system: midterm results. *J Endovasc Ther* 2002; 9: 1-13.

15 Criado FJ, Lingelbach JM, Ledesma DF, Lucas PR. Carotid artery stenting in a vascular surgery practice. *J Vasc Surg* 2002; 35: 430-434.

16 Wholey MH, Jarmoloski CR, Wholey M, Eles GR. Carotid artery stent placement: ready for the prime time? *J Vasc Interv Radiol* 2003; 14: 1-10.

17 Tan KT, Cleveland TJ, Berczi V et al. Timing and frequency of complications after carotid artery stenting: what is the optimal period of observation? *J Vasc Surg* 2003; 38: 236-243.

18 Howell M, Krajcer Z, Dougherty K et al. Correlation of periprocedural systolic blood pressure changes with neurological events in high-risk carotid stent patients. *J Endovasc Ther* 2002; 9: 810-816.

19 Wholey MH, Wholey MH, Tan WA et al. Management of neurological complications of carotid artery stenting. *J Endovasc Ther* 2001; 8: 341-353.

18

UNEXPECTED CAUSES OF
ACUTE LOWER LIMB ISCHEMIA

MAURI LEPÄNTALO, SAILARITTA VUORISALO, RIITTA LASSILA

Acute lower limb ischemia is an urgent condition requiring prompt diagnosis and treatment and is one of the most challenging problems encountered by the vascular surgeon. The ischemic process begins with thrombosis of a peripheral artery or bypass graft. The inciting event is most frequently embolism or thrombosis. The medical history of the patient, symptoms and signs are valuable indicators of the cause of acute ischemia. Embolism is of cardiac origin in 80%-96% of the cases and is mostly due to atrial fibrillation or other arrythmias, myocardial infarction with subsequent mural thrombus, cardiac aneurysm or dilatory cardiomyopathy. Emboli from artery to artery rarely occur.

Arterial thrombosis commonly develops on preexistent atherosclerotic changes in the vascular endothelium as a result of low blood flow, increased blood viscosity or a procoagulative state as already suggested by Virchow in the 19th century. Arterial thrombosis can also develop in arterial aneurysm or dissection. Thrombophilia as a cause of acute ischemia has been underestimated for a long period of time as adequate large-scale epidemiological data are still missing. The rare causes of acute lower ischemia may be related to anatomic causes, vasculitis, drugs, trauma and iatrogenic reasons.

The distinction between embolus and thrombus is not necessarily easy [1]. The assumption should be that the occlusion is caused by thrombus if not otherwise proven, as the straightforward treatment of embolus may cause problems in arteriosclerotic vessels. Thus embolectomy attempts are not to be made in conditions necessitating better work-up for the selection of therapy. Yet the main factor in that selection is the severity of acute ischemia.

There are multiple rare causes of acute ischemia, some of which are easier to diagnose than others. These causes have recently been well described and listed by Koelemay and Legemate [2] (Table I). This list represents many causes most vascular surgeons never see. As acute ischemia often warrants urgent treatment, those rare causes may surprise the unsuspecting vascular surgeon. The diagnosis and treatment of unexpected causes of acute ischemia is a true challenge and may necessitate an open mind and inventive approaches. Furthermore, the diagnosis may be delayed both in the pretreatment and postprocedural period.

Anatomic sources

CARDIAC

At present, vegetations associated with endocarditis and cardiac valve anomalies are a diminishing problem and source for embolism [3]. Paradoxical embolism is caused by the passage of a right-sided venous or cardiac thrombus into the arterial circulation by a patent foramen ovale or another intracardiac defect, most often at the atrial level. Despite the high incidence of patent foramen ovale, paradoxical embolization as a cause of acute limb ischemia is low, 0.4% according to a study by Travis et al. [4]. Every textbook warns about atrial myxoma as a cause of acute leg ischemia. Yet, together with pulmonary malignancy invading the left atrium or pulmonary vein, it is a very rare cause of acute leg ischemia [2].

AORTA

Aortic aneurysms, aortic dissection and aortic thrombosis are well-known sources of distal embolization causing acute leg ischemia [2]. Atheroembolism, the discharge of atheromatous debris from proximal arterial lesions, may cause repetitive occlusions of small arteries of the feet, i.e. the phenomenon known as *blue toe syndrome.* Nonaneurysmal mural thrombus attached to a diseased aortic wall may cause distal embolization, as documented in 80 cases in the literature [5]. The prevalence of this potential source of embolization is 0.45% according to a large autopsy series [6]. Primary malignancies of the aorta are rare. Most of them stay undetected unless they cause peripheral tumor embolism. Only 87 cases have been reported in the literature up to 1997 [7]. Angiosarcoma, sarcoma, leiomyosarcoma and malignant fibrous histiosytoma are the most frequently encountered types [2]. Even a normal aorta can be infected by bacteremia. Cardiac valve vegetations, seldom encountered anymore, used to be a frequent cause of infectious aortitis. Patients with a compromised immune system and aortic aneurysm are at risk for aortic infection [2]. Infectious aortitis may cause peripheral embolization, although its main complication is rupture of the aorta.

INFRAINGUINAL ARTERIES

A frequent complication of popliteal aneurysms is acute ischemia caused by thrombotic occlusion of the aneurysm. Gradual distal embolization may, however, cause diagnostic problems *(case 1).*

| Table I | UNEXPECTED CAUSES FOR ACUTE LOWER LIMB ISCHEMIA * |

Anatomic

Cardiac: patent foramen ovale, atrial defects, atrial myxoma, pulmonary or other malignancies, cardiomyopathy

Aorta: dissection, aneurysm thrombosis or thrombus, aortic tumors, infectious aortitis due to bacteremia

Infrainguinal arteries: popliteal entrapment, primary dissection, peripheral aneurysms, osteochondroma, persistent sciatic artery, extenal compression, endofibrosis

Vasculitis and immunological mechanisms

Thrombophilia and prothrombotic state
Malignancy nephrotic syndrome, inflammatory bowel disease

Drugs
Abused substances, especially cocaine, HCG used in in-vitro fertilization, anabolic steroids, heparin, chemotherapeutic agents, thrombin injection

Trauma
Blunt abdominal/aortic trauma, bullet embolism

Iatrogenic
Surgical interventions, endovascular procedures, aortic endoprosthesis, catherization, aortic cannulation, intra-aortic balloon pump, puncture sealing devices, hemostatic glue

* Modified from Koelemay and Legemate 2003 [2]

External compression of the popliteal artery is an underdiagnosed condition. Popliteal entrapment syndrome is an entity in which the popliteal artery may be displaced medially by the medial head of the gastrocnemius muscle (type I) or compressed by fibromusclular bands (type II) or the popliteus muscles (type III). Young patients with atypical claudication, paresthesia, or numbness of the foot deserve thorough investigation to avoid the problems related to acute thrombosis and rare distal embolization (case 2). Smooth hourglass stenosis can be provoked in angiography by active plantar flexion in conjunction with popliteal entrapment whereas this sign is more constant in cystic adventitial disease. Simultaneous occurrence of type I and III popliteal entrapment syndrome and cystic adventitial disease have been reported [8]. Physiological popliteal entrapment may occur due to gastrocnemius, soleus or plantaris muscle hypertrophy in athletes [9]. According to a more recent observation, repetitious compression of the artery by strong muscles may cause endofibrosis [10]. These mechanisms may lead to acute obstruction of the artery (case 3). Osteochondroma is a benign tumor of the metaphysis of long bones that can displace adjacent blood vessels, such as the superficial femoral and popliteal arteries [2,11]. External compression may also be caused by callus formation after bone fractures.

Primary dissection of the peripheral arteries should be considered in young patients with acute leg ischemia without preceding symptoms. This is a rare condition with male preponderance and hypertension as risk factors [2]. Marfan syndrome and fibromuscular dysplasia may be contributing factors.

Thrombophilia and procoagulative states

Thrombophilia may be defined as a propensity to thrombosis, secondary to abnormalities in the coagulation system. Its role as a contributing factor to arterial disease and thrombosis has long been underestimated, as highlighted by Burns et al. in their recent review [12]. In association with injured arterial walls by atherosclerosis, hypercoagulable blood enhances clinical problems by causing resistance to antithrombotic treatment and the risk of reoccurrence of thrombosis. Data related to peripheral arterial disease and specifically to acute ischemia are scarce, although indirect data may suggest up to 10-fold risk in conjunction with hyperhomocystenemia or protein C deficiency (Table II). Multiple coagulation abnormalities have a synergistic deletorious effect as reported by Ray et al. [13]. If thrombophilia is not diagnosed, repeated vascular interventions may be useless (case 1). Antiphospholipid syndrome, if undetected, may have a disastrous outcome and, even when diagnosed, cause difficult challenges for treatment (case 5).

Malignancies are known to provoke hypercoagulability and thus increase the risk of acute leg ischemia. Nephrotic syndrome is reported to have caused thrombosis of the superficial femoral artery, most likely due to urinary loss of natural anticoagulants, i.e. antithrombin and proteins C and S. Inflammatory bowel disease is associated with arterial thrombosis with an estimated prevalence of 0.5%-2% [2]. Patients with ulcerative collititis or

18
187

Table II	PREVALENCE OF THROMBOPHILIA IN PERIPHERAL ARTERIAL DISEASE (PAD) *	
	PAD %	Control population %
General coagulation activation	76	
Homocysteinemia	50-60	5
Antithrombin III deficiency		3
Hyperfibrinogenemia	50	
Antiphospholipid antibodies	26-45	
Protein C deficiency	1.7-15	
Activated protein C resistance/ factor V Leiden	18-26	0-3
Protein S deficiency	8-15	0.7
Prothrombin G20210A mutation	5.7	0.7

*Modified from Burns et al. [12]

Crohn's disease have increased risk for aortic and lower extremity thrombosis *(case 6)*. These patients present a therapeutic problem of how to balance between the risks of bleeding and thrombosis. Furthermore, myeloproliferative diseases, i.e. polycythemia vera and essential thrombocythemia, may be etiological factors to acute ischemia.

Vasculitis and immunological mechanisms

Nonspecific vasculitis of the aorta, such as Takayasu's disease and giant cell arteritis, may cause acute leg ischemia [14]. In Takayasu's disease, emboli originating from the aorta or its bifurcation may necessitate thrombolysis with repair by means of prosthetic grafting or thromboendarterectomy. Steroid therapy is the medical therapy of choice [2]. The role of immunological mechanisms in formation of arterial thrombosis and thrombotic microangiopathy is largely unexplored.

Drugs

Cocaine is a potent vasoconstrictor. The use of cocaine, whether taken intranasally or smoked as crack, has been reported to cause arterial thrombosis [15,16]. Cocaine induces a hyperadrenergic state and the unknown ingredients may contribute to coagulation activity. Anabolic steroids have been reported to cause diffuse arterial thrombosis or emboli from left-sided intraventricular thrombus [17-19]. The effect of the steroids may occur by platelet activation, activation of the coagulation cascade, decrease in fibrinolytic activity or through external compression [9]. The use of human chorionic gonadotropin (HCG) may increase not only the risk of venous but also of arterial thrombosis.

Unfractioned heparin may induce antibody formation against platelets causing thrombocytopenia five to ten days after the beginning of the heparin treatment. Contact of blood with artificial surfaces (perfusion, dialysis) and large operations increase exposure to heparin-induced trombosytopenia (HIT). There is a strong propensity towards thrombosis, but not towards bleeding, despite thrombocytopenia. Heparin should be immediately changed to lepirudin, bivalirudin or danaparoid infusion. Heparin-induced thrombocytopenic thrombotic syndrome (HITTS),

also called white dot disease, resembles disseminated intravascular coagulation (DIC) and may cause thrombosis in any artery or vein.

Chemotherapeutic agents may induce arterial thrombosis. Tamoxifen, used as an adjuvant chemotherapy for breast cancer in premenopausal patients, increased the risk of thrombosis [20]. Thrombin injections are increasingly used for treating pseudoaneurysms, typically at the inguinal region, but, in cases of accidental intra-arterial injection, arterial thrombosis may ensue [21]. Drug abuse may cause a number of vascular complications as a result of accidental arterial injection of the abused substance, direct arterial injury or infection. Acute limb ischemia may be due to intimal damage, thrombosis and emboli and is associated with compartment syndrome, rhabdomyolysis, vasopasm and *trash foot*.

Trauma

Vascular injuries are associated with a number of typical trauma mechanisms such as the fracture of the femur with injury of the superficial femoral artery, luxation of the knee or proximal tibial fracture with injury of the popliteal artery and crural fractures with injury of crural arteries. Blunt abdominal trauma by seat belt injury with subadventitial rupture of the common or external iliac artery can result in acute leg ischemia [22]. Seat belt injury or Heimlich maneuver may also dislodge thrombotic material from aneurysmal sacs [23]. Blunt trauma may also cause aortic dissections *(case 7)*. Delayed onset of arterial ischemia after gun shot injury may be due to the late migration of bullet fragments from large caliber arteries to peripheral arteries [24,25].

Iatrogenic

In European countries, vascular trauma is caused by iatrogenic mechanisms in 35%-46% [25]. Orthopedic surgery contains procedures with a risk of operative arterial trauma such as total knee arthroplasty, total hip replacement, lumbar disc surgery and retroperitoneal exposure of the spine. Osteosynthetic material may penetrate the artery or cause intimal damage. Surgery for inguinal hernia carries a risk for arterial injury as well.

An increasing number of iatrogenic complications are related to endovascular diagnostic and therapeutic procedures. Embolic complications are related to femoral artery catherization for diagnostic angiographies, percutaneous transluminal angioplasties and sealing femoral artery punctures with closure devices *(case 8)*. The use of intra-aortic balloon pumps is also reported to cause acute ischemia [2]. The limbs of endovascular devices for aortic aneurysm may also thrombose. Even dislodgement of hemostatic glue used to fix the separated layers in aortic dissection has been reported as a cause of distal ischemia [26]. Many endovascular complications can be treated with additional endovascular procedures, but sometimes damages may necessitate open repair.

Case presentations

The following eight clinical cases are described in order to illustrate the unexpected causes of acute lower limb ischemia mentioned above.

CASE 1. POPLITEAL ANEURYSM

A 68-year-old healthy man developed sudden calf pain during walking and was thereafter unable to move. Distal pulses were not palpable and no doppler signal could be detected. The angiogram revealed popliteal aneurysm with thrombus and distal embolization (Fig. 1). The patient was treated with thrombolysis with good results (Fig. 1C). The aneurysm was corrected by an interposition vein graft through a posterior S-shaped approach.

CASE 2. POPLITEAL ENTRAPMENT

A 40-year-old healthy man complained of gradually worsening pain in his right foot without any trauma. He was not known to have risk factors for atherosclerotic disease. His symptom was treated by the general practitioner as fasciitis and he received cortisone injections until the foot became so painful that he could not sleep anymore. With a six week delay from the onset of symptoms, he was sent to the vascular surgeon. The ankle brachial index

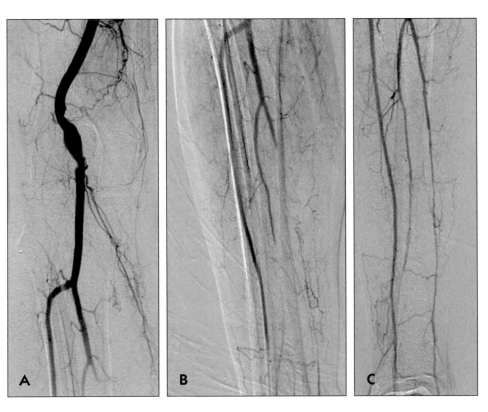

FIG. 1 Popliteal aneurysm with thrombus (A) and distal embolization (B) recanalized with thrombolysis (C).

(ABI) was 0.43. The angiogram showed normal arteries down to the knee level but the passage of the popliteal artery was occluded. After hydrolyser thrombectomy, the artery was still filled with clot and the distal run-off was mostly obstructed (Fig. 2). Distal embolization was treated with rtPA-trombolysis with local infusion into the thrombus. The popliteal artery was compressed between the medial head of the gastrocnemius muscle and the medial condyl of the femur. This popliteal entrapment type I was treated by cutting the medial insertion of the muscle, reconstructing the artery with vein interposition graft and rerouting it more laterally.

Case 3. External Compression

A 31-year-old enthusiastic winter sportsman complained of increasingly painful cramps in his left leg during exercise. Finally, he had claudication after walking 50 meters. The orthopedic surgeon referred the patient to the vascular surgeon. The popliteal and distal pulses were not palpable and the ABI was 0.49. The magnetic resonance angiogram revealed a long superficial femoral artery occlusion in the adductor canal (Fig. 3). The patient did not smoke, transthoracic echocardiography was normal, and no indicators for prothrombotic state was found. The patient was treated with autologous vein reconstruction. The cause of the occlusion seemed to be associated with strenuous exercise causing compression of the adductor canal. As no histological specimen of the artery is available, it remains unclear what kind of histological changes there were in the arterial wall but this case resembles a recently reported case with endofibrosis.

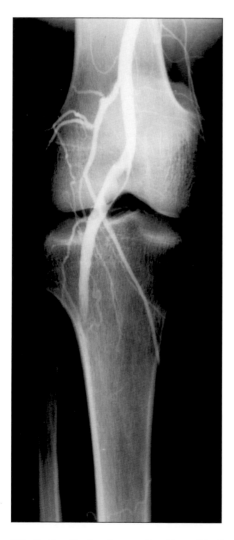

FIG. 2 Popliteal entrapment with residual thrombus after hydrolyser thrombectomy and with occluded outflow due to embolization.

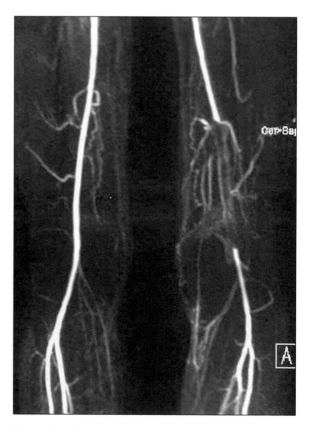

FIG. 3 Sudden occlusion of superficial femoral artery due to external compression.

Case 4. Thrombophilia

A 36-year-old healthy woman felt sudden numbness in her right leg. Rapidly evolving rest pain forced her to contact her general practitioner who referred her to the vascular surgeon. The right foot was colder than the left one and there were no palpable pulses in the right foot. Urgent angiography showed thrombosis in the distal popliteal artery and thrombolysis was started (Fig. 4). Following two days of thrombolysis, the result was not good and thrombectomy was done with subsequent rethrombosis. After five thrombectomies, the laboratory tests for thrombophilia disclosed that the patient had pro-

thrombin G20210A mutation. As rethrombosis occurred under administration of heparin, anticoagulation was switched to lepirudin. HIT was excluded by laboratory testing. Permanent combination treatment with clopidogrel 75 mg once a day and LMWH (enoxaparin 40 mg b.i.d. subcutaneously) was instituted. The patient did not have thrombotic recurrence nor bleeding complications during the 4-year follow-up.

Case 5. Repeated Graft Occlusions

A 42-year-old physically fit man presented with subacute right leg ischemia caused by superficial femoral artery occlusion. As the ischemia deteriorated to rest pain, femoropopliteal bypass was performed. The arteries appeared normal but despite antithrombotic therapy with acetylsalisylic acid and warfarin, the patient encountered repeated reocclusions and eventually ended up undergoing above knee amputation after six years. At that time, he also suffered from acute ischemia in the left leg. Large-scale thrombophilia testing was now available, revealing extremely severe antiphospholipid syndrome (lupus anticoagulant positive, cardiolipin antibody titer greater than 100 and beta2-glycoprotein I antibody greater than 100). A vicious circle followed with new acute occlusions (Fig. 5A), thrombolysis (Fig.5B), redo surgery and an increase in medication. During the following six years the patient underwent 13 interventions altogether (with thrombolysis 11 times) on the left leg and still has a functioning limb despite the need for repeated interventions. At present, the antithrombotic therapy contains aspirin 100 mg/day, clopidrogel 75 mg/day, enoxaparin 40 mg twice a day. The patient has also developed type II diabetes during the past year and receives glimepidine medication and ACE inhibitor for hypertension. He was able to quit smoking eleven years after the initial acute occlusion.

Case 6. Inflammatory Bowel Disease and Hypercoagulable State

A 67-year-old man who has diabetes, cardiomyopathy and colitis ulcerosa in active state suffered from acute leg ischemia of the left foot with discoloration and impending gangrene. After a delay of ten days, the patient sought help as the toes were gangrenous, the foot infected and the patient complained of excruciating pain. As the popliteal pulse was palpable, urgent angiography was performed. It disclosed occlusion of a crural vessel, but the occlusion of the anterior tibial artery above the ankle

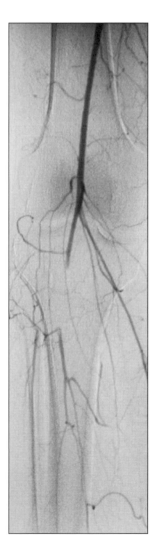

FIG. 4 Sudden occlusion of popliteal artery in a thrombophilic patient.

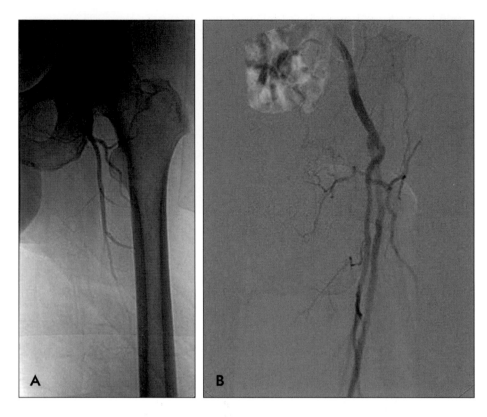

FIG. 5 Repeated graft thrombosis (A) after thrombolysis (B) but with short-term success.

was short (Fig. 6A). As the delay was considered too long for thrombolysis, balloon recanalization was performed (Figs. 6, B and C). Foot perfusion improved gradually after successful intervention allowing infection and edema to subside and gangrene to demarcate.

CASE 7. TRAUMA

A 61-year-old severely underweight man (BMI 15.3) was carring newspapers to the trash container and dropped his glove in it. He bent down over the edge of the container to catch his glove and he felt sudden pain in his lower back. He could hardly walk 50 meters back home to call an ambulance, which took him to the emergency trauma unit. The patient was complaining of pain in the lower back traveling to both legs. Physical examination revealed that the patient was hemodynamically stable, there was no palpable abdominal mass, no tenderness of spine and the patient could move his legs, but moving was painful. Bony structures

were normal at X-ray of lumbar spine. The abdominal aorta was calcified. Femoral and dorsalis pedis pulses were palpable, but the ultrasound study aroused suspicion of abdominal aortic dissection just above the aortic bifurcation. The patient was transferred to the vascular unit and a computed tomographic scan of the aorta demonstrated atherosclerotic changes in the infrarenal aorta and a free flap-like structure in the lumen of the distal aorta. The aortic lesion at the bifurcation was dissection (Fig. 7A) and it was repaired endovascularly by a self-expandable nitinol stent (60 x 20 millimeters) (Fig. 7B).

CASE 8. PUNCTURE SEALING DEVICE

An angiogram was done in a 66-year-old man with a tight anastomotic stenosis at the orifice of the femorotibial vein bypass in his left leg. The right femoral artery was punctured and the puncture hole was closed with a Vasoseal device. After the examination, the patient complained of pain in his

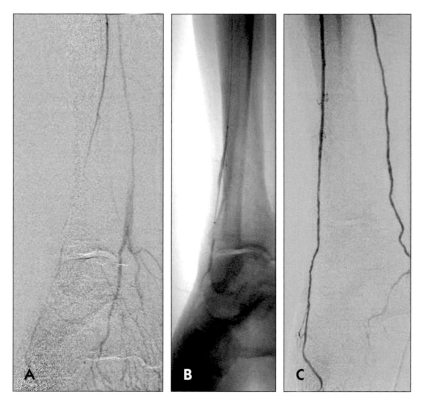

FIG. 6 Subacute ischemia with crural occlusion (A) and after recanalization of distal anterior tibial artery (B,C).

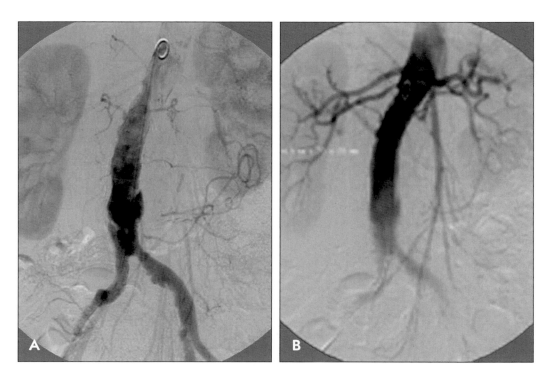

FIG. 7 Dissection at aortic bifurcation after blunt abdominal trauma (A) treated with stenting (B).

right leg which was cold. The duplex-doppler examination revealed monophasic flow in the common femoral artery. The patient was operated on and it was found that the Vasoseal device had pushed an atherosclerotic plaque into the lumen of the femoral artery, causing ischemia of the right leg. Femoral endarterectomy with patch and profundoplasty was done at the right side and the stenosis in the anastomosis area in left side was corrected with a patch plasty as well.

Conclusion

The majority of patients with acute lower limb ischemia suffer from an embolic or local thrombotic event. These mechanisms are well known to the vascular surgeon. However, several rare causes of acute lower limb ischemia exist and are related to anatomic reasons, vasculitis, drugs, trauma and iatrogenic causes.

REFERENCES

1 Kauhanen P, Peräkylä TK, Lepäntalo M. Clinical distinction between acute and acute on chronic leg ischemia. *Ann Chir Gynaecol* 1995; 84. 335-338.

2 Koelemay M, Legemate D. Rare causes of acute ischemia of the limbs. In: *Vascular emergencies*. Branchereau A, Jacobs M (Eds). Futura, an imprint of Blackwell Publishing 2003; pp 253-260.

3 Haimovici H. Arterial embolism of the extremities and technique of embolectomy. In: *Haimovici's vascular surgery, 5th edition*. Ascher E (Ed). Blackwell Publishing 2004; pp 388-408.

4 Travis JA, Fuller SB, Ligush J Jr et al. Diagnosis and treatment of paradoxical embolus. *J Vasc Surg* 2001; 34: 860-865.

5 Rossi PJ, Desai TR, Skelly CL et al. Paravisceral aortic thrombus as a source of peripheral embolization. Report of three cases and review of the literature. *J Vasc Surg* 2002; 36: 839-843.

6 Machleder HI, Takiff H, Lois JF, Holburt E. Aortic mural thrombus: an occult source of arterial thrombo-embolism. *J Vasc Surg* 1986; 4: 473-478.

7 Seelig MH, Klingler PJ, Oldenburg WA, Blackshear JL. Angiosarcoma of the aorta: report of a case and review of the literature. *J Vasc Surg* 1998; 28: 732-737.

8 Sipponen J, Lepäntalo M, Kyösola K et al. Popliteal artery entrapment. *Ann Chir Gynaecol* 1989; 78: 103-109.

9 Lepori M, Perren A, Gallino A. The popliteal artery entrapment syndrome in a patient using anabolic steroids. *N Engl J Med* 2002; 346: 1254-1255.

10 Ford SJ, Rehman A, Bradbury AW. External iliac endofibrosis in endurance athletes: a novel case in an endurance runner and a review of the literature. *Eur J Vasc Endovasc Surg* 2003; 26: 629-634.

11 Vasseur MA, Fabre O. Vascular complications of osteochondromas. *J Vasc Surg* 2000; 31: 532-538.

12 Burns PJ, Mosquera DA, Bradbury AW. Prevalence and significance of thrombophilia in peripheral arterial disease. *Eur J vasc Endovasc Surg* 2001; 22: 98-106.

13 Ray SA, Rowley MR, Loh A et al. Hypercoagulable states in patients with leg ischemia. *Br J Surg* 1994; 81: 811-814.

14 Greene GM, Lain D, Sherwin RM et al. Giant cell arteritis of the legs. Clinical isolation of severe disease with gangrene and amputations. *Am J Med* 1986; 81: 727-733.

15 Mirzayan R, Hanks SE, Weaver FA. Cocaine-induced thrombosis of common iliac and popliteal arteries. *Ann Vasc Surg* 1998; 12: 476-481.

16 Webber J, Kline RA, Lucas CE. Aortic thrombosis associated with cocaine use: report of two cases. *Ann Vasc Surg* 1999; 13: 302-304.

17 Falkenberg M, Karlsson J, Ortenwall P. Peripheral arterial thrombosis in two young men using anabolic steroids. *Eur J Vasc Endovasc Surg* 1997; 13: 223-226.

18 McCarthy K, Tang AT, Dalrymple-Hay MJ, Haw MP. Ventricular thrombosis and systemic embolism in bodybuilders: etiology and management. *Ann Thorac Surg* 2000; 70: 658-660.

19 Nieminen MS, Rämö MP, Viitasalo M et al. Serious cardiovascular side effects of large doses of anabolic steroids in weight lifters. *Eur Heart J* 1996; 17: 1576-1583.

20 Saphner T, Tormey DC, Gray R. Venous and arterial thrombosis in patients who received adjuvant therapy for breast cancer. *J Clin Oncol* 1991; 9: 286-294.

21 Sadiq S, Ibrahim W. Thrombo-embolism complicating thrombin injection of femoral artery pseudoaneurysm: management with intra-arterial thrombolysis. *J Vasc Interv Radiol* 2001; 12: 633-636.

22 Gupta N, Auer A, Troop B. Seat belt-related injury to the common iliac artery: case report and review of the literature. *J Trauma* 1998; 45: 419-421.

23 Mack L, Forbes TL, Harris KA. Acute aortic thrombosis following incorrect application of the Heimlich maneuver. *Ann Vasc Surg* 2002; 16: 130-133.

24 Adegboyega PA, Sustento-Reodica N, Adesokan A. Arterial bullet embolism resulting in delayed vascular insufficiency: a rationale for mandatory extraction. *J Trauma* 1996; 41: 539-541.

25 Fingerhut A, Leppäniemi AK, Androulakis GA et al. The European experience with vascular injuries. *Surg Clin North Am* 2002; 82: 175-188.

26 Guerrero MA, Cox M, Lumsden AB et al. Embolus of surgical adhesive to the extremities causing acute ischemia. Report of two cases. *J Vasc Surg* 2004; 40. 571-573.

19

OCCLUSION OF THE LEG ARTERIES DURING INFRAINGUINAL PTA

ANDREA STELLA, BERNADETTE AULIVOLA
GIAN LUCA FAGGIOLI, MAURO GARGIULO

Increasing experience and availability of new devices have greatly enhanced the endovascular treatment possibilities in infrainguinal peripheral arterial occlusive disease (PAD). This enhanced capability has moved the application of endovascular techniques towards more extensive disease, including sequential lesions, more calcified vessels and longer stenoses and occlusions. The use of percutaneous transluminal angioplasty (PTA) and subintimal angioplasty (SA) in the treatment of PAD is, however, accompanied by an unique set of potential complications. Early complications, including those ones associated with the puncture site, are described in 3%-19% of cases [1-3]. These complications range from minor hematomas and vessel perforation to limb-threatening distal embolization and acute vessel thrombosis. The techniques employed to remedy these situations are variable and include endovascular and, if required, surgical intervention. The majority of complications encountered have a minor impact, however, approximately 2%-3% of all patients undergoing angioplasty will require surgical intervention. A key component in the competence of the individual performing infrainguinal angioplasty is the ability to minimize the occurrence of associated complications, but also to recognize and treat such complications when they do occur.

During the last decade, treatment of vascular disease has gone through a major change, with a significant shift from surgery to endovascular techniques. Between 1980 and 2000, the overall number of catheter-based interventions increased by a remarkable thousand per cent. In contrast, the number of surgical infrainguinal reconstructions has remained constant over the same time period, increasing slightly during the first half and then decreasing over the second half of this period. Competence in catheter-based skills has become mandatory for vascular surgeons in the comprehensive treatment of critical limb ischemia. In addition to familiarity with the techniques available for the treatment of occlusive disease, the interventionalist must be fully acquainted with the techniques available for treating the complications encountered in this setting.

Classification of complications

For the purpose of comparing results in the literature, adhering to an established classification scheme is important when reporting the outcome of endovascular infrainguinal interventions. The interventionalist should be familiar with the recommended standards for reporting complications as elaborated in the *Transatlantic Intersociety Consensus* (TASC) document on PAD [4]. Change in clinical status associated with complications may be described using the widely accepted revised standards published by Rutherford et al. in 1997 [5]. In addition, the *Society of Cardiovascular and Interventional Radiology* (SCVIR) classification scheme is also available, utilizing six categories depending on the outcome of the complication. Level A includes minor complications requiring no therapy. Level B comprises minor complications requiring minor therapy, such as unplanned overnight hospital admission for observation only. Levels C through F consist of major complications requiring major therapy or unplanned short hospitalization (Level C); those requiring major therapy and higher level of care with longer hospitalization (Level D); and those associated with permanent adverse sequelae (Level E); and death (Level F) [6].

Several factors have been associated with higher complication rates in cases of infrainguinal angioplasty including: the indications for intervention (critical limb ischemia vs. claudication), the type of intervention (subintimal vs. intraluminal), the number of lesions, and the location of disease. It has been documented that the complication rate is higher after intervention for critical limb ischemia (23%) as compared to intermittent claudication (13%) [1]. This observation may be due in part to the higher incidence of multi-segment disease in patients with critical ischemia, as well as the more aggressive nature of the intervention necessary to improve blood flow. If the intervention fails, the risk of limb loss is obviously increased. A higher complication rate has also been observed following treatment of occlusive lesions as compared to stenotic pathology. Subsequently, subintimal procedures carry a higher risk than intraluminal angioplasty because they are more frequently used in cases of occlusion. Complications associated with peripheral angiography and infrainguinal angioplasty can basically be divided into three groups: puncture site, catheter-related, and systemic complications. This chapter focuses on early complications, including those occurring at the time of the intervention and within 24 hours after the procedure. Technical failures, restenosis and reocclusion (also considered as complications), are not discussed in this chapter.

Puncture site complications

Because improvements in technology allow the use of smaller diameter diagnostic and interventional catheters, puncture site complication rates have decreased. When only considering thrombotic complications that require treatment, a rate of 0.5% at femoral punctures and 1.7% at axillary punctures were reported in an early study [7]. More recent reports have documented lower rates of femoral puncture site complications requiring blood transfusion or surgical intervention [8].

PSEUDOANEURYSM
Iatrogenic pseudoaneurysms after arterial puncture for angioplasty are caused by failing local hemostasis. Essentially, pseudoaneurysms consist of a hematoma with liquid blood in its center, communicating with the arterial circulation. The incidence of puncture site pseudoaneurysms in most reports is less than 3% [9]. The highest rates of pseudoaneurysm formation are seen in cases with low puncture sites, located in the superficial femoral artery [10]. More than half of the detected pseudoaneurysms are self-limiting and will resolve spontaneously. This emphasizes the possibility for conservative management in selected cases [11].

Suspicion of a pseudoaneurysm in cases of a groin hematoma or pulsatile mass is best investigated by duplex examination, allowing diagnosis as well as treatment, if needed. Duplex scanning will detect pseudoaneurysms with almost 100% sensitivity and specificity. Absolute indications for operative treatment include active hemorrhage, impending skin necrosis, severe pain, groin infection, nerve compression, and limb ischemia. Relative indications for repair (either surgical or ultrasound-guided compression [12] and thrombin injection [13]) include: larger lesions (more than 3 centimeters), patients unable or unwilling to return for follow-up of small pseudoaneurysms, and patients requiring continued anticoagulation. Ultrasound guided compression and percutaneous thrombin injection are an accepted treatment option in patients without the above-mentioned absolute indications for surgical repair [13]. Ultrasound guided compression has been reported with a 90% success rate.

Prevention of pseudoaneurysms, as well as other hemorrhagic complications, is best achieved by adequate compression at the puncture site after sheath removal, either by manual or mechanical application of pressure.

Catheter-related complications

Complications related to catheter manipulation are documented in less than 2% of diagnostic arteriographies [7]. The complication rate is a little higher following angioplasty. Recent literature suggests that the majority of catheter-related complications encountered after infrainguinal angioplasty can be handled with endovascular solutions, limiting surgery to only 0.5% of cases [1].

DISSECTION
Arterial dissection is the principle mechanism of the SA-technique and therefore localized dissection is not considered as a complication when employing this method. Dissection during PTA is angiographically evident in less than 6% of cases, most of which are self-limiting and of no clinical significance. Small non-flow-limiting dissections may be treated conservatively. Dissection as a result of trauma during the initial puncture may be localized in the femoral or iliac artery. In these cases, sheath removal and re-puncturing may be necessary in order to perform balloon angioplasty of the dis-

sected vessel. Particularly below the inguinal ligament, stent placement should be reserved for cases of flow-limiting dissection only. The stent should be placed to cover the origin of the dissection when required. Rarely, dissection may lead to vessel thrombosis or more extensive chronic dissection.

ACUTE VESSEL THROMBOSIS OR OCCLUSION
Acute vessel thrombosis occurs in 0-7% of cases [14]. Risk factors for thrombosis during angioplasty are smaller vessel size, hypercoagulability and poor arterial run-off. The use of aspirin and intraprocedural systemic heparinization decrease the risk of vessel thrombosis. Immediate occlusion of a successfully treated intraluminal or subintimal channel, or thrombosis of the vessel at another location, requires immediate attention. When associated with a dissection, stent placement should be performed. If persistent vessel thrombosis is noted, suction thrombectomy should be performed as described below in the treatment of peripheral emboli. Thrombolytic therapy should be considered when thrombectomy is unsuccessful.

Although thrombolysis is very rarely applied in the setting of infrainguinal angioplasty, a wire and catheter can be placed across the entire thrombosed region, if necessary, and urokinase can be administered as a bolus of approximately 250.000 IU with a subsequent infusion of 60.000-120.000 IU/h. In addition, intravenous heparin should be administered at a rate sufficient to maintain the partial thromboplastin time prolonged at 1.5-2 times the normal rate. Follow-up arteriograms may then be performed at intervals to document thrombus resolution. In cases where thrombolysis fails or the extent of limb ischemia warrants prompt intervention, a full range of surgical options are available, including Fogarty catheter thrombectomy and bypass bridging of the thrombosed segment.

PERIPHERAL EMBOLIZATION
New occlusion of a vessel distal to the site of angioplasty should raise the suspicion of peripheral embolization. This finding is most commonly detected angiographically during the angioplasty procedure and may be associated with signs and symptoms of progressive ischemia. Peripheral embolization occurs in less than 3.7% [15]. Although its incidence is low, this complication requires routine performance of a completion arteriogram following angioplasty, assessing not only the site of angioplasty, but also the run-off arteries. The completion arteriogram should

be compared with the initial study if the precise location of an embolus is uncertain.

Emboli in small branch vessels or areas of poor run-off may be without clinical significance. In cases of important peripheral emboli, several techniques for immediate treatment should be considered. The simplest approach is the well-documented technique of aspiration embolectomy, first described in 1969 by Greenfield et al. in the setting of pulmonary embolus [16]. The technique generally requires an 8 French introducer sheath, a 5-8 French straight catheter with a tapered atraumatic tip, and a hydrophilic guide wire. The guide wire is passed across the proximal angioplasty site and directed to the area of the embolus. Localization of an embolus in the tibial vessels may require an angled catheter and/or guide wire. The suction catheter is then advanced over the wire until its tip reaches the embolus and the wire is subsequently withdrawn. Appropriate placement of the tip of the catheter against the embolus should result in cessation of free back-bleeding through the catheter lumen. While pushing the suction catheter into the embolus, manual aspiration is performed with a 50 ml Luer lock syringe. Small emboli may be aspirated into the lumen of the catheter, whereas larger emboli may require the application of continuous suction as the catheter is withdrawn into the sheath, with the embolus adhering to its tip. Several passes with the aspiration catheter may be required, depending on the embolus load. Atheroemboli may be accompanied by thrombus and the number of aspirations required will depend on the length of thrombus as well. After each aspiration and withdrawl, the catheter should be cleaned and flushed with heparinized saline to ensure that debris is not reintroduced into the vessel. The success rate of suction aspiration after peripheral embolization during angioplasty is reported to be 68%-80% [15].

If attempts of suction embolectomy are unsuccessful, alternate techniques are warranted. Conventional options include thrombolysis and surgical removal. Some argue against the efficacy of thrombolysis with atheroemboli. However, this technique remains a viable option if thrombus is suspected. An alternative method for treating peripheral emboli is the so-called *push and park* technique, initially described in 2001 by Higginson et al. [15]. This technique involves assessment of the run-off vessels distal to the level of the embolus for a location to *push and park* the embolus. In cases where collateral or multiple run-off vessels exist, the ves-

sel with the poorest distal run-off should be chosen. When all three calf run-off vessels are patent, an embolus proximal to the trifurcation may be pushed straight into the tibioperoneal trunk or distally into the peroneal artery, sparing the anterior and posterior tibial arteries. The technique requires application of the same catheter used for suction embolectomy. The catheter is engaged with the embolus, which is then pushed into the chosen distal vessel. If necessary, the guide wire may be advanced distal to the embolus, prior to the pushing maneuver, in an attempt to steer the embolus and catheter into the chosen run-off vessel. In its initial description, the *push and park* technique was associated with a 17% recurrent critical ischemia rate within the first 24 hours, requiring reintervention in 1 out of 6 patients. This technique is generally reserved for application in cases where suction embolectomy is unsuccessful.

Another endovascular option in treating a peripheral embolus unresponsive to suction embolectomy is to mold the embolus to the vessel wall. In this technique, the guide wire must be passed between the embolus and arterial wall. Balloon angioplasty is then performed at the site of the embolus to mold it into the surface of the vessel, thereby restoring blood flow. When endovascular options are exhausted, surgical embolectomy may be performed either via a remote cut down and passage of a Fogarty catheter, or by direct access at the site of the embolus.

ARTERIAL PERFORATION

In a recent study, it was documented that arterial perforation occurs twice as often following subintimal than after intraluminal angioplasty [17]. The overall incidence of vessel perforation in this series was 3.7%, with more than half resolving spontaneously and the remainder undergoing successful endovascular treatment. Another report on subintimal angioplasty documented a perforation rate of 17%, although all resolved spontaneously without treatment [2]. When arterial perforation occurs during intraluminal or subintimal angioplasty, complete radiologic evaluation of the area in question is essential. If persistent extravasation of contrast is observed, a second subintimal dissection plane should be developed proximal to and contralateral to the perforation. The new dissection track should then be dilated using standard balloon angioplasty techniques. The mechanism by which this technique seals the area of perforation is by diverting blood flow away from the perforation site through a new path of least resistance. The site of perforation is now also compressed by the atheroma shifted during the contralateral wall subintimal angioplasty. If balloon occlusion is unsuccessful in sealing the perforation, coil embolization of the site may be performed. When perforation occurs during the attempt to create a subintimal dissection, some investigators choose to use coil embolization as their first choice of treatment. In order to accomplish this, the initial subintimal dissection plane is used for deployment of a coil just proximal to the area of perforation. Needless to say, care must be taken to avoid deployment of the coil into the main lumen created by the contralateral wall subintimal angioplasty, as this may result in distal embolization of the coil. The appropriate coil size depends on the site of perforation, with larger coils used for perforations in the femoropopliteal region than the infragenicular area.

If perforation is not caused by the initial guide wire manipulation, but is the result of balloon dilatation, the first repair attempt should be balloon tamponade of the area lasting 2-3 minutes, with subsequent contrast injection to document resolution of the leak. This may be repeated up to three or four times and, if unsuccessful, coil embolization may be performed as described above.

A more severe form of vessel perforation, such as arterial rupture, may be associated with sudden pain and hypotension requiring patient resuscitation. Vessel rupture can be detected by rapid swelling, as well as contrast extravasation on the arteriogram. Rupture occurs more commonly during the balloon inflation phase of the angioplasty procedure than during guide wire manipulation and may be caused by an oversized balloon.

Treatment involves immediate reinflation of the angioplasty balloon at the site of rupture in order to arrest blood loss. Although rarely described in the literature on infrainguinal vessel rupture, covered stent repair can offer an alternative option to surgical repair. This technique has been widely described in the treatment of iliac vessel rupture where the hemodynamic consequences can be more profound, given the potential for retroperitoneal hemorrhage. Surgical repair is obviously a valid modality as well.

Systemic complications

The incidence of systemic complications during infrainguinal percutaneous interventions is less than 5%. Vasovagal hypotension may occur and present with lightheadedness, bradycardia and hypotension. For the purpose of classification, hypotension is considered as a complication of angioplasty if the systolic pressure falls below 90 mmHg and treatment is required. So-called *allergic* reactions to contrast media occur in less than 3% of arteriographic procedures and may present with facial edema, urticaria, and wheezing. Lower osmolality contrast agents are associated with even fewer reactions and should be considered, especially in patients with a history of contrast reaction or risk factors for reaction (such as allergies or asthma). A randomized trial using high- vs. low-osmolality contrast media demonstrated an adverse reaction rate of 3.9% with high- and 0.9% with low-osmolality contrast [18]. This study concluded that, although uncommon, 67% of systemic contrast reactions could be avoided with the routine use of non-ionic contrast in patients at risk for reaction.

Contrast-induced nephrotoxicity has had varying definitions in the literature and, therefore, its incidence is difficult to determine. Different degrees of nephrotoxicity as a major complication should be distinguished as delayed hospital discharge, unexpected but required hospital admission or occurrence of permanent renal impairment. Preexisting renal failure is the leading risk factor for the development of contrast-associated nephropathy, although dehydration, insulin-dependent diabetes, and large contrast load may play a role as well.

Personal experience with occlusive complications following tibial artery PTA

We believe that PTA is the technique of choice in patients with rest pain and/or tissue loss and arterial disease with limited occlusion (smaller than 3 centimeters), or isolated or multiple stenosis of one ore more tibial vessels with open run-off to the pedal arteries. In our setting, the PTA procedures are performed in the operating room under locoregional anesthesia (spinal anesthesia for patients with rest pain, epidural anesthesia for patients with tissue loss requiring surgical debridment) and antegrade femoral access. In general, our femoral access is percutaneous but a surgical approach with a 3 centimeter oblique inguinal incision is used in obese patients, in patients with a difficult approach to the superficial femoral artery and in patients in whom surgical treatment of the common femoral artery or the femoral bifurcation is necessary. After insertion of a 5 or 7 F introducer in the femoral artery, 5000 IU of heparin are infused systemically. A 0.035 guide wire and a 5 F catheter are then inserted in the popliteal artery to perform selective angiography of the tibial arteries and the foot arteries. On the basis of the angiography, the target tibial artery is cannulated with a hydrofile 0.018 guide wire *(Boston Scientific-Meditech)* and a balloon - catheter *(Symmetry, Boston Scientific-Meditech)* of adequate dimension (1.5-3.5 millimeter diameter and 2-10 centimeter length). Completion angiography is always performed at the end of the procedure.

From January to December 2002, we performed tibial artery angioplasty in 43 limbs of diabetic patients with critical ischemia. A complication (thrombosis, dissection) or failure (residual stenosis) occurred in 9 limbs (20.9%) and required the use of a stent. The stent was deployed in 2 cases (4.6%) for focal thrombosis, in 2 (4.6%) for focal arterial dissection and in 5 (11.7%) for residual stenosis. In one patient with chronic renal failure and hemodialysis, the focal thrombosis was the result of thrombolytic treatment for acute femoro-popliteal-tibial thrombosis following tibial artery PTA and the presence of a local thrombosis at the origin of the anterior tibial artery was underestimated. Stents were deployed in the proximal tibial artery in six cases, in the tibio-peroneal trunk in two cases and in the proximal peroneal artery in one case.

Thrombosis is a rare event during tibial artery PTA and is usually due to plaque rupture with subsequent stenosis. Dissection is, therefore, a complication that should be noted and treated accordingly to prevent subsequent thrombosis (Fig. 1).

Thrombolytic treatment is not always indicated. In the case showed in Fig. 2, thrombolytic therapy would have prolonged ischemia time with muscular damage. The presence of a target vessel in the foot should lead to immediate surgical revascularization.

In our experience, the total local complication rate was 20.9%. In two patients we have observed a local dissection and a non-occlusive focal thrombosis in another two. Both types of complications occurred in the proximal tibial artery; more specifically, the dissection occurred in the segment of the artery below the interosseous membrane and the thrombosis occurred at the tibial artery origin. Those two segments are at risk during transluminal angioplasty. The anterior tibial artery is submitted not only to the endoluminal damage, but also to external pressure from the interosseous membrane. Angioplasty can determine rupture of a popliteal artery plaque extending in the tibial artery.

Because of the high thrombotic risk of transluminal angioplasty in the crural arteries, we anticoagulate all patients systemically.

General considerations

Infrainguinal angioplasty has become one of the mainstays in the treatment of lower limb PAD and its application has dramatically increased over the past two decades. Techniques to avoid and treat the associated complications must be part of the armamentarium of the vascular interventionalist. The reported complication rates associated with infrainguinal angioplasty vary considerably in the published literature and this can be partially attributed to the varying used definitions. Effective self-assessment includes adherence to the published classifications which mainly address type and severity of the complication. Fortunately, the majority of complications are minor and do not require treatment. Only few patients will require a surgical procedure in the setting of complications following angioplasty. Advances in endovascular technology not only extend the possibilities to treat more complex lesions of peripheral occlusive disease, but also allow the use of catheter-based modalities to solve complications.

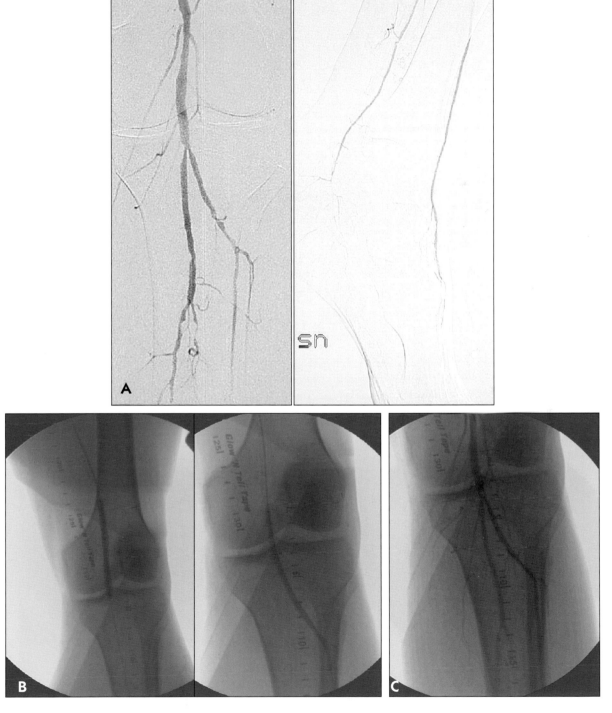

FIG. 1 A - Preoperative angiogram: multiple stenoses of the popliteal and tibial arteries. B - Percutaneous transluminal angio-plasty (PTA) of popliteal and tibial arteries. C - Completion angiography after the endoluminal procedure. *(to be continued)*

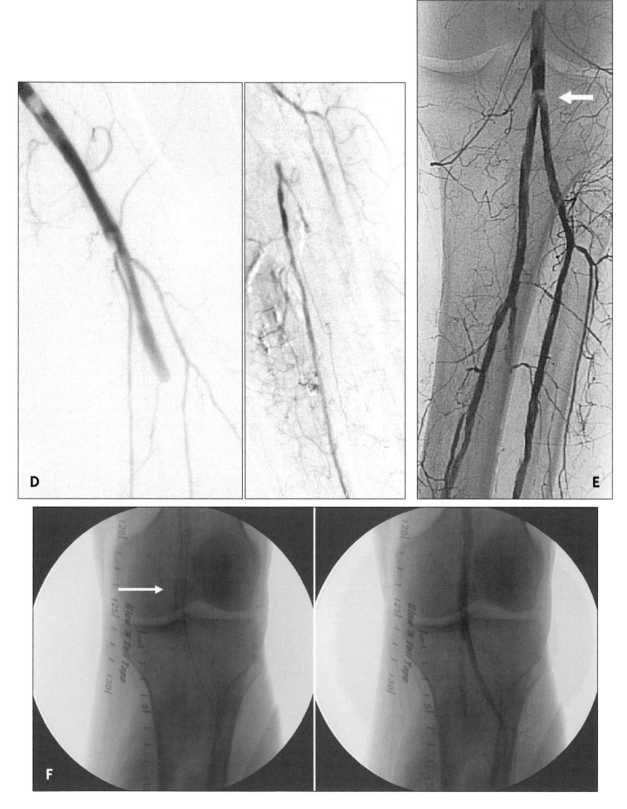

FIG. 1 D - Thrombosis six hours after the procedure. E - Recanalization after locoregional urokinase infusion. F - Completion angiography of popliteal stenting procedure.

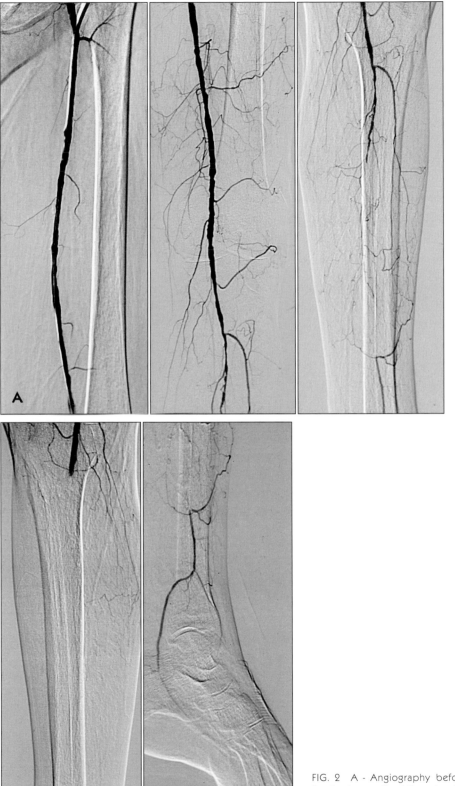

FIG. 2 A - Angiography before treatment.
B - Acute popliteal thrombosis as a consequence of PTA. Only the distal peroneal and the posterior tibial artery at the ankle are still patent.

REFERENCES

1 Papavassiliou VG, Walker SR, Bolia A et al. Techniques for the endovascular management of complications following lower limb percutaneous transluminal angioplasty. *Eur J Vasc Endovasc Surg* 2003; 25: 125-130.

2 Desgranges P, Boufi M, Lapeyre G et al. Subintimal angioplasty: feasible and durable. *Eur J Vasc Endovasc Surg* 2004; 28: 138-141.

3 Salas CA, Adam DJ, Papavassiliou VG et al. Percutaneous transluminal angioplasty for critical limb ischemia in octogenarians and nonogenarians. *Eur J Vasc Endovasc Surg* 2004; 28: 142-145.

4 Anonymous. Transatlantic Intersociety Consensus. Complications of endovascular procedures. *Eur J Vasc Endovasc Surg* 2000; 19: S32.

5 Rutherford RB, Baker DJ, Ernst C et al. Recommended standards for reports dealing with lower extremity ischemia: revised version. *J Vasc Surg* 1997; 26: 517-538.

6 Singh H, Cardella JF, Cole PE et al. Quality improvement guidelines for diagnostic arteriography. *J Vasc Interv Radiol* 2002; 13: 1-6.

7 Hessel SJ, Adams DF, Abrams HL. Complications of angiography. *Radiology* 1981; 138: 273-281.

8 Waugh JR, Sacharias N. Arteriographic complications in the DSA era. *Radiology* 1992; 182: 243-246.

9 Soder HK, Manninen HI, Matsi PJ et al. Prospective trial of infrapopliteal artery balloon angioplasty for critical limb ischemia: angiographic and clinical results. *J Vasc Interv Radiol* 2000; 11: 1021-1031.

10 Kim D, Orron DE, Skillman JJ et al. Role of superficial femoral artery puncture in the development of pseudoaneurysm and arteriovenous fistula complicating percutaneous transfemoral catheterization. *Cathet Cardiovasc Diagn* 1992; 25: 91-97.

11 Toursarkissian B, Allen BT, Petrinec D et al. Spontaneous closure of selected iatrogenic pseudoaneurysms and arteriovenous fistulae. *J Vasc Surg* 1997; 25: 803-808.

12 Coley BD, Roberts AC, Fellmeth BD et al. Postangiographic femoral artery pseudoaneurysms: further experience with US-guided compression repair. *Radiology* 1995; 194: 307-311.

13 Kang SS, Labropoulos N, Mansour MA et al. Percutaneous ultrasound guided thrombin injection: a new method for treating post-catheterization femoral pseudoaneurysms. *J Vasc Surg* 1998; 27: 1032-1038.

14 Belli AM, Cumberland DC, Knox AM et al. The complication rate of percutaneous peripheral balloon angioplasty. *Clin Radiol* 1990; 41: 380-383.

15 Higginson A, Alaeddin F, Fishwick G et al. "Push and park". An alternative strategy for management of embolic complication during balloon angioplasty. *Eur J Vasc Endovasc Surg* 2001; 21: 279-282.

16 Greenfield LJ, Kimmel GO, McCurdy WC III. Transvenous removal of pulmonary emboli by vacuum-cup catheter technique. *J Surg Res* 1969; 9: 347-352.

17 Hayes PD, Chokkalingam A, Jones R et al. Arterial perforation during infrainguinal lower limb angioplasty does not worsen outcome: results from 1409 patients. *J Endovasc Ther* 2002; 9: 422-427.

18 Barrett BJ, Parfrey PS, McDonald JR et al. Nonionic low-osmolality vs. ionic high-osmolality contrast material for intravenous use in patients perceived to be at high risk: randomized trial. *Radiology* 1992; 183: 105-110.

20

CRITICAL LIMB ISCHEMIA
WITH TOTALLY CALCIFIED ARTERIES

JESPER SWEDENBORG

The existence of diffuse arterial calcifications can be considered as a marker for the severity of atherosclerosis. In practice, we must distinguish between two different processes: intimal calcifications, due to the well known atherosclerotic mechanism, and mediasclerosis or Moenckeberg's disease, which represents a metabolic disorder and is most often encountered in patients suffering from diabetes and renal failure. In vascular reconstructive surgery, severe arterial calcifications always pose two problems: safe interruption of circulation and performance of the anastomosis in a calcified arterial wall. These problems become even more apparent in lower leg arteries because of their small diameter and the required accuracy to perform arterial reconstructions. The aim of this chapter is to describe the pathophysiology of arterial calcifications, to assess calcifications as a risk factor and to elaborate on surgical techniques in patients with severe calcified lower leg arteries.

Mechanisms of arterial calcification

Calcification of atherosclerotic arteries is an event determined by several factors and regulated by various proteins and signalling substances. Inflammation is an integral part of atherosclerosis and there is a link between inflammation and calcification of the extracellular matrix. This is dependent upon se-cretion of signalling substances from macrophages, T-lymphocytes and leucocytes, which contribute to calcification. These signalling substances are already found in atherosclerotic vessels before calcification occurs [1]. One such substance, osteopontin, facilitates the adhesion of osteoblasts to the bone matrix and also of smooth muscle cells to the matrix in the process of atherosclerosis [2]. The mechanism that has received most attention is matrix GLA protein, a mineral binding protein in the extra cellular matrix. This protein inhibits calcification in arteries and mice lacking it die from vascular rupture caused by complete calcification of their arteries [3].

There are two major types of vessel calcification associated with atherosclerosis. Calcification of the intima is the true atherosclerotic calcification. Medial or Monkeberg's sclerosis is a component of vessel disease in diabetes mellitus and end stage renal disease, but can also occur in patients at high age without these diseases. Both systemic factors and cellular components influence the calcification in both types. Inflammatory cells facilitate the calcification in the intima and vascular smooth muscle cells are the principal cause of calcification in the media.

Intimal calcification generally starts with a patchy calcification, macroscopically reminiscent of crushed egg shells. It has been demonstrated that high cholesterol levels, particularly low-density lipoproteins, cause an increased calcification whereas high-density lipoproteins are protective [4]. This may explain why statins prevent calcification [5]. Another illustration of the importance of lipids for calcification is that delipidation of bioprosthetic heart valves decreases the risk of calcific degradation [6].

Medial calcification occurs in older patients and the calcium is seen on plain X-ray, an observation which had already been made in 1950 [7]. It is distinct from intimal calcification and is associated with elastin fibres [8]. In younger patients it is observed in connection with diabetes mellitus and end stage renal disease. No association with lipids or inflammatory cells has been shown for medial calcification. In diabetic patients, it occurs predominantly in those with neuropathy. Medial calcification can, in its most extreme forms, produce a circumferential layer of calcium crystals in the media. It is probable that this type of calcification is the one that is referred to when vascular surgeons encounter *rock-like* arteries. In both diabetic patients and patients with end stage renal disease, vascular smooth muscle cells turn into osteoblast-like cells, a process which is probably facilitated by high glucose levels and inorganic phosphate. The elastic fibres then serve as a nidus for the calcification [9]. This is why medial sclerosis is mostly confined to elastic arteries. In patients with end stage renal disease, calcification in the media is closely associated with hyperphosphatemia [10] and, in diabetic patients, it is influenced by high glucose levels [11].

Calcification as a risk factor for future events

Vascular calcification can be imaged with special computed tomography techniques like electron beam computed tomography. This provides a *calcium score* which correlates closely with the degree of atherosclerosis [12]. A high coronary calcium score has been shown to be a predictor of myocardial infarction and/or death from coronary heart disease [13]. The rigidity of the arterial wall causes increased arterial stiffness which influences cardiac work when it is localized in the aorta and the great vessels, as there is an increase in pulse pressure. This may contribute to the increased risk of myocardial infarction and cardiovascular death in patients with heavily calcified arteries [14]. Medial calcification in diabetic patients is an independent predictor of cardiovascular mortality [15]. Also, in patients with end stage renal disease, the effect of arterial stiffness on cardiac work causes an increased risk for cardiac morbidity and mortality [16]. A 1.5-fold increase in mortality and 5.5-fold increased risk of amputation was seen among diabetic patients with medical calcification as compared to diabetic patients without medial arterial calcification [17].

Technical considerations

Totally calcified incompressible arteries present various technical difficulties. Regular vascular clamps should be avoided since they are not effective and, if they are used for complete inflow and outflow control, severe vascular damage may be caused by crushing the artery. This can cause dissection leading to distal occlusion. Therefore, a bloodless field is recommended, using tourniquets or intraluminal occlusive devices.

The use of tourniquets is widely adopted by other specialists but seems to have a lower acceptance rate in vascular surgery despite having already been reported in 1980 [18]. It has long been known that tourniquet occlusion can be life-saving in trauma and it has a wide acceptance in orthopedic surgery. One reason for the reluctance of vascular surgeons to adopt the techniques is the fear of nerve and muscle injury. Such injuries have been reported when applying pressures of 500-1000 mmHg but not with a pressure of 250 mmHg for less than two hours [19]. When using tourniquet occlusion in clinical materials, no signs of nerve and muscle injury have been reported [20, 21].

The mostly frequently used technique includes application of an Esmarch bandage after elevation of the leg in order to empty it of blood. Once this has been done, a pneumatic cuff is applied to the lower thigh or upper calf as needed (Fig. 1). We have found a roll on cuff more useful. This type of cuff is inflated and then rolled on to the leg, thus emptying the leg of blood during the procedure of the application of the cuff.

The advantages of using a bloodless field are several. It avoids the necessity to dissect the outflow vessel completely and consequently lowers operating time and diminishes the risk of injury to the adjacent veins. Only the anterior surface of the recipient vessel needs to be dissected free. When performing a femorodistal procedure, the upper anastomosis is usually created first. In cases of reversed saphenous vein bypass or synthetic grafts, some authors have advocated construction of the distal anastomosis first with the aid of the bloodless field and then creating the proximal anastomosis after releasing the cuff. When performing an in-situ saphenous vein bypass, creating the proximal anastomosis first is generally recommended. The inflation pressure should be 250-350 mmHg. If a completely bloodless field cannot be achieved, a proximal vessel clamp in the groin can be added. The disadvantages with a tourniquet is that some muscle and venous bleeding can still be disturbing. If in a distal bypass using the distal femoral or popliteal artery as an inflow is performed and the patent superficial femoral artery is heavily calcified, the procedure should not be used. First, the cuff pressure is usually unable to occlude the artery and second, if it does, it can cause a crushing injury to the artery.

An alternative method for proximal and distal control of a totally calcified artery is intraluminal devices, such as balloons or vessel occluders with a fixed diameter. A number 2 or 3 Fogarty catheter with an attached three-way stopcock and syringe can be used (Fig. 2). This method, however, is technically somewhat difficult since the catheters tend to obscure the operative field. Also, side branches can be difficult to control if they are close to the arteriotomy. T-shaped vessel occluders with a fixed diameter can also be used (Fig. 3). These, however, have the disadvantage that a completely bloodless field is often difficult to obtain and have to be supplemented with encircling silicone tapes. Needless

to say, this can also be unsuccessful as the artery is difficult to compress.

The suturing technique in heavily calcified arteries has to be meticulous. When the calcification is mainly affecting the intima, a dissection plane is often created inadvertently between the intima and the media. The use of stay sutures, which include both the intima and the media, may be helpful in such cases, both by widening the arteriotomy and keeping the two layers together. It is also helpful to use cutting cardiovascular needles which are resistant to bending. The tip of the needle should be placed close to the tip of the needle holder in order to guide the needle in a more controlled manner.

By adopting these rules, most calcified arteries can be used as a recipient vessel. However, should this be impossible, there is no solution other than ligation of the vessel after crushing it with a clamp. Such a procedure will, of course, result in a high risk of amputation.

Surgical results

Vascular reconstructive surgery to heavily calcified recipient arteries was initially considered to be associated with poor short- and long-term results [22, 23]. Recent publications, however, have indicated that saphenous vein bypass to circumferentially calcified arteries can be done with acceptable results, not significantly different from results obtained with non-calcified arteries. However relatively few series have been published. Ascer et al. [24] reported a three-year patency rate of 45% in patients with non-calcified vessels, compared to 47% in those with heavy circumferential calcification in patients operated on for limb salvage. The corresponding limb salvage rates were 75% and 66%, with no significant difference between the results [24]. This group used local endarterectomy and plaque fracturing when needed. Later series have avoided such techniques and used intraluminal occluders and cardiovascular cutting needles in the construction of the distal anastomosis. In a study from the Deaconess Hospital in Boston, Misare et al. [25] reported a comparison between a patient group with heavily calcified recipient arteries and those without any calcification. Cases with varying intermediate degrees of calcification were excluded. There were no significant differences in patency and limb salvage at long-term follow-up, although patients with severe calcification

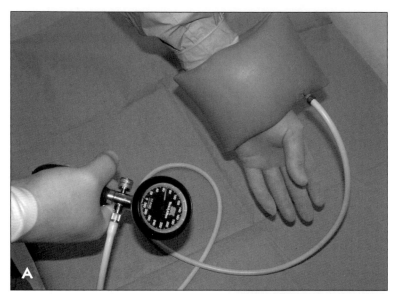

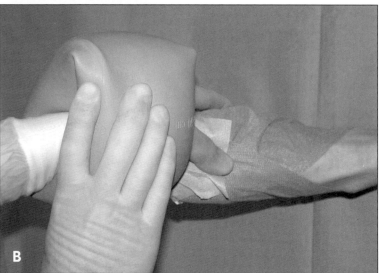

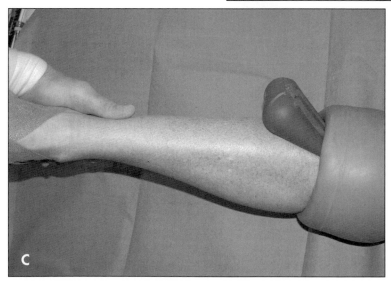

FIG. 1 Device for blood less field. A - The roll on cuff is inflated while applied to the surgeons lower arm. B - The tubing for inflation is removed and the device is rolled on to the leg of the patient. C - The cuff is secured at preferred level with a wedge.

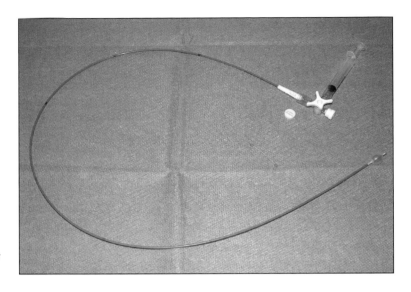

FIG. 2 A n° 2 Fogarty catheter with a 3 way stop cock.

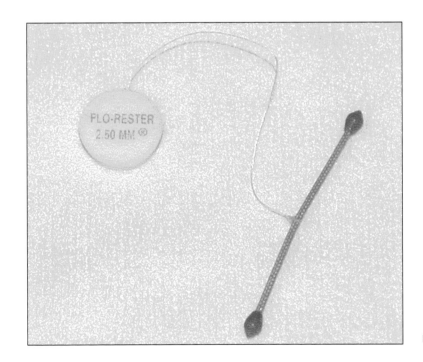

FIG. 3 Device with fixed size occluders.

tended to have a lower degree of patency after the first year. The same was true for limb salvage, but again in this case the difference was not statistically significant [25]. In a recent study by Ballotta et al. [26], the follow-up was five years. In this series, primary patency seemed to be worse in the group with heavily calcified arteries over time but did not reach a p-value of 0.05 at five years. The tendency towards a worse outcome in terms of patency could be reversed when looking at secondary patency rates

[26]. The latter two studies also confirm that more patients with diabetes and end stage renal disease are represented in the group with heavy calcification.

The question about postoperative medical adjuvant therapy has not been addressed in a prospective manner for patients with heavily calcified recipient arteries in the lower leg. It must be concluded that this patient group had a somewhat worse outcome, but that in most series this was not significantly worse. Accordingly, postoperative adjuvant therapy should be considered. The majority of these patients receive vein grafts and can be classified as having a high risk for occlusion. It has been suggested that such patients benefit from treatment with oral anticoagulants [27].

Conclusion

Heavily calcified distal arteries are mostly found in patients with diabetes and end stage renal disease. In these groups as well as in older patients, the calcification is confined to the media. The presence of heavily calcified arteries could be a prognostic sign of decreased longevity. After an initial pessimistic attitude towards lower limb revascularization, recent reports have stated good results. Relatively few reports have been published on this issue. Presence of circumferential calcification in the recipient artery should not be a contraindication to vascular reconstructive surgery in limbs with critical ischemia.

20
210

REFERENCES

1 Wallin R, Wajih N, Greenwood GT, Sane DC. Arterial calcification: a review of mechanisms, animal models, and the prospects for therapy. *Med Res Rev* 2001; 21: 274-301.

2 Gravallese EM. Osteopontin: a bridge between bone and the immune system. *J Clin Invest* 2003; 112: 147-149.

3 Luo G, Ducy P, McKee MD et al. Spontaneous calcification of arteries and cartilage in mice lacking matrix GLA protein. *Nature* 1997; 386: 78-81.

4 Parhami F, Basseri B, Hwang J et al. High-density lipoprotein regulates calcification of vascular cells. *Circ Res* 2002; 91: 570-576.

5 Callister TQ, Raggi P, Cooil B et al. Effect of HMG-CoA reductase inhibitors on coronary artery disease as assessed by electron-beam computed tomography. *N Engl J Med* 1998; 339: 1972-1978.

6 Shen M, Kara-Mostefa A, Chen L et al. Effect of ethanol and ether in the prevention of calcification of bioprostheses. *Ann Thorac Surg* 2001; 71: S413-416.

7 Lindbom A. Arteriosclerosis and arterial thrombosis in the lower limb; a roentgenological study. *Acta Radiol Suppl* 1950; 80: 1-80.

8 Proudfoot D, Shanahan CM. Biology of calcification in vascular cells: intima versus media. *Herz* 2001; 26: 245-251.

9 Trion A, van der Laarse A. Vascular smooth muscle cells and calcification in atherosclerosis. *Am Heart J* 2004; 147: 808-814.

10 London GM, Guerin AP, Marchais SJ et al. Arterial media calcification in end-stage renal disease: impact on all-cause and cardiovascular mortality. *Nephrol Dial Transplant* 2003; 18: 1731-1740.

11 Chen NX, Moe SM. Arterial calcification in diabetes. *Curr Diab Rep* 2003; 3: 28-32.

12 Agatston AS, Janowitz WR. Ultrafast computed tomography in coronary screening. *Circulation* 1994; 89: 1908-1909.

13 Wayhs R, Zelinger A, Raggi P. High coronary artery calcium scores pose an extremely elevated risk for hard events. *J Am Coll Cardiol* 2002; 39: 225-230.

14 Madhavan S, Ooi WL, Cohen H, Alderman MH. Relation of pulse pressure and blood pressure reduction to the incidence of myocardial infarction. *Hypertension* 1994; 23: 395-401.

15 Lehto S, Niskanen L, Suhonen M et al. Medial artery calcification. A neglected harbinger of cardiovascular complications in non-insulin-dependent diabetes mellitus. *Arterioscler Thromb Vasc Biol* 1996; 16: 978-983.

16 London GM, Marchais SJ, Guerin AP et al. Inflammation, arteriosclerosis, and cardiovascular therapy in hemodialysis patients. *Kidney Int Suppl* 2003: S88-93.

17 Everhart JE, Pettitt DJ, Knowler WC et al. Medial arterial calcification and its association with mortality and complications of diabetes. *Diabetologia* 1988; 31: 16-23.

18 Bernhard VM, Boren CII, Townc JB. Pneumatic tourniquet as a substitute for vascular clamps in distal bypass surgery. *Surgery* 1980; 87: 709-713.

19 Ochoa J, Fowler TJ, Gilliatt RW. Anatomical changes in peripheral nerves compressed by a pneumatic tourniquet. *J Anat* 1972; 113: 433-455.

20 Treiman GS. Tourniquet occlusion technique for tibial artery reconstruction. *Semin Vasc Surg* 2000; 13:40-43.

21 Ciervo A, Dardik H, Qin F et al. The tourniquet revisited as an adjunct to lower limb revascularization. *J Vasc Surg* 2000; 31: 436-442.

22 Dardik H, Ibrahim IM, Dardik, II. The role of the peroneal artery for limb salvage. *Ann Surg* 1979; 189: 189-198.

23 Karmody AM, Leather RP, Shah DM et al. Peroneal artery bypass: a reappraisal of its value in limb salvage. *J Vasc Surg* 1984; 1: 809-816.

24 Ascer E, Veith FJ, Flores SA. Infrapopliteal bypasses to heavily calcified rock-like arteries. Management and results. *Am J Surg* 1986; 152: 220-223.

25 Misare BD, Pomposelli FB Jr, Gibbons GW et al. Infrapopliteal bypasses to severely calcified, unclampable outflow arteries: two-year results. *J Vasc Surg* 1996; 24: 6-15.

26 Ballotta E, Renon L, Toffano M et al. Patency and limb salvage rates after distal revascularization to unclampable calcified outflow arteries. *J Vasc Surg* 2004; 39: 539-546.

27 Tangelder MJ, Lawson JA, Algra A, Eikelboom BC. Systematic review of randomized controlled trials of aspirin and oral anticoagulants in the prevention of graft occlusion and ischemic events after infrainguinal bypass surgery. *J Vasc Surg* 1999; 30: 701-709.

21

CT ANGIOGRAPHY OF THE AORTA AND LOWER LIMB ARTERIES

PIERRE GOUNY, MICHEL NONENT
ANTOINE VERHAEGHE, GILDAS GUERET, ALI BADRA

To perform a revascularization without conventional angiography is a challenge but it is possible thanks to all the acquired knowledge on vascular pathology. All available information provided by the medical history, physical examination and duplex scanning should be used. Also, other basic observations should be taken into account:
- the relationship between the level of intermittent claudication and the vascular lesion
- confirmation of critical ischemia related to the duration of pain or trophic changes
- distal pressures expressed as absolute values (mmHg), instead of using the ankle-brachial index.

If angiography is not available, it is necessary to follow a strict and cautious diagnostic process, which by itself can be considered as an advantage. It certainly eliminates the oculo-surgical *reflex.*

Clinical assessment of the level of the arterial lesions

The level of the disease should be assessed based on the medical history indicating the existence of occlusive arterial pathology. Suprainguinal and inguinal lesions should be differentiated first (absent femoral pulse, buttock claudication, pain in the groin, absence of ulcerations, previous aortoiliac or iliofemoral surgery), in addition to infrainguinal pathology (skin ulcerations, present femoral pulse, calf or foot claudication). Aortic or bilateral iliac artery involvement can be suspected in cases of more or less symmetrical bilateral claudication, the absence of femoral pulses and calcifications on a plain X-ray or computer tomography (CT) without contrast. Uni- or bilateral iliac artery disease can be assessed by duplex scanning following exercise. The latter can be achieved by walking, flexion-extension movements or on a moving walkway. In all cases, the pressure drop at the ankle following exercise and decreased femoral flux will indicate the level of the disease.

Skin ulcerations depict critical ischemia requiring below-knee revascularization in most patients. Pre-operative duplex scanning allows assessment of blood flow in the crural arteries. In critical ischemia, the posterior tibial artery is affected first and most severely, followed by the anterior tibial artery. The peroneal artery is most often preserved. In case magnetic resonance angiography (MRA) does not visualize the distal arteries, selective arteriography via common or profunda femoral artery puncture with delayed images should be performed prior to surgery.

CT and MR angiography

Conventional angiography by arterial puncture is no longer a prerequisite. CT and MR angiography are currently high-performing vascular imaging alternatives. Multislice scanning constitutes an important technique for assessing the anatomy of veins and arteries. The helical technique was an indispensable precondition in allowing rapid acquisition during apnoe and optimizing the contrast injection to assess the vessels selectively. The field of visualization was limited when using the previous generation monodetector scanners. Because of insufficient tube and generator power, it was not possible to study the aorta during a single apnoe or to assess the lower limb arteries during a single acquisition. In addition, the rotation speed did not allow the assessment of moving structures and the spatial resolution was too limited to visualize small diameter vessels. The principle advantages of multislice acquisition are: increased acquisition time (4-16 slices per rotation of 0.5 second), improvement of the longitudinal spatial resolution by using thin slices, and the possibility of choosing the slice thickness afterwards [1,2]. The reduced acquisition time allows us to optimize the vascular contrast and to limit the volume of injected dye. The possibility of obtaining thin collimations (0.625-0.75 millimeters) on a greater length is certainly an asset but still has to be developed further because excessive irradiation is a potential risk. A posteriori determination of slice thickness allows a wide range in the choice of reconstructions which necessarily overlap in the setting of vascular evaluation.

SUPRAINGUINAL CT ANGIOGRAPHY

If endoluminal angioplasty is considered, it is necessary to determine the following as well as the level of the lesion: whether it concerns a stenosis or an occlusion, the presence of calcifications, the length of the lesion, and whether the aortic and iliac bifurcation are involved. CT angiography allows these assessments. In any case, intraprocedural angiography will detect possible inaccuracies if endovascular treatment is planned. Conventional angiography actually provides information about the visceral and renal arteries as well as the femoral bifurcation and profunda femoral artery.

Duplex scanning does not always depict aortoiliac pathology because of obesity, digestive gas or superpositions. However, assessment of the femoral bifurcation and profunda femoral artery is easy.

The images of the renal and visceral arteries obtained by CT angiography are most often sufficient in the setting of assessing occlusive arterial disease of the lower limbs. By means of reconstructions, CT angiography allows us to visualize these arteries under different angles in such a way that it is accurate enough to identify and quantify possible lesions. Conventional angiography can be justified if surgical repair of a visceral artery is considered and the CT or MR images are unclear. In case aortic and iliac lesions are difficult to interpret due to calcifications, CT angiography should be red using specific procedures at the workstation:
- reading the reconstructions using the *transparency* technique, which allows us to vary the calcified zones with different transparency and, therefore, see the arterial lumen under and through the calcified plaques
- reading the millimeter slices one after another, thereby imitating angiographic endoscopy and evaluating the stenoses observed from the lumen
- choosing the area to be reconstructed. As in conventional angiography it is important that the field of imaging for which the analyses are crucial (such as the femoral bifurcation) is not cut off at the point of interest.

INFRAINGUINAL CT ANGIOGRAPHY
In general, CT angiography provides reliable images of the lower limb arterial system. The femoropopliteal occlusion is often the best visualized arterial lesion, irrespective of the applied diagnostic

method. However, the vascular surgeon is more interested in the distal outflow and, at present, CT angiography does not always allow visualization of the crural and foot arteries.

Limitations of CT angiography

Several problems can contribute to mediocre results of CT angiography, such as the area of interest (i.e. distal extremities), the lesion itself or artefacts caused by the technique.

INSUFFICIENT CONTRAST OF THE TARGET ARTERIAL SEGMENT

Contrast difficulties in the calf and inframalleolar area are mainly encountered in two situations. In the presence of severe aortoiliac or femoral disease, the distal flow might be significantly reduced with subsequent insufficient local contrast to allow accurate assessment of the arteries below the knee. This problem might be solved by using longer acquisition times (45-60 seconds).

In cases of compromised cardiac function, the distal arterial bed can be insufficiently opaque if the delay was empirically chosen not taking the hemodynamic alterations into account. Using an automatic detector is recommended as it senses the arrival of the contrast and starts acquisition if the arterial visualization is optimal.

EARLY VENOUS RETURN (FIG. 1)

Distal early venous return can occur in patients with infected ulcers or inflammatory lesions and is specifically present in diabetics. Early venous return can mask the distal arterial network and, therefore, might not allow visualization of the outflow. In these circumstances, MR angiography with gadolinium injection probably provides better information, as the use of multiphased sequences avoids venous superposition.

INSUFFICIENT SPATIAL RESOLUTION

This limitation is directly related to the technical capacity of the equipment. The spatial resolution is determined by the thickness of the nominal slices and is specifically important when assessing small diameter arteries. The smaller the vessel diameter, the smaller the acquisition slice thickness has to be. The new generation scanners [3] can perform slice acquisition of millimeters on much larger volumes, such as an entire lower limb. The spatial resolution

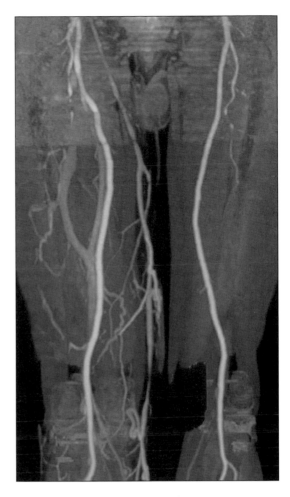

FIG. 1 Maximum intensity projection (MIP) reconstruction showing artefacts which hinder analysis of the proximal segments of the right superficial and profunda femoral arteries.

governs the quantification of the degree of the stenosis (Figs. 2A and B). This quantification should differentiate between significant and non-significant lesions because it plays an important role in decision-making. In practice, severe stenoses (larger than 70%) are relatively easy to detect. However, moderate stenoses with diameter reduction from 40% to 60% are difficult to assess. Limited spatial resolution carries the risk of overestimating the degree of stenosis and can even cause confusion between a very tight stenosis and an occlusion.

MODALITIES OF RECONSTRUCTION

CT image reconstructions have also become an essential integral part of arterial assessment because

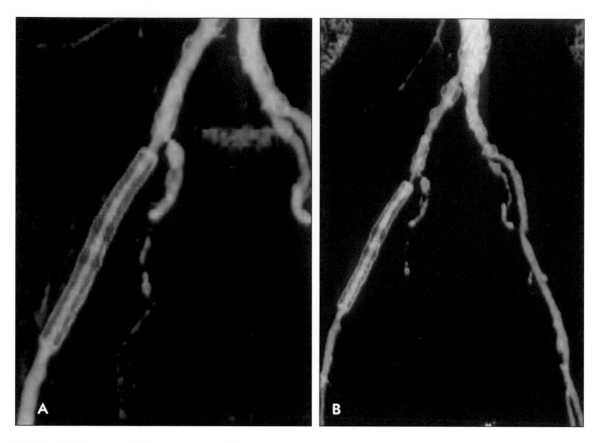

FIG. 2 A - Volume rendering technique (VRT) with transparency showing a moderate stenosis at the origin of the right external iliac artery. B - By slightly modifying the selected densities, the VRT reconstruction with transparency now depicts an incorrect image of the tight stenosis at the origin of the right external iliac artery.

they are easy to read and, therefore, amenable to all clinicians. It is not necessary to provide all native axial slices anymore, except maybe on CD-roms (replacing the traditional film) as part of the patient file. The radiologist, however, should be able to use the axial slices for interpretation at the workstation and to compare them with the acquired reconstructions. Nowadays these workstations constitute a crucial part of the diagnostic process and should therefore be fast, be interactive, have a large storage capacity and contain the software capable of providing the highest quality reconstructions. They should be connected to acquisition consoles with high data throughput to receive a large number of images, allowing storage on CT and DVD. The vascular reconstructions are variable: MPR, MIP, 3D surface shading, 3D rendered volume and virtual angioscopy [4].

MULTIPLANAR RECONSTRUCTIONS (MPR)

Two dimensional multiplanar reconstructions can be derived from native axial slices, 3D reconstruction or by automatic selection of a plane through the center of the artery. The latter allows assessment of the vascular structure and makes measuring the length, diameter and degree of the stenosis easier.

MAXIMUM INTENSITY PROJECTION (MIP)

MIP consists of image projection with maximal pixel density and is not a 3D reconstruction. The main drawback of MIP reconstructions is the potential inability to distinguish two structures when they have a density which is higher than the threshold of the selected maximal density. Therefore, a bone structure or calcification can completely mask the lumen of an artery. Fortunately, the different angles of view will allow us to distinguish the structures.

3D Reconstructions: 3D Surface Shading and Rendered Volume 3D

Three dimensional surface shading provides a nice quality image but is misleading. Depending on the chosen threshold, small diameter vessels might not be recognized and stenoses could be over- and underestimated. Rendered volume 3D reconstructions, or the volume rendering technique (VRT), are more interesting [5]. On image workstations in general, the rendered volume provides more information on the composition of the structures and their spatial relationship. VRT depicts a much wider scale of information and also visualizes structures in different layers. In this technique, minimal and maximal values on a scale of density histograms are chosen. It is, therefore, possible to select structures with high density (bone, calcifications) and vascular structures made opaque by iodized contrast independently. The 3D VRT reconstructions allow segmentations of a specific volume, do not loose information and solve the problem of calcifications by means of the transparency technique in which calcified densities receive minimal contrast. There is an obvious complement between VRT and MIP, which are actually the most often used techniques.

Arterial Wall Calcifications

The advantage of MIP is the ability to depict the allocation and extent of arterial wall calcifications (Fig. 3). VRT offers additional information on the patent arterial lumen because the technique allows us to visualize the calcifications under transparency [4,5], which is an indispensable part of CT angiography in the assessment of lower limb arteries.

Visualizing arterial wall calcifications is an advantage for the surgeon because it allows appropriate selection of levels to anastomose and, therefore, it is necessary to integrate the MIP and VRT reconstructions. VRT reconstructions with transparency can be considered equivalent to conventional angiography, with the additional advantage that they visualize the target lesions from different angles,

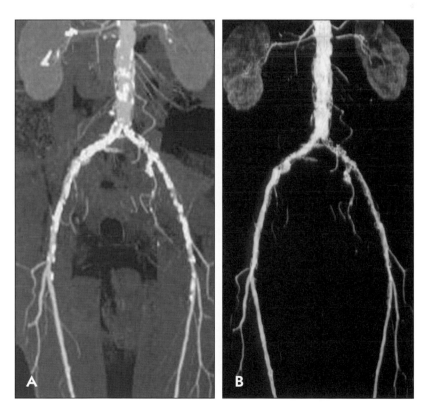

FIG. 3   A - MIP reconstruction showing the arterial wall calcifications. Because of extensive calcifications, the arterial lumen cannot be assessed. B - VRT reconstruction with transparency technique showing the patent lumen despite wall calcifications. The left iliac artery shows significant stenoses and an irregular arterial wall.

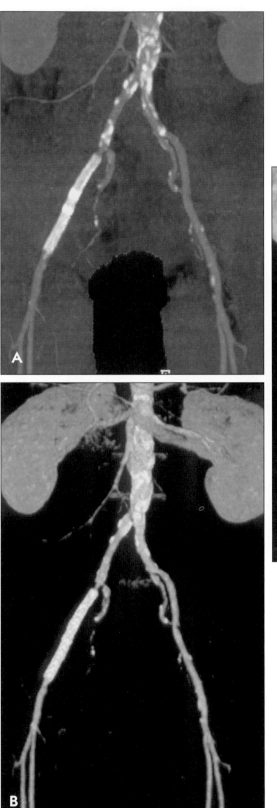

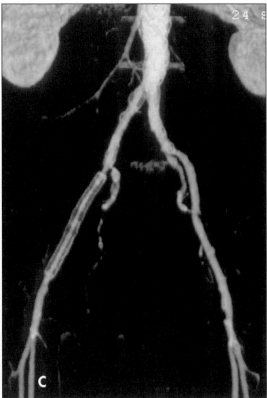

FIG. 4 A - CT angiography with MIP reconstruction. The right external iliac stent masks the arterial lumen. B - CT angiography with VRT reconstruction in the same patient. The stent obviously masks the lumen. C - CT angiography with VRT reconstruction and transparency, which now allows visualization of the lumen through the stent.

whereas MIP allows assessment of calcifications which are often not visible on conventional angiography.

VRT, however, is an operator-dependent technique because the final images depend on the choice of density thresholds. Therefore, it is possible to under- or overestimate the degree of stenosis.

ENDOGRAFTS AND METALLIC ARTEFACTS

Like calcifications, endografts have an increased density and on MIP reconstructions (Fig. 4A, p. 216) they completely mask the arterial lumen and prevent assessment of restenosis or intimal hyperplasia. Only VRT-derived reconstructions (Fig. 4B) with transparency (Fig. 4C) or multiplane reconstructions on the axis of the artery can visualize the lumen within the stent or endoprosthesis.

Metallic prostheses of the hip or knee also cause large artefacts on CT scanning, making analysis of adjacent arteries very difficult (Fig. 5). The same phenomenon is observed on MR angiography. The hip prostheses are less disruptive than the knee prostheses, which totally mask the popliteal arteries. Similarly, external fixators on the lower limb disturb distal artery assessment using CT angiography and often result in the use of conventional angiography, which itself might also be difficult to perform in such a way that usable images are produced.

Risks of CT angiography

CONTRAST NEPHROTOXICITY

Like conventional angiography, CT angiography requires injection of iodized contrast, and, therefore, carries the same risk of allergic reaction and nephrotoxicity. However, the amount of contrast to be injected for CT angiography is less than that needed for arteriography: on average 140-150 ml low osmolality non-ionic contrast for CT angiography vs. more than 200 ml for conventional arteriography. These volumes will be further decreased using the multidetector scanner.

In patients at risk (iodine allergy, renal failure) administering gadolinium as a contrast agent should be considered, although its application is still experimental and not officially agreed upon [6,7].

IRRADIATION

The multislice CT scanners comprise a higher irradiation risk, especially if thin slices on larger volumes are used [8]. Rubin et al. [9] have measured the effective doses received by the patients at the level of the abdomen and pelvis while CT- and conventional angiography are performed to assess the aorta and lower limbs. They reported an effective dose index of 0.93 cSv and 3.62 cSv for CT angiography and conventional angiography, respectively, showing a 3.9 higher rate required for intra-arterial arteriography.

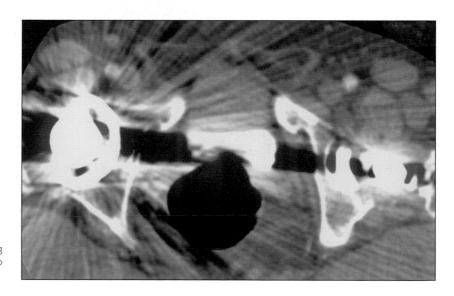

FIG. 5 CT angiography showing the metallic artefacts of a hip prosthesis.

Personal experience

In order to show the value of CT angiography in the pretherapeutic assessment of lower leg ischemia, we studied 93 scannings in 85 patients. Two groups were defined according to the level of revascularization: 52 angioscans were made prior to suprainguinal revascularization and 41 prior to infrainguinal reconstruction. Two decision attitudes were chosen by two different teams, each consisting of a radiologist and vascular surgeon, but all were members of the same team. The attitudes where then compared in order to evaluate the value of CT angiography. The first attitude was a pragmatic strategy based on the images as interpreted by the first team and on the intraoperative information including surgical treatment and, if necessary, angiography. This indicates that the results of this attitude cover the performed revascularizations. The second "virtual" attitude was chosen by the second team a posteriori, based solely on the medical file. They determined the therapeutic strategy on the basis of the same CT angiography images and the clinical information of the patient. These two strategies were compared in order to assess the agreement on the level of the lesion and the choice of revascularization. In 72 CT angiographies (77.5%), analysis of the lesions and the proposed strategies were identical. In 12 scans (12.9%), the analysis of the lesions and the choice of lesions to be treated were identical but there was a difference in the chosen revascularization technique. In 9.6% of scans, the strategies were not comparable because the lesions were interpreted differently or the scans were difficult to read. The sensitivity of CT angiography in detecting lesions and guiding the therapeutic strategy was 96% and its positive predictive value was 93%. Follow-up was reported according to the life-table method to assess the overall outcome and the results in both groups. The overall survival rate at 12 months for 85 patients was 90%. Primary patency rate at 12 months was 81%; secondary patency rate was 87%. Secondary patency rates at 12 months in the group of patients who underwent a suprainguinal and infrainguinal revascularization were 98% and 71% respectively. Overall limb salvage at 12 months was 94%.

In this setting, CT angiography allowed us to select adequate treatment in the majority of cases.

Our results with regard to patency rate, limb salvage and survival following supra- or infrainguinal revascularization based on CT angiography are comparable to the outcome as published in the literature obtained following conventional angiography.

General considerations

The goal of CT angiography is to provide at least as much as informations as conventional angiography generates. Therefore, radiologists developed specific protocols in order to allow the surgeons to determine the severity of the disease and decide on the therapeutic strategy.

In order to validate the technique of CT angiography, comparative studies with conventional angiography have been performed. These studies mainly rely on examinations performed by means of single-slice scanners [9-16] (Table) and show an acceptable agreement between both techniques. Rieker et al. [12] showed a sensitivity ranging between 94% and 100% (with a specificity of 98%-100%) in assessing arterial occlusion and a sensitivity of 73%-88% (with an associated specificity of 94%-100%) in diagnosing severe stenoses (greater than 75%) according to the level of disease.

Although there are certain discrepancies between the series, the overall outcome is very acceptable. The observed differences among the studies are related to the type of lesions: some authors only searched for occlusions or severe stenoses whereas others tried to quantify stenoses more accurately.

There was evidently less agreement when assessing smaller diameter arteries, such as lower limb, hypogastric and profunda femoral branches [15, 16]. CT angiography is superior to conventional angiography when studying popliteal pathology because the technique also assesses adjacent structures and, therefore, provides better images of aneurysms and cysts.

Rubin et al. [9] studied 378 arterial segments (aorta, common iliac, external iliac, common femoral, superficial femoral, popliteal, anterior tibial, posterior tibial, peroneal, pedal and inframalleolar posterior tibial arteries) and found a 100% agreement between CT- and conventional angiography. This study clearly illustrates the progress obtained with multislice scanners.

Table COMPARISON OF CONVENTIONAL ANGIOGRAPHY AND CT ANGIOGRAPHY

First author [ref.]	Year	Number of patients	Pathology	Scanner and reconstruction	Comparison	Results %
Lawrence [10]	1995	N = 6 134 arterial segments	PVD (aorta + LLA)	Single slice MIP, axial slices	Conventional angiography DSA	Sensitivity: 92.9 Specificity: 96.2
Raptopoulos [11]	1996	N = 39 18 comparison CT/angio	PVD and aneurysms (aorta + IA)	Single slice MIP, MPR, SSD, axial slices, cine	Conventional angiography	*Stenoses (85-99) and aneurysms:* agreement: 90 sensitivity: 93 specificity: 96
Rieker [12]	1996	N = 50	PVD (aorta + LLA)	Single slice MIP, axial slices, cine	DSA	*Occlusions:* sensitivity: 94-100 specificity: 98-100 *Stenoses:* sensitivity: 73-88 specificity: 94-100
Beregi [13]	1997	N = 26 52 popliteal arteries	Popliteal arteries	Simple slice, axial slices, MPR, SSD	Conventional angiography DSA	Agreement: 100
Kramer [14]	1998	N = 20	PVD (aorta + LLA)	Multislice, MIP, axial slices	DSA	*Sensitivity: 94* decreased to 65 if only MIP assessment
Walter [15]	2001	N = 22 24 comparison CT/angio	PVD (aorta + LLA)	Single slice, VRT, axial slices, cine	DSA	Iliac: agreement 64-66 SFA: agreement 77 Profunda: agreement 36 LLA: agreement 50-72
Tins [16]	2001	N = 35	PVD + IA	Single slice MPR, axial slices	Conventional angiography	Agreement: 84
Rubin [9]	2001	N = 24 18 comparison CT/angio 378 arterial segments	PVD (aorta + LLA)	Multislice (4), MIP, VRT, MPR, axial slices	Conventional angiography	Agreement: 100
Personal experience	2002	N = 85 93 CT	PVD (aorta + LLA)	Multislice MIP, VRT, axial slices	Two therapeutic strategies	Sensitivity: 96

CT : computer tomography
DSA: digital substraction angiography
IA : iliac arteries
LLA: lower limb arteries
MIP: maximum intensity projection

MPR: multiplanar reconstruction
PVD: peripheral vascular disease
SFA : superficial femoral artery
SSD : surface shading display
VRT: volume rendering technique

Conclusion

Conventional angiography remains an essential modality for visualizing distal arteries in the lower limb, especially in intraoperative circumstances. The arrival of the multislice scanners performing millimeter slices, associated with automated detection of contrast arrival, should provide accurate visualization of ankle and foot arteries. CT angiography of the aorta and lower limb arteries represents a valuable alternative to conventional arteriography as a modality for detecting the pathology involved and guiding the necessary therapeutic strategy.

REFERENCES

1 Blum A, Walter F, Ludig T et al. Multislice CT: principles and new CT-scan applications. *J Radiol* 2000; 81: 1597-1614.

2 Rubin GD. MDCT imaging of the aorta and peripheral vessels. *Eur J Radiol* 2003; 45 suppl 1: S42-49.

3 Cordoliani YS. Multi-detector helical CT: increased pitch does not mean decreased exposure. *J Radiol* 2000; 81: 587-588.

4 Remy-Jardin M, Bonnel F, Masson P, Remy J. Reconstruction techniques in spiral CT angiography. *J Radiol* 1999; 80: 988-997.

5 Marcus C, Ladam-Marcus V, Bertini C et al. Volume rendering technique in 3D vascular imaging. *J Radiol* 1997; 78: 481-484.

6 Gierada DS, Bae KT. Gadolinium as a CT contrast agent: assessment in a porcine model. *Radiology* 1999; 210: 829-834.

7 Kawano T, Ishijima H, Nakajima T et al. Gd-DTPA: a possible alternative contrast agent for use in CT during intraarterial administration. *J Comput Assist Tomogr* 1999; 23: 939-940.

8 McCollough CH, Zink FE. Performance evaluation of a multi-slice CT system. *Med Phys* 1999; 26: 2223-2230.

9 Rubin GD, Schmidt AJ, Logan LJ, Sofilos MC. Multi-detector row CT angiography of lower extremity arterial inflow and runoff: initial experience. *Radiology* 2001; 221: 146-158.

10 Lawrence JA, Kim D, Kent KC et al. Lower extremity spiral CT angiography versus catheter angiography. *Radiology* 1995; 194: 903-908.

11 Raptopoulos V, Rosen MP, Kent KC et al. Sequential helical CT angiography of aortoiliac disease. *AJR Am J Roentgenol* 1996; 166: 1347-1354.

12 Rieker O, Duber C, Schmiedt W et al. Prospective comparison of CT angiography of the legs with intraarterial digital subtraction angiography. *AJR Am J Roentgenol* 1996; 166: 269-276.

13 Beregi JP, Djabbari M, Desmoucelle F et al. Popliteal vascular disease: evaluation with spiral CT angiography. *Radiology* 1997; 203: 477-483.

14 Kramer SC, Gorich J, Aschoff AJ et al. Diagnostic value of spiral-CT angiography in comparison with digital subtraction angiography before and after peripheral vascular intervention. *Angiology* 1998; 49: 599-606.

15 Walter F, Leyder B, Fays J et al. Value of arteriography scanning in lower limb artery evaluation: a preliminary study. *J Radiol* 2001; 82: 473-479.

16 Tins B, Oxtoby J, Patel S. Comparison of CT angiography with conventional arterial angiography in aortoiliac occlusive disease. *Br J Radiol* 2001; 74: 219-225.

22

ARTERIAL DISSECTION AND RUPTURE DURING ENDOVASCULAR PROCEDURES

VINCENT RIAMBAU, CLARISMUNDO PONTES, XAVIER MONTAÑÁ

Several reports on iatrogenic vascular injuries have been published in the medical literature. The introduction of intravascular diagnostic techniques and endovascular devices, as well as vascular trauma induced by some orthopedic procedures and tumor resections, has caused an exponential increase in adverse vascular events.

Arterial rupture and perforation have been reported following simple Fogarty embolectomies from the beginning of their use [1]. Arterial dissections have been well documented since the first angiographic experiences with the Seldinger technique. During the 1970s, the incidence of arterial dissection after retrograde femoral arteriography [2] was 6% but the incidence has been reduced to 0.04% [3]. Although open vascular surgery can create an arterial dissection or rupture, endovascular interventions are more prone to generating these vascular complications [4-6]. However, clear information about the incidence of arterial dissections and ruptures is lacking in this actual endovascular era. In this chapter, we will address the most common clinical scenarios related to these complications occurring during endovascular procedures. We will also recommend some tips and tricks to prevent and treat specific disasters.

Endovascular injury of the iliac artery

Iliac arteries can be injured when used as an endovascular access or during local treatment of stenotic or aneurysmal disease. This explains why iliac injuries are most commonly caused by arterial accidents related to endovascular diagnostic and therapeutic procedures. Femoral access is the most commonly used endovascular approach but retrograde dissections have been underreported because they have a benign evolution, especially when no re-entry tear occurs [3]. Surveillance with duplex scan or computed tomography (CT) is strongly recommended. In contrast, anterograde dissections can persist and cause stenosis and subsequent arterial thrombosis (Fig. 1). If this type of complication is detected during the endovascular procedure, it should be repaired with simple balloon angioplasty or, if necessary, additional stenting. Furthermore, secondary complications, such as arterial thrombosis or pseudoaneurysm formation, can be detected during surveillance and often require additional vascular or endovascular repair [6]. In the majority of cases, the problem can be solved by endovascular techniques [4,5].

Arterial dissection can originate at the puncture site or may occur some centimeters higher up if preexisting atherosclerotic plaques (with or without calcium or additional tortuosities) are present in

the way of access. Moreover, iliac plaque dissections can occur as a consequence of balloon angioplasty. It is widely accepted that stenting the dissected plaque is a good solution and leaving a guide wire in place through the lesion until a final completion angiogram is performed, is recommended. The wire allows new and easy access in case an additional endovascular procedure is needed.

It is well known that difficult iliac anatomy can facilitate a dissection accident, although it may also appear even within apparently healthy iliac arteries [7]. Some practical recommendations to avoid this sometimes catastrophic complication can be outlined as follows. First of all, it is mandatory to perform clean arterial punctures. Secondly, the wire should be advanced under fluoroscopic control. A manual contrast injection can be useful in establishing the presence of an iliac dissection. Any resistance and loop shapes should be avoided. Hydrophilic wire is preferable when a puncture plastic sheath is used. Hydrophilic wires should not be used through metal needles because the sharp end can act as a blade and scratch the external hydrophilic film, with the result that some fragments might embolize. If these steps are not successful, a second puncture and attempt is a safer solution. An angiographic catheter could be a helpful tool (i.e. multipurpose catheter) in facilitating wire navigation in very tortuous arteries. The guide wire should never be pushed by means of a mechanical force. Alternatively, an anterograde approach can be used: approaching from the contralateral groin and performing a crossover technique. Also, the brachial approach with aortic pass way can be considered; the left arm is easier because of a less angulated subclavian-aortic curve. However, by using these alternatives, the endovascular procedure becomes more complex and a large amount of endovascular experience is needed in order to avoid major iatrogenic events.

Iatrogenic rupture of an iliac artery is a serious problem, specifically concerning tortuosity, if aortic endografts are used. Iliac atherosclerotic narrowing, tortuosity, calcified arteries, small iliac arteries (such as those in female or young patients) and thoracic endograft procedures are all predisposing factors for iliac ruptures. In our personal experience with aortic endografts, we encountered 3 iliac ruptures in 400 procedures (0.7%). All 3 cases were related to a thoracic endograft procedure (2.5% of all thoracic endografts) and occurred in 1 male and 2 female patients. When iliac rupture is suspected

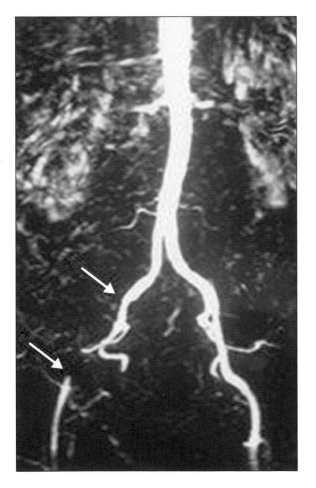

FIG. 1   Angio-MR showing an occlusion of the right external iliac artery following angiography *(white arrows).*

during an endovascular procedure, the first maneuver should aim to achieve hemorrhagic control. The quickest hemostatic control is achieved by balloon catheter occlusion of the afferent artery. If the rupture is limited and caused by a balloon angioplasty procedure, prolonged balloon dilation could be effective [5], although a covered stent is recommended in order to avoid later pseudoaneurysm formation. Where a large rupture is suspected, usually as a result of aortic endograft procedures, endoclamping with balloon catheters is effective in avoiding exsanguination, allowing hemodynamic control, and providing time to decide on the next strategy. Usually the rupture can be treated with an endograft (Fig. 2), using the same wire and access and modifying the endoclamp position using a contralateral femoral or arm access. In contrast, if the rupture is too large or a convenient endograft is not available, open surgery should be performed, leaving the endoclamp during the surgical dissection.

Obviously, the best idea is to avoid this life-threatening complication, which indicates avoidance of those with important predisposing factors, such as atherosclerotic iliac stenosis, severely calcified and tortuous small arteries (female and young patients). Additional attention is required during thoracic endografting procedures. Accurate morphologic examination is performed before the procedure by means of CT, angiography and, if possible, intravascular ultrasound. In case of any doubt concerning the iliac access, it is much better to perform a retroperitoneal approach using a transient regular vascular conduit attached to a common iliac or distal aorta. In cases of localized iliac stenosis, it can be useful to perform a balloon angioplasty just prior to introducing the sheath. Also, a simulation could be made using an equivalent introducer sheath with the same caliber of the delivery endograft system but without the endograft. This action allows for testing the quality of the iliac access without damage and with less manipulation of the delivery system. If there are no other options, or the navigation through the iliac access was done with friction and difficulties despite excellent endograft deployment, special attention should be given to the iliac axis. Removal of the big sheath should be done carefully with the dilator inside and the wire should be left inside until the final angiogram excludes suspected iliac injuries. Leaving the guide wire in place allows the opportunity of applying additional endovascular devices as well as a balloon catheter. Even if a thoracic endograft could be placed with a single arterial approach, it is recommended that at least two arterial accesses are maintained until the procedure is finally complete: the wire is the lifeline for quick endovascular control.

Other optional arterial routes for endovascular purposes, such as radial, brachial and axillary arteries, can be complicated with dissections and

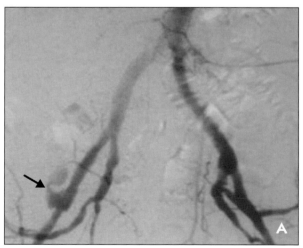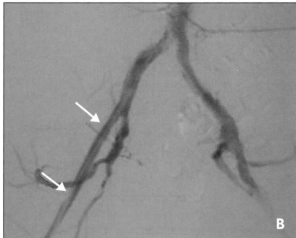

FIG. 2   A - Rupture of right external iliac artery *(black arrow)*. B - Its correction with a covered stent *(between white arrows)*.

ruptures. Unfortunately, there is no reliable information available about the incidence of these iatrogenic accidents. Nerve and vein injuries are also limiting the use of these approaches. In any of these cases, the same treatment as described above can be applied. The *body floss, through-through* or axillary-femoral access is a technique which has been used in aortic endografting procedures in order to advance in very tortuous iliac arteries. An infrequent but very dangerous accident is subclavian ostium rupture due to wire friction in the subclavian-aortic angle. Using protection by means of a short angiographic catheter crossing the subclavian ostium is recommended, thereby limiting the maneuvers as much as possible in a careful and gentle way. Again, an angiographic check is strongly recommended just before removing the protective catheter.

Endovascular injury of the abdominal aorta

Aortic injuries can be caused by diagnostic and therapeutic endovascular procedures. During the last three decades, aortic iatrogenic injuries have been related to diagnostic angiographies and retrograde dissection was the most common finding. However, the introduction of aortic endografting of thoracic and abdominal lesions would theoretically increase the incidence of catheter-related aortic injury, both in number and in severity.

Fortunately, retrograde abdominal aortic dissection due to endovascular procedures is a rare complication. Short reports can be derived from the medical literature but the incidence is very low: less than 4/10 000 [3,8]. Despite the increasing use of arterial catheterization for endovascular procedures and radiologic examinations, iatrogenic dissections of the abdominal aorta are paradoxically much rarer than spontaneous dissections. In an old review, only 2% to 4% of all aortic dissections occurred in the abdominal portion of the aorta [9]. The majority of iatrogenic abdominal aortic dissections were related to the famous translumbar aortography introduced by Dos Santos in the 1950s [10]. However, these lesions were underestimated because most iatrogenic dissections of the abdominal aorta are asymptomatic, especially if the entry is small and the re-entry is absent. In some cases, however, clinical manifestations appear and depend on the

extension or progression of the dissection. The clinical findings are comparable to those of spontaneous dissections. Acute abdominal aortic dissections may be suspected if severe chest or abdominal pain occurs immediately after contrast injection, associated with arterial hypotension and diminution or abolition of lower extremity pulses. Chronic dissections may be revealed by the onset of intermittent lower extremity claudication after angiography, or by the development of an aortic aneurysm. Duplex scanning can detect an intimal flap inside a dilated aorta, but CT is more accurate in confirming dissection and assessing its extent. Angiography is the best technique for locating the sites of entry and re-entry and assists in planning the appropriate repair (Fig. 3). The evolution of iatrogenic abdominal aortic dissection involves two risks: thrombosis of the true lumen or persistent patency of the false lumen with compression of the true lumen or rupture, especially if no re-entry tear is present.

Indications for treatment depend on the presence of complications, such as lower limb ischemia, rupture of the false lumen or the dilatation of the false lumen leading to saccular false aneurysms. All iatrogenic abdominal aortic dissections, even the asymp-

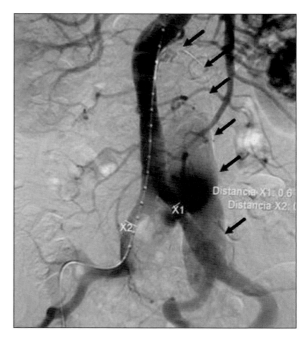

FIG. 3 Angiogram of aorto-iliac dissection with aneurysm formation *(black arrows)*.

tomatic ones, should be monitored with CT scanning or magnetic resonance to assess any changes in the dissection features. The surgical management of these lesions has a wide spectrum and includes prosthetic replacement of the aorta, surgical fenestration or extra-anatomic bypass without aortic repair. Endovascular treatment includes fenestration, balloon angioplasty (with or without stents) and aortic endografting [11,12]. The problem is substantially worse if the suprarenal aorta is also affected by the dissection. This situation requires more complex open surgery or endovascular repair with fenestrated or branched endografts. Selective visceral stenting has been suggested for some special cases.

The occurrence of iatrogenic rupture of the abdominal aorta during endovascular procedures is extremely rare. There are some anecdotal reports addressing this event during elective endovascular repair of abdominal aortic aneurysms. A fast therapeutic response is needed when this life-threatening situation occurs and the endovascular team must act as it if were a ruptured aneurysm; this implies application of an aortic balloon above the renal arteries and completing the endovascular repair as usual. If the patient remains unstable the retrograde flow can be controlled with additional iliac balloons. If the endovascular treatment cannot be applied for any reason, conversion to open repair should be performed.

Endovascular injury of the thoracic aorta

An interesting review of the IRAD (The *International Registry of Acute Aortic Dissection*) [13] demonstrated that iatrogenic dissection of the thoracic aorta was surprisingly common. Although proximal iatrogenic aortic dissection (type A) most often followed cardiac surgery, distal dissections (type B) were more likely to follow cardiac catheterization or interventional procedures. Compared with spontaneous aortic dissection, patients with iatrogenic dissections were older and tended to have a higher incidence of arteriosclerosis. In addition, the diagnosis of iatrogenic dissections was difficult to make due to its atypical presentation and the relative lack of classic signs of aortic dissection on imaging studies. This report concluded that mortality for iatrogenic dissections is high, specifically in cases of

type B iatrogenic dissections, and exceeds mortality for spontaneous dissection.

The incidence of iatrogenic thoracic aortic dissection has probably increased during the past few years as a result of the incorporation of the new endovascular procedures, particularly thoracic endografting. Unfortunately, reliable information about the incidence and prevalence of these vascular complications is lacking. Many case reports about retrograde type A dissection following endovascular treatment of type B dissection or aneurysm have recently been published [14-17]. In our study of 120 thoracic endografts, we have 2 cases of retrograde type A dissection; one case following endovascular treatment of an arch aneurysm (Fig. 4) and another following repair of an acute symptomatic type B dissection. Anecdotal cases on iatrogenic type B dissection have been described following different endovascular procedures, such as endovascular repair of an abdominal aneurysm [18] or balloon angioplasty of native aortic coarctation [19].

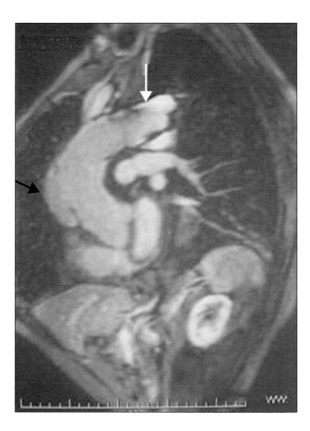

FIG. 4 Type A dissection *(black arrow)* following endovascular repair of a saccular arch aneurysm *(white arrow)*.

Treatment of these thoracic aortic complications does not differ from the management of spontaneous dissection. Iatrogenic type A dissection requires emergent surgical correction and type B dissection can be treated medically or, if necessary, by means of open or endovascular techniques, depending on morphology and symptoms.

Iatrogenic thoracic aortic rupture is a very rare consequence of endovascular treatment, although it may occur in the context of endovascular repair of aortic dissection, aneurysm or traumatic lesions. Endovascular treatment of this catastrophic event is potentially the best and fastest solution. Again, a balloon catheter and maintenance of the wire are crucial in trying to avoid a fatal outcome. For centers with a high volume of aortic endografting, having thoracic endografts on the shelf is recommended.

As for the rest of endovascular injuries, prevention is the most practical recommendation. Careful manipulations of wires and catheters is important. Appropriate stiff wires should be used and lateral movements with big sheaths should be avoided. Ballooning in dissected aortas should also be avoided. Gentle oversized long endografts, which cover enough aortic surface above and below the lesion, are preferred. Further aortic endograft designs will perhaps play a role in preventing these complications.

Miscellaneous arterial endovascular injuries

Any vascular field amenable to endovascular therapy has a potential risk of iatrogenic dissection or rupture. Therefore, lower limb, renal [20], mesenteric [21], celiac axis [22], pulmonary and supra-aortic arteries [23,24] can all be areas for adverse events. Fortunately, the prevalence of such complications seems to be low, although reliable data are not available. Dissection or rupture of these vessels can lead to an occlusion, pseudoaneurysm formation or hemorrhage. Endovascular treatment can be applied using bare or covered stents and even balloon fenestration could be useful [22]. In small vessels, endovascular embolization with coils is an acceptable solution.

In conclusion, even with the explosion of endovascular therapy, iatrogenic arterial dissection and ruptures rarely occur. However, the situation can be catastrophic when these complications occur. All endovascular specialists must be aware of these circumstances and their management. Endovascular complications should be repaired by endovascular techniques as a first choice because of their speed and effectiveness. Prevention is, nevertheless, the best advice.

REFERENCES

1 Stoney RJ, Ehrenfeld WK, Wylie EJ. Arterial rupture after insertion of a Fogarty catheter. *Am J Surg* 1968; 115: 830-831.

2 Bryk D, Yound RS, Roska JC, Moadel E. Arterial dissection with use of catheter needle in retrograde femoral arteriography. *J Can Assoc Radiol* 1979; 30: 46-47.

3 Sakamoto I, Hayashi K, Matsunaga N et al. Aortic dissection caused by angiographic procedures. *Radiology* 1994; 191: 467-471.

4 Murphy TP, Dorfman GS, Segall M, Carney WI Jr. Iatrogenic arterial dissection: treatment by percutaneous transluminal angioplasty. *Cardiovasc Intervent Radiol* 1991; 14: 302-306.

5 Berger H, Steiner W, Waggershauser T et al. The percutaneous treatment of surgical and catheter-angiographic vascular complications. *Rofo* 1995; 162: 506-513.

6 Giswold ME, Landry GJ, Taylor LM, Moneta GL. Iatrogenic arterial injury is an increasingly important cause of arterial trauma. *Am J Surg* 2004; 187: 590-592.

7 Tillich M, Bell RE, Paik DS et al. Iliac arterial injuries after endovascular repair of abdominal aortic aneurysms: correlation with iliac curvature and diameter. *Radiology* 2001; 219: 129-136.

8 Bariseel H, Batt M, Rogopoulos A. Iatrogenic dissection of the abdominal aorta. *J Vasc Surg* 1998; 27: 366-370.

9 Hirst Ae Jr, Johns Vj Jr, Kime Sw Jr. Dissecting aneurysm of the aorta: a review of 505 cases. *Medicine* (Baltimore) 1958; 37: 217-279.

10 Gaylis H, Laws JW. Dissection of aorta as a complication of translumbar aortography. *Br Med J* 1956; 12: 1141-1146.

11 Johnson MS, Lalka SG. Successful treatment of an iatrogenic infrarenal aortic dissection with serial Wallstents. *Ann Vasc Surg* 1997; 11: 295-299.

12 Gorog DA, Watkinson A, Lipkin DP. Treatment of iatrogenic aortic dissection by percutaneous stent placement. *J Invasive Cardiol* 2003; 15: 84-85.

13 Januzzi JL, Sabatine MS, Eagle KA et al. Iatrogenic aortic dissection. *Am J Cardiol* 2002; 89: 623-626.

14 Modine T, Lions C, Destrieux-Garnier L et al. Iatrogenic iliac artery rupture and type A dissection after endovascular repair of type B aortic dissection. *Ann Thorac Surg* 2004; 77: 317-319.

15 Fanelli F, Salvatori FM, Marcelli G et al. Type A aortic dissection developing during endovascular repair of an acute type B dissection. *J Endovasc Ther* 2003; 10: 254-259.

16 Urbanski PP. Retrograde extension of type B dissection after endovascular stent-graft repair. *Eur J Cardiothorac Surg* 2002; 21: 767-768.

17 Bethuyne N, Bove T, Van den Brande P, Goldstein JP. Acute retrograde aortic dissection during endovascular repair of a thoracic aortic aneurysm. *Ann Thorac Surg* 2003; 75: 1967-1969.

18 Haulon S, Greenberg RK, Khwaja J et al. Aortic dissection in the setting of an infrarenal endoprosthesis: a fatal combination. *J Vasc Surg* 2003; 38: 1121-1124.

19 Aydogan U, Dindar A, Gurgan L, Cantez T. Late development of dissecting aneurysm following balloon angioplasty of native aortic coarctation. *Cathet Cardiovasc Diagn* 1995; 36: 226-229.

20 Morris CS, Bonnevie GJ, Najarian KE. Nonsurgical treatment of acute iatrogenic renal artery injuries occurring after renal artery angioplasty and stenting. *AJR Am J Roentgenol* 2001; 177: 1353-1357.

21 Desgranges P, Bourriez PA, d'Audiffret A et al. Percutaneous stenting of a iatrogenic superior mesenteric artery dissection complicating suprarenal aortic aneurysm repair. *J Endovasc Ther* 2000; 7: 501-505.

22 So YH, Chung JW, Park JH. Balloon fenestration of iatrogenic celiac artery dissection. *J Vasc Interv Radiol* 2003; 14: 493-496.

23 Galli M, Goldberg SL, Zerboni S, Almagor Y. Balloon expandable stent implantation after iatrogenic arterial dissection of the left subclavian artery. *Cathet Cardiovasc Diagn* 1995; 35: 355-357.

24 Finlay DJ, Sanchez LA, Sicard GA. Subclavian artery injury, vertebral artery dissection, and arteriovenous fistulae following attempt at central line placement. *Ann Vasc Surg* 2002; 16: 774-778.

23

EXPANSION OF THE ANEURYSMAL NECK AND PROXIMAL STENT-GRAFT MIGRATION

LINA LEURS, GUIDO STULTIËNS, JUR KIEVIT, JAAP BUTH

It is now understood that the configuration of the aortoiliac vascular anatomy may change significantly after endovascular abdominal aortic aneurysm repair (EVAR). One of the morphologic changes concerns the increase of the diameter of the proximal neck. Late neck dilatation may be caused by a number of mechanisms including: continued aneurysmal degeneration of segments adjacent to the aneurysm; shortening of the neck in case of incomplete aneurysm exclusion, with expansion of the sac; and radial force exerted by the proximal fixation stent.

The position of the implanted endograft may also be subject to changes during follow-up. This may occur either in response to progressive enlargement of the aneurysm neck or independently. Migration of the proximal stent-graft, because of destabilized fixation is an important complication of EVAR, with recognized associations with late aneurysm rupture, proximal endoleak, graft kinking and graft limb thrombosis [1,2].

Movement of the endograft occurs when the displacement forces on the endograft exceed the strength of fixation at the proximal attachment zones (Fig. 1). With early generations of endografts, migration was a frequent event, the incidence of which increased progressively with time. Cumulative rate of migration in these older series was as high as 75% after 7 years of follow-up [3,4].

This report is based on an assessment of the EUROSTAR database (European Stent-graft Treatment of Abdominal Aortic Aneurysms Registry) and has the objective to study the prevalence of aneurysmal dilatation, proximal migration of the stent-graft and the correlation between these two phenomena (Fig. 1). Implications of these findings for post-EVAR surveillance will be discussed.

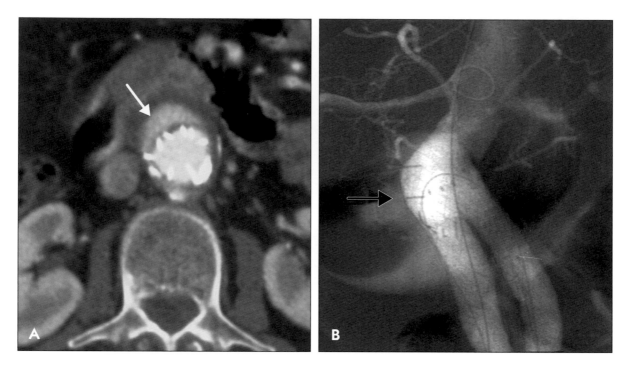

FIG. 1   A - Example of neck dilatation with proximal endoleak indicated by white arrow.   B - Stent-graft migration indicated by black arrow.

Methods

This chapter summarizes the experience collated in the EUROSTAR-database, with the data of 4403 patients operated over a 10-year period between 1994 and 2004, constituting the basis of this analysis. The experience was obtained in 147 centers in Europe. All patients had a minimal follow-up of one month. Patients with an aneurysm smaller than 4 centimeters in diameter, including those with large iliac aneurysms, were excluded from this study group. In addition, patients in whom neck diameters were measured on less than two occasions were excluded from analysis. Only migration of the proximal stent-graft was considered for this analysis. This selection involved checking free text fields of case record forms with recorded migration to distinguish proximal from distal stent-graft migration and component dislocation.

Baseline data, including comorbidity, estimate of unfitness for open repair, anatomic aspects and operative details were recorded by the participating institutions on case record forms and submitted for inclusion to the Data Registry Center. Findings at follow-up visits, which involved clinical examination, CT-assessment or (in 5% of the visits) angiographic, MRI or ultrasound follow-up studies were recorded in data forms and returned at regular intervals to the Data Registry Center for processing and analysis. Since 2002 all data transmission is by Internet connection (*KIKA Medical Communications, Nancy, France*).

Growth of the infrarenal aneurysm neck was determined on the recording of an increase of the diameter measured 3 millimeters distally from the lower renal artery. The measurement was performed from outer wall to outer wall across the minor diameter on the axial CT-slice. Growth of the aneurysm neck was defined as a diameter increase of at least 4 millimeters relative to the preoperative measurements on CT. The maximum-recorded neck diameter during follow-up was taken to identify neck expansion. The diagnosis of migration was made entirely on the judgement of the management team of any individual patient. Although in the majority of cases details regarding the site of the migration was provided on the follow-up form, the extent of the migration was rarely quantified as device displacement in millimeters.

Standard statistical methods were used as in previous EUROSTAR-publications [5-7]. In addition, a multivariate analysis with adjustment for follow-up time was used to determine variables, with an independent correlation with neck growth and device migration respectively as the outcome event.

Results

The 4403 patients, 4122 (93.6%) male and 281 (6.4%) female, ranged in age from 37 to 101 years. The average diameter of the aneurysm sac was 5.8 centimeters (4-1centimeters) in minor dimension. Patient characteristics grouped according to general/systemic factors, morphologic factors and procedural/device-related factors are summarized in Table I.

Of the entire patient group, 2804 had neither neck dilatation or device migration. Neck dilatation without migration was observed in 1400 patients. The group that had device migration, but no dilatation was 87 (3% of all migrators). The group with migration and dilatation was 112 (7% of all migra-

tors). The correlation between migration and dilatation of the neck was statistically significant (p < 0.0001). In order to examine the relation between the two phenomena in the study further, the timing was assessed in the 112 patients that had dilatation as well as migration (Fig. 2). The proportion in whom neck dilatation preceded the migration was 36%, migration was identified first in 27%, and dilatation and migration occurring at the same follow-up visit in 37%.

A number of general clinical, morphologic and procedural/device-related factors were entered into the multivariate Cox-model in order to examine the independent influence of clinical variables further (Table II). Neck dilatation had a positive correlation (occurred more frequently) when the proximal oversizing was 20% or greater and with increasing device main diameter. A negative correlation (less frequent neck dilatation) was observed in patients with smaller necks and a device category that had no supra-renal bare stent or hook fixation (the combined category of AneuRx®, Excluder®, Vanguard® and Stentor® devices). Most importantly, migration, when entered as a variable in the model, had no

Table I DEMOGRAPHIC CHARACTERISTICS, MORPHOLOGIC AND PROCEDURAL DETAILS IN 4403 PATIENTS

	Patients number	%
General and systemic factors		
Gender	4122	93.6
Hypotension	2738	62.2
Smoking	1028	23.4
Morphologic factors		
Neck length	23.4 +/- 3.0	
Neck diameter	27.6 +/- 12.9	
Significant neck angulation	1016	
Aneurysm diameter	57.6 +/- 10.5	
Device/neck diameter ratio ≥ 1.20%	1129	
Procedure and device-related factors		
Use of aortic extension cuff	144	3.3
Intraoperative proximal endoleak	1849	42.0
Absence of proximal bare stent fixation	124	2.8

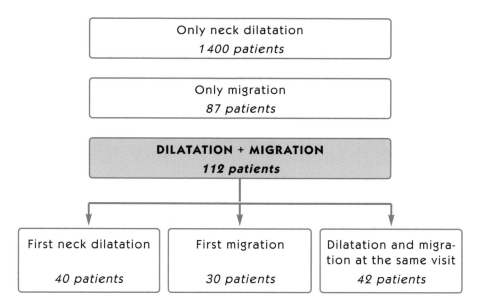

FIG. 2 Findings regarding neck dilatation and device migration. Relation with time of identification of these findings.

Table II	RISK FACTORS OF DILATATION, MULTIVARIATE COX-ANALYSIS OF 4403 PATIENTS		
	Hazard ratio	*95% Confidence limits*	*p-value*
Hypertension	-		
Smoking	-		
Neck diameter	0.83	0.80 - 0.86	< 0.0001
Aneurysm diameter	-		
Neck length	-		
Neck angulation	-		
Device/neck diameter ratio ≥ 20%	-		
Device main diameter	1.13	1.09 - 1.17	< 0.0001
Use of aortic extension cuff	-		
Intraoperative proximal endoleak	-		
No suprarenal fixation system or hooks	0.58	0.52 - 0.66	< 0.0001
Device migration	**0.90**	**0.73 - 1.11**	**0.3**

statistical influence on the occurrence of neck dilatation.

Similarly, a multivariate analysis with device migration as the outcome event using the same variables demonstrated a weak, but negative, influ-ence of hypertension and a positive association of neck diameter, aneurysm diameter and absence of a suprarenal fixation system. A shorter neck length was associated with increased tendency of migra-tion (Table III). Finally, and most importantly, neck dilatation had an independent statistically significant positive effect on the occurrence of device migration.

The various endograft types were compared in an univariate analysis with the frequency of the two outcome events (Table IV). Two main categories

Table III RISK FACTORS OF MIGRATION, MULTIVARIATE COX-ANALYSIS OF 4403 PATIENTS

	Hazard ratio	95% Confidence limits	p-value
Hypertension	0.74	0.55 - 0.98	0.03
Smoking	-		
Neck diameter	1.09	1.03 - 1.15	0.002
Aneurysm diameter	1.005	1.001- 1.009	0.02
Neck length	0.98	0.966- 0.994	0.005
Neck angulation	-		
Device/neck diameter ratio ≥20%	-		
Device main diameter	-		
Use of aortic extension cuff	-		
Intraoperative proximal endoleak	-		
No suprarenal fixation system or hooks	2.12	1.52 - 2.96	< 0.0001
Infrarenal neck dilatation	**1.48**	**1.09 - 2.01**	**0.01**

23
233

Table IV UNIVARIATE COMPARISON OF DIFFERENT DEVICE BRANDS WITH NECK DILATATION AND DEVICE MIGRATION IN 4403 PATIENTS

Devices	Number of patients *	% with dilatation	% with migration
With suprarenal fixation or hooks	**2554**	**33**	**2.4**
Talent	932	34	3.8
Zenith	1237	35	0.9
Lifepath	69	27	5.8
EVT/Ancure	144	17	1.4
Others	172	25	5.8
Without suprarenal fixation or hooks	**1849**	**36**	**7.4**
Vanguard/Stentor	670	44	11.0
AneuRx	693	38	8.4
Excluder	486	22	1.6

* The device brand was not recorded in 17 patients.

were distinguished: devices with suprarenal fixation or anchoring hooks (Talent®, Zenith®, Lifepath®, EVT/Ancure® and others), and devices without suprarenal fixation or hooks (Vanguard®, Stentor®, AneuRx®, Excluder®). It is obvious from this table that suprarenal fixation may not protect so much from dilatation of the neck (33% vs. 36% for patients with suprarenal fixation and hooks and without respectively, p = 0.02), but does protect against device migration (prevalence 2.4% in patients with suprarenal fixation or hooks vs. 7.4% in patients without suprarenal fixation or hooks, p < 0.0001).

Discussion

Neck dilatation has been described as a continuous process by several investigators [8, 9,10]. In a provoking article, May et al. presented evidence to suggest that endografts positioned correctly immediately below the renal arteries may protect the infrarenal aortic segment from further dilatation in a manner that does not occur after open repair of an abdominal aortic aneurysm (AAA) [11]. In this study, several factors have been associated with proximal neck dilatation after endovascular AAA repair including smoking, initial wide-size neck and large stent-graft diameter, and absence of suprarenal or hook fixation. The influence of smoking could not be established in our study. In addition, large diameter aneurysms and aneurysm sac expansion have been linked to shortening of the infrarenal neck. Cao et al. found significant dilatation of the infrarenal neck in 20% of patients with a positive correlation with wide preoperative necks, mural thrombus in the neck, and large size aneurysm diameter [12]. No correlation with neck dilatation in their and our analysis was found with regard to neck angulation, neck length, excessive proximal oversizing, early endoleak or suprarenal fixation. Nevertheless, in Cao's experience, significant proximal neck dilatation was a harbinger of risk as 20% either had a proximal extension cuff or a conversion, and 13.8% demonstrated device migration. This compared unfavorably with the 2.0% of non-dilators who had a cuff or conversion and 0.8% who had a migration.

Mohan et al. [13] have indicated increased systolic blood pressure, reversed conical infrarenal necks (increase of diameter from proximally to distally) and significant angulation of iliac arteries as

significant downward displacement forces. Although in our analysis neck dilatation correlated statistically significant with proximal migration, there is a large proportion that demonstrates no adverse consequences from widening of the neck. This may be due to improvements in graft design and technology including increased radial force ascertained by self-expanding stents, hooks, barbs and most importantly suprarenal fixation. Another factor that has impacted favorably upon the issue of proximal migration is the tendency of interventionalists to oversize the stent-graft relative to the proximal neck by 15% to 20%, more than the 5% to 10% advocated originally. When commercial devices became available, the incidence of migration of the proximal stent (5 millimeters as distal movement) decreased to 3% and, in a recent study relating to a second generation endograft, evidence of clinically significant migration was observed in just 1% of cases at two years after the operation [13,14].

Opinions about the mechanisms of late migration vary. Some authorities have reported progressive enlargement of the aneurysm neck and claim that this may destabilize fixation. Patients with larger aneurysms appear to be at significantly higher risk from neck dilatation [12,15]. This observation was confirmed in this study. There is agreement that careful patient selection, by excluding patients with necks that are excessively angulated or too short, and accurate placement of the graft adjacent to the renal arteries both help to minimize the risk of distal migration [11,15]. As a general principle, maximal overlapping of all healthy tissue until the acknowledged anatomical boundaries of the renal arteries proximally should be the aim.

Excessive endograft oversizing (more than 20% diameter) may accelerate the process of neck dilatation and, perhaps, thereby migration [16]. As in our own study, neck angulation was not a risk factor for migration in the study of Conners et al. [15].

There are reasons to believe that migration can lead to sudden loss of "seal" with immediately disastrous consequences. Therefore, it is advisable that secondary intervention, usually by placement of an extension cuff, should be undertaken sooner rather than later when migration has been identified. Thus, vigorous endograft surveillance may prevent aneurysm-related death by identifying infrarenal neck dilatation and/or endograft migration [17]. Vigorous surveillance using CT-scanning and plain abdominal X-rays according to a standardized protocol is a proven method to detect migration [18,

23

234

19]. In this study, it was documented that migration may be caused by neck dilatation. However, other mechanisms, such as progressive wall degeneration, are also likely to play a role. Accepted criteria of neck dimensions should be adhered to in order to obtain acceptable results from EVAR.

REFERENCES

1 Resch T, Ivancev K, Brunkwall J et al. Distal migration of stent-grafts after endovascular repair of abdominal aortic aneurysms. *J Vasc Interv Radiol* 1999; 10: 257-264.

2 Harris PL, Vallabhaneni SR, Desgranges P et al. Incidence and risk factors of late rupture, conversion and death after endovascular repair of infrarenal aortic aneurysms: the EUROSTAR experience. *J Vasc Surg* 2000; 32: 739-479.

3 Alric P, Hinchliffe RJ, Wenham PW et al. Lessons learned from the long-term follow-up of a first-generation aortic stent graft. *J Vasc Surg* 2003; 37: 367-373.

4 Resch T, Malina M, Lindblad B, Ivancev K. The impact of stent-graft development on outcome of AAA-repair: a 7-year experience. *Eur J Vasc Endovasc Surg* 2001; 22: 57-61.

5 Peppelenbosch N, Buth J, Harris PL et al. Diameter of abdominal aortic aneurysm and outcome of endovascular aneurysm repair: does size matter? A report from EUROSTAR. *J Vasc Surg* 2004; 39: 288-297.

6 Torella F. Effect of improved endograft design on outcome of endovascular aneurysm repair. *J Vasc Surg* 2004; 40: 216-221.

7 Leurs LJ, Hobo R, Buth J. The multicenter experience with a third-generation endovascular device for abdominal aortic aneurysm repair. A report from the EUROSTAR database. *J Cardiovasc Surg* 2004; 45: 293-300.

8 Wever JJ, Blankensteijn JD, Th M Mali WP, Eikelboom BC. Maximal aneurysm diameter follow-up is inadequate after endovascular abdominal aneurysm repair. *Eur J Vasc Endovasc Surg* 2000; 20: 177-182.

9 Resch T, Malina M, Lindblad B et al. The impact of stent design on proximal stent-graft fixation in the abdominal aorta: an experimental study. *Eur J Vasc Endovasc Surg* 2000; 20: 190-195.

10 Matsumura JS, Chaikof EL. Continued expansion of aortic necks after endovascular repair of abdominal aortic aneurysms. EVT Investigators, EndoVascular Technologies, Inc *J Vasc Surg* 1998; 28: 422-430.

11 May J, White GH, Ly CN et al. Endoluminal repair of abdominal aortic aneurysm prevents enlargement of the proximal neck: a 9-year life table and 5-year longitudinal study. *J Vasc Surg* 2003; 37: 86-90.

12 Cao P, Verzini F, Parlani G et al. Predictive factors and clinical consequences of proximal aortic neck dilatation in 230 patients undergoing abdominal aorta aneurysm repair with-self-expandable stent-graft. *J Vasc Surg* 2003; 37: 1200-1205.

13 Mohan IV, Harris PL, van Marrewijk CJ et al. Factors and forces influencing stent-graft migration after endovascular aortic aneurysm repair. *J Endovasc Ther* 2002; 9: 748-755.

14 Matsumura JS, Brewster DC, Makaroun MS, Naftel DC. A multicenter controlled clinical trial of open versus endovascular treatment of abdominal aortic aneurysm. *J Vasc Surg* 2003; 37: 262-271.

15 Conners MS, Sternbergh WC, Carter G et al. Endograft migration one to four years after endovascular abdominal aortic aneurysm repair with the AneuRx device: a cautionary note. *J Vasc Surg* 2002; 36: 476-484.

16 Sternbergh WC, Money SR, Greenberg RK, Chuter TA. Influence of endograft oversizing on device migration, endoleak, aneurysm shrinkage, and aortic neck dilatation: results from the Zenith multicenter trial. *J Vasc Surg* 2004; 39: 20-26.

17 Cao P, Verzini F, Zannetti S et al. Device migration after endoluminal abdominal aortic aneurysm repair: analysis of 113 cases with a minimum follow-up of 2 years. *J Vasc Surg* 2002; 35: 229-235.

18 Beebe HG, Jackson T, Pigott JP. Aortic aneurysm morphology for planning endovascular aortic grafts: limitations of conventional imaging methods. *J Endovasc Surg* 1995; 2: 139-148.

19 Murphy M, Hodgson R, Harris PL et al. Plain radiographic surveillance of abdominal aortic stent-grafts. The Liverpool/Perth protocol. *J Endovasc Ther* 2003; 10: 911-912.

ENDOVASCULAR AIDS
FOR CONTROLLING
OPEN SURGICAL BLEEDING

WILLEM WISSELINK, JAN RAUWERDA

In the situation of open surgical bleeding, traditional means of hemostatic control such as clamping, remote or direct compression usually require additional surgical dissection and/or preclude adequate exposure for vascular repair. Extensive vascular dissection in the face of active bleeding is technically difficult, time-consuming, and may aggravate the bleeding problem due to poor visualization. Use of endovascular aids such as occluding balloons, shunts and stent-grafts may avoid the need for additional dissection and at the same time provide adequate exposure for vascular repair. The literature on this subject is scattered and anecdotal, probably due to its obviousness: "when it works it works". In this chapter, endoluminal hemostatic techniques, from the neck down, are reviewed and are interspersed with tricks and tips from personal experience which the authors hope will benefit those entering the field.

Endovascular aids
to control bleeding in the
neck and thoracic outlet

Balloon catheter tamponade can be a useful technique to control intraoperative hemorrhage from inaccessible or fragile vascular structures in the neck and thoracic outlet. Such inaccessible structures include: the internal carotid artery and the internal jugular vein at the base of the skull; the internal maxillary artery and its deep branches; and the vertebral artery (except its proximal segment which is surgically accessible). Feliciano et al. [1] described intraoperative placement of No.3 to No.8 Fogarty embolectomy catheters with a three-way stopcock directly into the bleeding artery or vein. Inflation of the balloon led to control of hemorrhage in most cases, allowing for subsequent surgical repair and control at the site of injury. An even more expeditious approach is transcutaneous balloon catheter tamponade which has been advocated for selected cases of penetrating vascular trauma in the neck and clavicular region. DiGiacomo et al. [2] described placement of 18F Foley catheters directly in the gunshot track or stab wound in tow patients, following exsanguinating hemorrhage resulting from penetrating injury in the infraclavicular area. Bleeding ceased immediately following inflation of the balloon with 10 ml of sterile saline. No arterial injuries were identified by angiography, whereas venography demonstrated balloon tamponade of the axillary vein with filling of the subclavian vein via collaterals. Three to four days later, the balloon was deflated and the wound loosely packed without recurrent bleeding. Alternatively, this method can be used temporarily, allowing time for further workup and transportation to the operating room for definitive control and vessel repair.

Endovascular aids to control bleeding in the chest

During thoracoabdominal aortic aneurysm repair, especially in the presence of a dissection, profuse bleeding usually occurs from multiple patent intercostal arteries upon opening the thoracic aorta. Immediate, temporary control of back-bleeding from intercostal arteries is mandatory in order to maintain collateral perfusion pressure to the spinal cord until reperfusion is established [3]. Use of Fogarty embolectomy catheters towards this goal is a simple, direct, atraumatic and reversible technique. Many different techniques for balloon occlusion in penetrating cardiac trauma have been described elsewhere [1].

Endovascular aids to control bleeding in the abdomen and pelvis

Embolization of pelvic vessels for bleeding after pelvic fractures, and also in cases where laparotomy is indicated for bleeding from other sources, has been well reported in the trauma literature and is beyond the scope of this chapter [4,5].

During suprarenal aortic clamping for repair of juxtarenal aneurysm, endoluminal occlusion of the renal arteries with 9 French Pruitt infusion catheters offers, besides hemostasis, the option for perfusion of the kidneys with cold saline. Although there is no evidence to support renal protection in this setting and many authors claim they perform the proximal anastomosis routinely in less than 15 minutes, we have found this technique of renal cooling and occlusion to provide extra time and ease in a teaching situation [6].

In the face of ruptured abdominal aortic aneurysm, several authors have described placement of supraceliac or suprarenal aortic occlusion balloons (Reliant®, *Medtronic, Santa Rosa, CA, USA*) over a guidewire via a transfemoral or transbrachial approach [7,8]. This procedure has been proved effective in a set up for emergency endovascular aneurysm repair, where it can provide the extra time necessary to achieve definitive hemostasis. Although conceptually elegant, the technique may be time-consuming and therefore has never found common acceptance for the hemodynamically unstable patient who is to undergo open aortic repair. Alternatively, supraceliac aortic clamping in order to avoid emergent dissection of the proximal aneurysm neck, with its inherent risk of venous injury, is a valid and time proven method to obtain proximal control. However, in certain cases, the surgeon is faced with a situation of complete hemodynamic collapse occurring just before or at the time of laparotomy. On those occasions, bulging of the retroperitoneal hematoma may render even supraceliac dissection cumbersome and too time-consuming. Obviously, immediate control of the aorta, as proximally as possible, is the only chance of restoring coronary and cerebral perfusion. Faced with this dramatic situation we have resorted to the following technique. The retroperitonal hematoma is entered by pushing one's fingers towards the left psoas muscle, from where the aneurysm sac then can be palpated. When absence of pulsatility is confirmed, the aneurysm sac can be entered simply by pushing the index-finger through the wall which at this site is invariably weak or absent. From here, the aortic neck can then be easily palpated and immediate proximal control is obtained with the index-finger as a cork into the proximal aortic lumen. A soft-tipped large balloon catheter (20 charriere Foley catheter with a 30 ml balloon) should be prepared with two strong clamps to occlude the central lumen. After the aneurysm sac is opened further, with the scissors if necessary, the catheter is inserted more or less blindly over the index-finger into the proximal aorta and advanced over its entire length. The balloon is then inflated with 30 ml of sterile saline resulting in occlusion of the mid-to-lower thoracic aorta (Fig. 1). In cases where no time was available for preoperative imaging and the ruptured aneurysm turns out to extend juxta- or suprarenally, this technique may be valuable as a last resort when everything else has failed. Obviously, thoracic aortic occlusion should be maintained for as short a duration as possible and dissection of the proximal aortic neck should be performed immediately, which at this time is facilitated by collapse of the aneurysm. Back-bleeding from the iliacs may be controlled with insertion of Fogarty embolectomy

catheters. If at this time, with maximal fluid and cardiac resuscitation, no measurable blood pressure returns, the procedure should be abandoned. However, high thoracic occlusion frequently leads to the return of cardiac function and, if the surgeon is careful not to let the pressure drop too far, the balloon can be partly deflated and allowed to drift down slowly while an aortic clamp is held on stand-by on the infra-or suprarenal aorta. Admittedly, our experience is anecdotal and a detailed analysis of results of this technique is simply not available. Interestingly, comparable techniques have been described since the early 1950s but somehow seem never to have entered the regular vascular curricula. Robicsek and Pruitt [9] described a modification of the technique because, as they stated, *"opening*

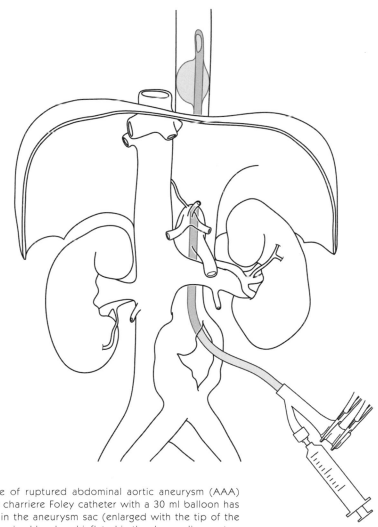

FIG. 1 Bail-out procedure in case of ruptured abdominal aortic aneurysm (AAA) with absent blood pressure. A 20 charriere Foley catheter with a 30 ml balloon has been passed through the rupture in the aneurysm sac (enlarged with the tip of the index-finger), advanced into the proximal level and inflated in the descending aorta.

of the aneurysm without proximal control certainly takes some nerve and occasionally is associated with considerable blood loss". These authors used an introducer with a "peel-away" sheath *(Cook Inc., Bloomington, IN, USA)* which was inserted directly into the aneurysmal sac and advanced in a 45 degree angle upward toward the proximal aorta until return of blood indicated the needle tip's free position past the clot in the lumen. They then entered a specially designed double lumen balloon catheter *(Ideas for Medicine Inc., Tampa, FL, USA)* into the proximal aorta. Although an elegant technique, with difficult tortuous aortic necks and the presence of a large hematoma, passage of the balloon catheter into the proximal aorta may be difficult and, especially in the situation of absence of blood pressure, we prefer the index-finger technique described above.

Another application for soft-tipped large balloon catheters, such as a Foley bladder catheter, is in injuries of the inferior vena cava (IVC). Obviously, proven methods of simple compression against the spine with sponge sticks, with or without lateral clamping with vascular or Babcock clamps, will allow ample exposure for the repair of simple (iatrogenic) injuries. With large lacerations, however, hemostasis by compression alone may be insufficient and (clamp-occluded) Foley catheters may be inserted into the IVC directly through the laceration and carefully inflated as described by Ravikumar and Stahl [10]. It should also be mentioned that IVC wounds that have spontaneously stopped bleeding should be left unexposed, especially when the retrohepatic IVC is involved. In situations of intraoperative bleeding where extensive IVC repair is needed, prolonged occlusion of the IVC in the face of hypovolemic shock may not be tolerated hemodynamically and use of a shunt is recommended. Several techniques towards this goal have been described in the literature and in an earlier issue of this book series [11-13]. We have used a slightly different approach whereby thoracotomy may be avoided in cases of penetrating trauma and renal cell tumor with IVC involvement. An endotracheal tube *(Mallinckrod, I.D 9.0 mm, O.D. 12.1 mm)* is cut to the appropriate length to match the distance from the diaphragm to 10 centimeters below the injury approximately. In very extensive, low lesions cutting may not be necessary but we have never found the tube to be too short. If prosthetic repair is necessary, a PTFE tube graft is placed around the shunt prior to insertion. Tourniquets are placed

around the IVC below and, if possible, above the injury. The shunt is then inserted balloon-side-up through the IVC defect and advanced proximally into the right atrium until it meets resistance. At this time, any excessive tube length may be removed, in order that it matches the lower extent of the injury. The balloon is inflated in the atrium and the lower end of the shunt is advanced into the distal IVC until the balloon is felt to reach the intrapericardial IVC. The tourniquet is tightened around the shunt and IVC repair is performed as indicated (Fig. 2).

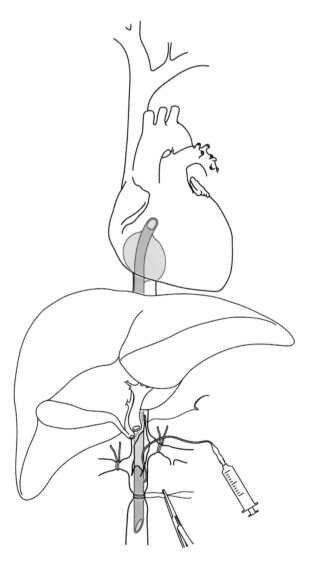

FIG. 2 An endotracheal tube provides both hemostasis and inferior vena cava (IVC) shunting in case of large IVC injuries or need for IVC replacement.

Endovascular aids to control bleeding in the extremities

For repair of anastomotic aneurysms in the groin, control of back-bleeding from the deep femoral artery (Fig. 3) by means of insertion of a Fogarty embolectomy catheter precludes additional surgical dissection in a previous operative field, with its inherent risk of arterial or venous injury. Likewise, in cases of (ruptured) popliteal or femoral aneurysms, proximal and distal control may be obtained by means of Fogarty embolectomy catheters.

Blunt arterial injury is associated with high morbidity and amputation rates, especially when the popliteal artery is involved. Delay of arterial and/or venous repair until stabilization prolongs the ischemic period, whereas repair before may render the vascular reconstruction vulnerable during repositioning of the musculoskeletal parts. Alternatively, a temporary shunt (Sundt carotid shunt) providing both hemostasis and flow may be secured proximally and distally with small tourniquets, thereby providing enough slack for skeletal manipulation [14].

Conclusion

Long before cathetcr-based techniques such as percutaneous transluminal angioplasty, stent placement and endovascular aneurysm repair had become mainstream therapeutic modalities, vascular surgeons had applied endovascular techniques to control bleeding during open surgical procedures. These methods, under represented in the literature, generally are passed on to next generations in the operating room and this chapter is an attempt to document some of the most useful.

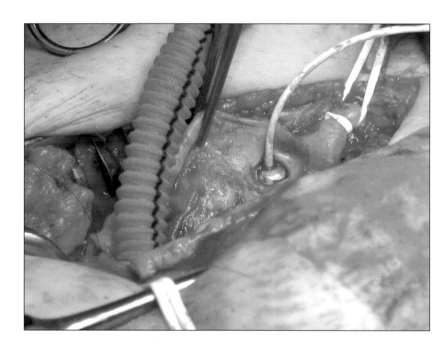

FIG. 3 Repair of a femoral artery aneurysm. A 4 French Fogarty thrombectomy catheter has been placed in the orifice of the deep femoral artery, providing control of back-bleeding without the need for further surgical dissection.

REFERENCES

1 Feliciano DV, Burch JM, Mattox KL et al. Balloon catheter tamponade in cardiovascular wounds. *Am J Surg* 1990; 160: 583-587.

2 DiGiacomo JC, Rotondo MF, Schwab CW. Transcutaneous balloon catheter tamponade for definitive control of subclavian venous injuries: case reports. *J Trauma* 1994; 37: 111-113.

3 Jacobs MJ, Elenbaas TW, Shurink GW et al. Assessment of spinal cord integrity during thoracoabdominal aortic aneurysm repair. *Ann Thorac Surg* 2002; 74: S1864-1866.

4 Velmahos GC, Toutouzas KG, Vassiliu P et al. A prospective study on the safety and efficacy of angiographic embolization for pelvic and visceral injuries. *J Trauma* 2002; 53: 303-308.

5 Valmahos GC, Chahwan S, Falabella A et al. Angiographic embolization for intraperitoneal and retroperitoneal injuries. *World J Surg* 2000; 24: 539-545.

6 Allen BT, Anderson CB, Rubin BG et al. Preservation of renal function in juxtarenal and suprarenal abdominal aortic aneurysm repair. *J Vasc Surg* 1993 May; 17: 948-958.

7 Ohki T, Veith FJ. Endovascular graft and other image-guided catheter-based adjuncts to improve the treatment of ruptured aortioiliac aneurysms. *Ann Surg* 2000; 232: 466-479.

8 Greenberg RK, Srivastava SD, Ouriel K et al. An endoluminal method of hemorrhage control and repair of ruptured abdominal aortic aneurysms. *J Endovasc Ther* 2000; 7: 1-7.

9 Robicsek F, Pruitt C. Transaneurysmal aortic balloon tamponade. *J Cardiovasc Surg* 1987; 28: 549-551.

10 Ravikumar S, Stahl WM. Intraluminal balloon catheter occlusion for major vena cava injuries. *J Trauma* 1985; 25: 458-460.

11 Chiche L, Kieffer E. Traumatic injury of the vena cava and its major branches. In Branchereau A, Jacobs M (eds) *Vascular Emergencies.* Elmsford, Futura, an imprint of Blackwell Publishing, 2003: pp 193-206.

12 Klein SR, Baumgartner FJ, Bongard FS. Contemporary management stragety for major inferior vena caval injuries. *J Trauma* 1994: 37: 35-41.

13 Blute ML, Leibovich BC, Lohse CM et al. The Mayo Clinic experience with surgical management, complications and outcome for patients with renal cell carcinoma and venous tumour thrombus. *BJU Int* 2004; 94: 33-41.

14 Hossny A. Blunt popliteal artery injury with complete lower limb ischemia: is routine use of temporary intraluminal arterial shunt justified? *J Vasc Surg* 2004; 40: 61-66.

25

STEAL SYNDROME: THE SWORD OF DAMOCLES OF ARTERIOVENOUS ACCESS SURGERY

VOLKER MICKLEY

Depending on the type of arteriovenous access for hemodialysis, the risk of steal syndrome varies from 1% to 2% (in forearm arteriovenous fistulae) to up to 5% to 15% (in elbow fistulae and upper limb graft access) [1-4]. For thigh access the risk may be even higher [5]. About 30% of steal syndromes occur immediately or early after access creation [4]. Women, diabetics and patients with coronary and peripheral arterial occlusive disease (PAOD) are believed to be at higher risk than the remaining hemodialysis population [6-10], but there is no specific preoperative test to determine an individual patient's risk potential. Although a digital/brachial blood pressure index (DBI) of less than 0.6 was shown to help identify patients at risk of developing symptoms of steal syndrome following access creation [11,12], steal can also occur in patients with normal preoperative values [10]. Despite thorough preoperative evaluation, steal syndrome remains the sword of Damocles of arteriovenous access surgery.

Depending on the extent of arterial steal, signs and symptoms of steal syndrome may vary in strength: mild (pale and cold hand, pain during exertion or exercise); severe (pain during hemodialysis; or limb-threatening (rest pain, acral necrosis). Monomelic ischemic neuropathy (MIN) is a special manifestation of access-induced ischemia mainly found in patients with preexisting (diabetic) neuropathy [13].

When severe symptoms of peripheral arterial steal develop following arteriovenous access creation, urgent and consequent action is necessary with the twin aims of preventing ischemic damage to the affected limb and preserving the patient's vascular access for hemodialysis whenever possible.

Pathophysiology

Arteriovenous fistulae for hemodialysis are usually created suturing a side-of-artery to end-of-vein anastomosis. The proximal artery will of course provide the main part of access flow but, due to the high peripheral arterial resistance in muscle-feeding arteries, retrograde inflow coming from the distal artery can appear during diastole. This *physiologic* steal phenomenon has been reported to occur in 73% of native arteriovenous fistulae and in 91% of arteriovenous grafts [14]. In normal arteries, peripheral steal is compensated by dilatation of the arteries proximally and distally to the arteriovenous anastomosis and of collaterals around it [15].

In the first weeks and months after creation, the arteriovenous fistula will maturate: the fistula vein dilates as a consequence of the high shear stress because the arterial inflow exerts on its wall; rising vein diameter (= falling venous resistance) allows for enhanced arterial inflow; and the subsequent rising shear stress exerted on the arterial wall causes successive arterial dilatation, compensating for the enhancement of arteriovenous flow volume. When a bridge graft is implanted connecting an artery and a draining vein, the same adaptive processes will occur in the native vessels, however, it is frequently counteracted by a progressive stenosis developing at the graft-to-vein anastomosis. Consequently, the late onset of steal symptoms (after some months or years) is a rare event in grafts, but it is frequently observed in autogenous fistulae [4,16].

The amount of distal arteriovenous steal depends on several variables:
- a feeding artery capable to dilate sufficiently will reduce peripheral steal,
- arterial collaterals around the arteriovenous anastomosis capable of dilation will enhance peripheral blood supply and also enhance retrograde drainage (thus enhancing net arteriovenous access flow and reducing the risk of steal syndrome),
- elevated venous resistance (caused by a hemodynamically significant stenosis) will reduce retrograde drainage,
- a feeding artery not capable of sufficient dilation and/or elevated peripheral arterial resistance (arteriosclerosis, media sclerosis, vasculitis) will enhance retrograde drainage.

Clinical findings

Steal syndrome can be classified according to Leriche and Fontaine's classification of peripheral arterial occlusive disease (PAOD) as shown in Table I [17]. Diastolic retrograde flow in the artery distal to the arteriovenous anastomosis (steal phenomenon) without any signs or symptoms of steal syndrome (Stage 0) is frequently observed in newly created and mature arteriovenous accesses and can easily be visualized by color-coded duplex-ultrasound. Digital blood pressures (DBI) and transcutaneous pO_2 measurements ($tcpO_2$) are normal in most of the patients.

Only in cases of enhanced peripheral arterial resistance and/or central arterial stenosis, will more or less pronounced signs and symptoms of peripheral ischemia (Table I) occur. Digital blood pressures inferior to 50 mmHg, a DBI of less than 0.6 and $tcpO_2$ values of less than 20 mmHg to 30 mmHg indicate critical ischemia. During compression of the arteriovenous access, the otherwise pale or bluish hand shows reactive hyperemia and digital blood pressures, as well as $tcpO_2$, values rise significantly (but not always to normal levels) [14]. These tests help distinguish steal syndrome from other conditions causing pain, dystrophy and necrosis (carpal tunnel syndrome, Sudeck's syndrome, calciphylaxis). In PAOD patients, critical leg ischemia can cause a predominantly sensory neuropathy often obscured

Table I	CLASSIFICATION OF STEAL SYNDROME (ACCORDING TO [17])
Stade 0	Retrograde flow in the distal artery (demonstrated by color-coded duplex-ultrasound) without any signs and symptoms of ischemia (= steal phenomenon)
Stade I	Pale/blue and/or cold hand without pain
Stade II	(Arm) claudication; pain during exercise, on exertion, and/or during hemodialysis
Stade III	Rest pain
Stade IV	Ulceration / Necrosis / Gangrene

by the effects of ischemia on other tissues [18]. In diabetic hemodialysis patients, however, access-induced and otherwise mild ischemia can induce rapid deterioration of preexisting diabetic neuropathy. Symptoms of this MIN comprise not only sensory disturbances but also loss of motor function and these do not necessarily improve after successful correction of steal syndrome [13].

Angiography is an important tool to demonstrate eventual arterial stenoses proximal to or at the arteriovenous anastomosis (Figs. 1A, 2) and to determine the distal arterial anatomy, which is necessary when planning a corrective procedure [14,19]. In case of severe steal syndrome, when virtually all blood is drained into the access, digital access compression can be helpful in improving the ability to opacify the peripheral arteries (Figs. 3B, 4B). Color-coded

duplex-ultrasound cannot be a complete substitute for diagnostic angiography because stenoses at the origin of the subclavian artery can be missed (there is already a positive diastolic flow in the brachial artery above the arteriovenous anastomosis) and severely calcified peripheral arteries produce artifacts making the distinction between stenosis and occlusion difficult. Ultrasound, however, should be used to measure access flow (see below).

Prevention

Several groups of patients have been identified to be at higher risk of developing access-induced steal syndrome than the average hemodialysis population: diabetics, women, patients with PAOD, and those

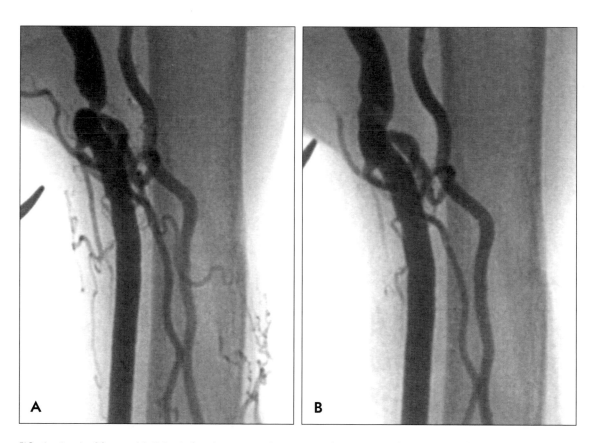

FIG. 1 A - An 86-year-old diabetic female presented two years after creation of a brachiobasilic arteriovenous fistula with stage II steal syndrome (pain during hemodialysis) and insufficient fistula flow (less than 150 ml/min). Angiography showed this high-grade proximal brachial artery stenosis and another stenosis in the fistula vein close to the arteriovenous anastomosis (not shown). B - Stenoses were simultaneously corrected by retrograde dilatation of the brachial artery and PAVA procedure (5 mm ePTFE interposition graft). Steal syndrome completely resolved despite significantly enhanced arteriovenous flow (600 ml/min).

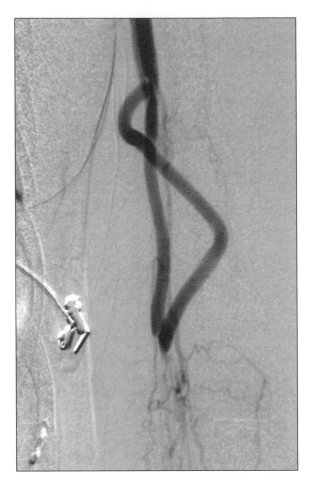

FIG. 2 A 46-year-old diabetic female presented two days after an atypical upper arm curved graft had been implanted at another institution. She complained of severe rest pain, dysesthesia and weakness of her left hand which had started immediately following the operation. Transfemoral angiography showed suture-induced high-grade stenoses of the brachial artery at the proximal and distal ends of the anastomosis. Resection of the arterial graft anastomosis with patch angioplasty to the brachial artery and conversion into a forearm looped graft resulted in complete resolution of symptoms.

with preceding access procedures on the same extremity [6-10]. In other words, in the great majority of instances, the hemodialysis patient is at risk. Consequently, the access surgeon has to be aware of this impending complication during each and every access procedure. This is especially true, because there is no reliable preoperative test to predict the relative risk of an individual patient. A preoperative DBI of less than 0.6 was demonstrated to be associated with a higher incidence of postoperative steal

syndromes. Using 0.6 as threshold level, the sensitivity of DBI measurement was 100%, its specificity, however, only 59% to 76%, and its positive predictive value 19% to 46% [11,12]. On the other hand peripheral ischemia can occur in patients with normal preoperative DBI values [10]. Thus DBI measurements may help identify patients at higher risk of developing postoperative steal syndrome, but they are not suitable for excluding an individual patient (or limb) from arteriovenous access surgery.

Several strategies may help to reduce the risk of postoperative steal syndrome occuring. Peripheral arteriovenous fistulae at the wrist are associated with the lowest frequency of access-induced ischemia (1% to 2% [3, 4]). When a wrist fistula cannot, or can no longer be created, due to the bad quality of peripheral arteries and/or veins, before going to the level of the elbow, a mid-forearm fistula should be considered. When an elbow fistula is the only option, the (cephalic, basilic, or median antecubital) vein need not necessarily be sutured to the brachial artery. It is very often possible to create an anastomosis with the origin of the radial or ulnar artery. This technique preserves the other forearm artery as a valuable *collateral* to the hand. In order to further reduce arteriovenous flow in elbow fistulae and to prevent excessive dilatation of the anastomosis, it has been advised to use the often small perforating vein for the anastomosis [8] and to perform short arteriotomies (6 to 7 millemeters) [17]. When a graft has to be implanted, a rectangular arterial anastomosis and/or the usage of tapered grafts may add to a greater anastomotic resistance and thereby to limitation of flow [17].

Treatment

BASIC CONSIDERATIONS

Even a mild steal syndrome can rapidly deteriorate to tissue loss or to severely disabling MIN. Timely diagnosis and consequent treatment are of utmost importance in order to achieve the twin aims of therapy: to preserve the affected limb and to keep the access functioning. Some of the surgical options for the correction of arteriovenous access-induced steal syndrome have already been discussed shortly in an earlier EVC textbook [20]. Their adjustment to the patient's individual vascular anatomy and flow conditions, eventually in combination with endovascular procedures, is crucial for the successful therapy of the often complex pathophysiology of steal.

Arterial inflow obstructions (Fig. 1A) and arterial anastomotic stenoses (Fig. 2) should be treated irrespective of the stage of steal syndrome, as they do impair not only peripheral circulation but also access function and, thereby, reduce the quality of renal replacement therapy. When access-induced steal syndrome is associated with peripheral arte-

rial disease, the indication for treatment depends on the severity of symptoms and on the type of vascular access (fistula or graft).

In autogenous fistulae, blood flow tends to rise over time due to maturation. Therefore fistula patients presenting with stage II disease deserve the permanent attention of their nephrology team to

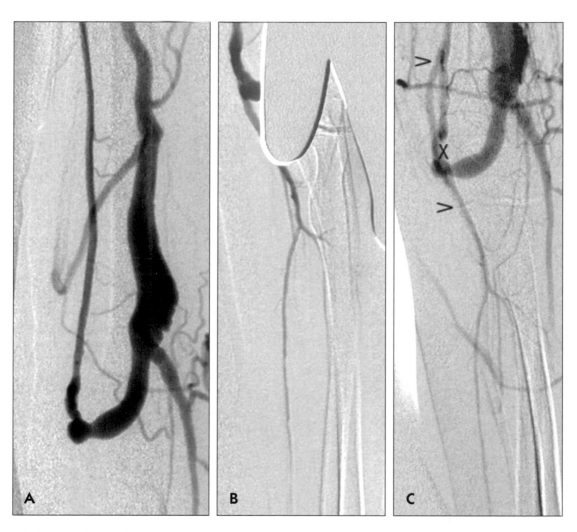

FIG. 3 A - A 32-year-old diabetic male presented nine months after creation of a brachiocephalic arteriovenous fistula with rest pain and acral necroses of the three radial fingers of his left hand. Fistula flow was measured to be 400 ml/min. Transfemoral angiography showed drainage of virtually all arterial blood into the access vein. B - Forearm arteries could be visualized only with digital compression of the access vein. Complete occlusion of the radial artery and distal stenoses of the ulnar artery were visible. C - A DRIL procedure was performed: the brachial artery was ligated immediately distal to the arteriovenous anastomosis (X), and a vein bypass (reversed greater saphenous vein) was implanted from 5 centimeters above the anastomosis to below the ligation (arrow heads marking proximal and distal anastomosis). Postoperative angiography showed spontaneous opacification of forearm arteries. Rest pain subsided and necroses healed subsequently. The patient is still free from symptoms of ischemia two and a half years after the operation. (Reprinted with kind permission from: Mickley V. Surgical alternatives to central venous catheters in chronic renal replacement therapy. Nephrol Dial Transplant 2003; 18: 1045-1051).

detect progression to stage III or to stage IV early. However, in diabetic hemodialysis patients with significant neuropathy, early correction of stage II steal syndrome should be considered in order to prevent the development of MIN. Progressive stenosis of the venous anastomosis of access grafts frequently causes flow reduction due to enhanced venous resistance. When stage II steal syndrome occurs early after graft access creation, after exclusion of technical errors (Fig. 2), watchful waiting is justified because symptoms of steal are most likely to disappear in time. However, once such a stenosis has to be treated later on, simultaneous pro-

phylactic correction of steal should be considered, especially in patients at risk of MIN.

Steal syndrome causing critical limb ischemia (stage III or stage IV) or MIN should be reason enough for urgent imaging and treatment irrespective of the type of arteriovenous access.

TREATMENT OPTIONS
Ligation. Access ligation will lead to immediate improvement of steal syndrome, but also to loss of the access with the need for creation of another one, again with the risk of steal syndrome. It may be performed in severe ischemia or MIN to gain

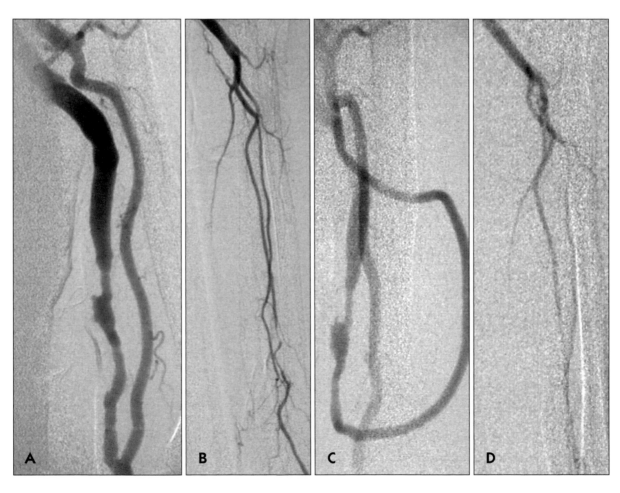

FIG. 4   A - A 74-year-old diabetic male presented with rest pain a year after creation of a left brachiobasilic arteriovenous fistula. The basilic vein was difficult to needle because it had not been transposed. B - Severely diseased forearm arteries could be visualized only with access compression. C - A PAVA procedure was performed using a 7 millimeter standard wall ePTFE graft connecting the proximal brachial artery with the basilic vein, transforming the brachiobasilic fistula into an easy accessibly upper arm looped graft. D - Rest pain completely resolved and forearm arteries were opacified on postoperative angiography without compression of the access.

time for thorough diagnostic work-up and preferably in a way that later reactivation of the access with simultaneous treatment of steal syndrome is possible. Access ligation can of course be performed when steal syndrome develops after successful kidney transplantation and it must be done when other corrective procedures are not suitable or have failed.

Banding. Surgical banding of the access is usually performed close to the arterial anastomosis. Arteriovenous fistulae can be banded by non-absorbable sutures, a small caliber interposition graft, or by narrowing the vein with a tight Dacron or PTFE cuff. In prosthetic access, interposition of a short tapered graft segment has been suggested [2,3,19,21]. All these procedures create a reduction in blood flow up the fistula and steal syndrome will disappear after a sufficient reduction in fistula blood flow or cessation of diastolic retrograde inflow from the distal artery. This can be achieved only when access resistance at least approaches the level of peripheral arterial resistance. Sufficient surgical banding thus means suturing a high grade anastomotic stenosis with the risk of insufficient flow or even access thrombosis [14,19]. Therefore, banding should be attempted only with intraoperative monitoring of access flow, as well as peripheral circulation (pulse oximetry, tcpO$_2$ measurement, digital photoplethysmography, pulse volume recordings or DBI measurement [3,11,21]).

Arteriovenous access patency rates are correlated with access flow. Hemodialysis quality is correlated with the flow achieved in the dialyser which, of course, is limited by access flow. Flow reduction caused by suturing a hemodynamically significant stenosis compromises access survival and hemodialysis quality. Therefore access banding should only (if ever) be considered in high flow accesses (more than 1500 ml/min, [17]). Despite subtle technique, access banding results in high rates of thrombosis or recurring steal (Table II).

Table II SUCCESS RATES OF DIFFERENT TREATMENT OPTIONS

First author [ref.]	Year of publication	Number of patients	Success %	Access patency %
Banding				
Odland et al. [3]	1991	16	100	40
DeCaprio et al. [19]	1997	11	91	10
Morsy et al. [2]	1998	6	100	33
DRIL				
Schanzer et al. [9]	1992	14	93	82
Haimov et al. [26]	1996	23	96	73
Katz et al. [27]	1996	6	83	100
Berman et al. [6]	1997	21	100	94
Lazarides et al. [1]	1998	7	94	NA
Stierli et al. [28]	1998	6	100	100
Knox et al. [7]	2002	52	90	83
PAVA				
Zanow et al. [4]	2001	56	88	88

DRIL: Distal Revascularization Interval Ligation
PAVA: Proximalization of the Arteriovenous Anastomosis
NA: not available

Ligation of distal radial artery. The easiest way to block retrograde arterial inflow into a distal access at the wrist is to ligate (or embolize) the artery distally to the anastomosis. In radio-cephalic (or ulnar-basilic) fistulae, the effect can be preoperatively simulated by digital compression of the respective artery at the wrist below the anastomosis. In 1971, Bussell et al. [22] demonstrated an increase in pulse amplitude of the thumb averaging 80% in compressing the radial artery distal to the anastomosis, thus impairing retrograde inflow. Before ligation or interventional embolization of the artery, temporary balloon blockade can also be used to predict the effect of treatment. Pulse oximetry, $tcpO_2$ measurement or digital photoplethysmography prior to and after definitive treatment are helpful in quantifying the problem and assessing the improvement in hand circulation [23].

DRIL procedure. Arterial ligation distal to the arteriovenous fistula can also be performed successfully in elbow fistulae to treat steal syndrome. Ligation of the brachial artery, however, was felt to enhance the risk of forearm ischemia. Therefore Distal Revascularization was added to Interval Ligation of the artery [24]. In this so-called DRIL procedure, the artery is ligated distally to the access anastomosis, and a vein bypass from proximal to the anastomosis to distal to the ligation is inserted (Fig. 3). It is recommended that construction of the proximal anastomosis should be at a reasonable distance (more than 5 centimeters) proximal to the access, in order to prevent diastolic retrograde flow and, thereby, recurrence of steal syndrome within the bypass. DRIL is as effective as banding in the treatment of ischemia and obviously superior to banding as far as access patency is concerned (Table II).

PAVA procedure. Steal syndrome can occur at any access flow. In one series, 14 out of 22 patients with peripheral ischemia had access flows below 250 ml/min [25]. In such cases, banding would further compromise access function (and dialysis quality) or even result in access thrombosis, whereas DRIL does not have any influence on access flow. In order to enhance access flow and at the same time treat ischemia, Proximalization of the Arteriovenous Anastomosis (PAVA) can be performed. The arteriovenous anastomosis in the antecubital fossa is disconnected and a venous or prosthetic interposition graft is used to connect the access with the artery at the axillary-brachial junction (Fig. 4). Although access flow is significantly enhanced, PAVA is otherwise hemodynamically very similar to DRIL (retrograde inflow out of forearm arteries is blocked) and, consequently, success rates of PAVA are comparable to those of DRIL (Table II).

Conclusion

The surgical treatment of hemodialysis access-induced steal syndrome must be individualized according to the patient's vascular pathology, the type of access and the amount of access flow. Banding the access leads to significant reduction in access flow with the risk of access thrombosis and should therefore be considered only in high-flow situations. Intraoperative control of peripheral perfusion is mandatory to achieve satisfying results. Steal associated with normal-flow access is best treated by DRIL, which does not have any influence on access function. PAVA gives the opportunity to enhance otherwise low access flow and at the same time enhance peripheral perfusion. Ligation can be performed after successful kidney transplantation, or as last resort when other treatment options have failed.

REFERENCES

1 Lazarides MK, Staramos DN, Panagopoulos GN et al. Indications for surgical treatment of angioaccess-induced arterial steal. *J Am Coll Surg* 1998; 187: 422-426.
2 Morsy AH, Kulbaski M, Chen C et al. Incidence and characteristics of patients with hand ischemia after a hemodialysis access procedure. *J Surg Res* 1998; 74: 8-10.
3 Odland MD, Kelly PH, Ney AL et al. Management of dialysis-associated steal syndrome complicating upper extremity arteriovenous fistulas: use of intraoperative digital photoplethysmography. *Surgery* 1991; 110: 664-669.
4 Zanow J, Petzold M, Petzold K et al. Diagnosis and differentiated treatment of ischemia in patients with arteriovenous vascular access. In: Henry ML (ed). *Vascular access for hemodialysis - VII.* Chicago, Precept Press 2001: pp 201-208.
5 Gradman WS, Cohen W, Haji-Aghaii M. Arteriovenous fistula construction in the thigh with transposed superficial femoral vein: our initial experience. *J Vasc Surg* 2001; 33: 968-975.
6 Berman SS, Glickman MH, Mills JL et al. Distal revascularization - interval ligation for limb salvage and maintenance of dialysis access in ischemic steal syndrome. *J Vasc Surg* 1997; 26: 393-402.

7 Knox RC, Berman SS, Hughes JD et al. Distal revascularization - interval ligation: a durable and effective treatment for ischemic steal syndrome after hemodialysis access. *J Vasc Surg* 2002; 36: 250-255.

8 Konner K, Hulbert-Shaeron TE, Roys EC, Port FK. Tailoring the initial vascular access for dialysis patients. *Kidney Int* 2002; 62: 329-338.

9 Schanzer H, Skladany M, Haimov M. Treatment of angioaccess-induced ischemia by revascularization. *J Vasc Surg* 1992; 16: 861-864.

10 Valentine RJ, Bouch CW, Scott DJ et al. Do preoperative finger pressures predict early arterial steal in hemodialysis access patients? A prospective analysis. *J Vasc Surg* 2002; 36: 351-356.

11 Goff CD, Sato DT, Bloch PH et al. Steal syndrome complicating hemodialysis access procedures: can it be predicted? *Ann Vasc Surg* 2000; 14: 138-144.

12 Papasavas PK, Reifsnyder T, Birdas TJ et al. Prediction of arteriovenous access steal syndrome utilizing digital pressure measurements. *Vasc Endovascular Surg* 2003; 37: 179-184.

13 Hye RJ, Wolf YG. Ischemic monomelic neuropathy: an under-recognized complication of hemodialysis access. *Ann Vasc Surg* 1994; 8: 578-582.

14 Schanzer H, Eisenberg D. Management of steal syndrome resulting from dialysis access. *Semin Vasc Surg* 2004; 17: 45-49.

15 Wixon CL, Hughes JD, Mills JL. Understanding strategies for the treatment of ischemic steal syndrome after hemodialysis access. *J Am Coll Surg* 2000; 191: 301-310.

16 Lazarides MK, Staramos DN, Kopadis G et al. Onset of arterial "steal" following proximal angioaccess: immediate and delayed types. *Nephrol Dial Transplant* 2003; 18: 2387-2390.

17 Tordoir JH, Dammers R, van der Sande FM. Upper extremity ischemia and hemodialysis vascular access. *Eur J Vasc Endovasc Surg* 2004; 27: 1-5.

18 Weinberg DH, Simovic D, Isner J, Ropper AH. Chronic ischemic monomelic neuropathy from critical limb ischemia. *Neurology* 2001; 57: 1008-1012.

19 DeCaprio JD, Valentine RJ, Kakish HB et al. Steal syndrome complicating hemodialysis access. *Cardiovasc Surg* 1997; 5: 648-653.

20 Mickley V. Acute complications of arteriovenous fistula for hemodialysis. In: Branchereau A, Jacobs M (eds). *Vascular emergencies*. Elmsford, Futura, an imprint of Blackwell Publishing 2003: pp 217-229.

21 Rivers SP, Scher LA, Veith FJ. Correction of steal syndrome secondary to hemodialysis access fistulas: a simplified quantitative technique. *Surgery* 1992; 112: 593-597.

22 Bussell JA, Abbott JA, Lim RC. A radial steal syndrome with arteriovenous fistula for hemodialysis. Studies in seven patients. *Ann Intern Med* 1971; 75: 387-394.

23 Chemla E, Raynaud A, Carreres T et al. Preoperative assessment of the efficacy of distal radial artery ligation in treatment of steal syndrome complicating access for hemodialysis. *Ann Vasc Surg* 1999; 13: 618-621.

24 Schanzer H, Schwartz M, Harrington E, Haimov M. Treatment of ischemia due to "steal" by arteriovenous fistula with distal artery ligation and revascularization. *J Vasc Surg* 1988; 7: 770-773.

25 Meyer F, Müller JS, Grote R et al. Fistula banding - success-promoting approach in peripheral steal syndrome. *Zentralbl Chir* 2002; 127: 685-688.

26 Haimov M, Schanzer H, Skladani M. Pathogenesis and management of upper-extremity ischemia following angioaccess surgery. *Blood Purif* 1996; 14: 350-354.

27 Katz S, Kohl RD. The treatment of hand ischemia by arterial ligation and upper extremity bypass after angioaccess surgery. *J Am Coll Surg* 1996; 183: 239-242.

28 Stierli P, Blumberg A, Pfister J, Zehnder C. Surgical treatment of steal syndrome induced by arteriovenous grafts for hemodialysis. *J Cardiovasc Surg* 1998; 39: 441-443.

26

LIGATURE AND REMOVAL OF THE FEMORAL VEIN AND OTHER DISASTERS IN VARICOSE VEIN SURGERY

MARKUS ENZLER

The oldest reference to the treatment of varicose veins goes back to Hippocrates (Kos, 460-377 BC) who counseled patients with venous ulcers to avoid a sedentary life style. The Roman physician Cornelius Celsus (Alexandria, 3-64 AD) introduced hook phlebectomy around 45 AD. Claudius Galenus of Pergamon (129-199 AD) modified the Celsus technique. The Arab physician Al-Zahrawi (Cordoba, 931-1013 AD, also called Albucasis) described the removal of the long saphenous vein using interrupted sequential longitudinal incisions. In modern times, Friedrich Trendelenburg (Berlin, 1844-1924) described mid-thigh ligation of the varicose great saphenous vein for the first time, although this concept had been known since the 7th century. His disciple Georg Clemens Perthes (1869-1927) recommended an incision in the groin followed by ligation of the sapheno-femoral junction.

At the beginning of the twentieth century, various techniques of vein stripping were developed. We owe the first publication in this field to William Keller [1] from Chicago who described an invaginating stripping technique in 1905. In 1906, Charles Mayo communicated an alternative method using a ring at the head of the stripper. In 1907, Stephen Babcock contributed the now widespread technique of using a stripper with an olive at its tip.

Case reports

ARTERIAL INJURIES

The oldest report on complications of varicose vein treatment known to this author was published by Luke and Miller in 1948 [2]. It describes two cases of inadvertent injection of sclerosing agents into the superficial femoral artery. Both resulted in major amputations.

In 1964, Natali [3] reported five patients who had sustained inadvertent ligation of the superficial femoral artery. All ligations were removed within less than twelve hours, and the outcome was uneventful in all patients. Further similar cases were reported by Buri in 1971 [4] and by Hagmüller [5]. Their patients also remained free of adverse symptoms.

In 1975, Liddicoat et al. [6] reported two patients who had inadvertent *surgical interruption* of the femoral arterial system, both requiring vascular reconstruction. In 1998, Ramsheyi et al. [7] reported 3 cases of *iatrogenic arterial injuries*. Two patients had sustained acute severe ischemia and required prompt revascularization but had no severe sequelae. The third patient suffered from persistent claudication.

In 1979, Largiadèr and Brunner [8] reported two patients with tears of the superficial femoral artery. Both tears were repaired successfully without major sequelae.

Single occurrences of inadvertent excision of the superficial femoral artery were further reported by Morton et al. [9], Eger et al. [10] and Leitz and Schmidt [11]. In the latter case, a segment of the deep femoral artery had also been excised. In the report from Eger et al., the limb was successfully salvaged by a composite graft. In the two cases reported by Morton et al. and Leitz et al., attempts at vascular reconstruction were futile and resulted in amputation.

A number of reports describe extensive removals using strippers, where arteries have been mistaken for veins. Hagmüller [5] in 1992 gave an account of a patient in whom the superficial femoral artery was stripped. The reconstruction with a vein graft was successful and the outcome was good. Further articles report at least five further total strippings of the superficial femoral and popliteal artery plus one leg artery [5,12,13,14]. This latter was in most instances the posterior tibial artery. One of these cases was reported by Becker [12]. The limb was successfully revascularized with a vein graft. Denck et al. [13] communicated two cases. In one of them, no attempt at reconstruction was made, which resulted in above-knee amputation. In the second case, the limb was salvaged by revascularization using a composite graft. Another patient reported by Hagmüller [5] underwent revascularization using a vein graft and the limb was also salvaged. However, in both of the latter two cases the limbs developed drop foot (equinus) due to ischemic muscle damage.

VENOUS INJURIES

Largiadèr and Brunner [8] reported five injuries of great veins during varicose vein surgery. Of these, two patients had sustained tearing of the common femoral vein (CFV). In two other patients, the CFV had been divided and in one it had been ligated. The tears were sutured and the follow-up was uneventful. The ligation led to thrombosis which was not diagnosed until four weeks later and then managed conservatively with anticoagulants. This patient was lost to follow-up. One divided CFV was reanastomosed which led to a good result. The second devided CFV prompted reanastomosis and two attempts at venous thrombectomy which were ultimately futile. Nevertheless, only moderate swelling persisted.

Denck et al. [13] reported two patients with iatrogenic stenosis of the CFV associated with chronic swelling. The same author communicated the case of a patient who had sustained division of the CFV. It was re-anastomosed and the patient became free of symptoms. In a further patient reported by Denck, the CVF had been stripped. It was successfully replaced by a segment of the ipsilateral long saphenous vein.

Flis [15] reported a patient who had sustained stripping of the superficial femoral and the popliteal vein. In addition, the origin of the deep femoral vein had been ligated. This led to massive venous congestion and critical ischemia with paralysis in the lower leg. Reconstruction included a venous bypass using the intact long saphenous vein. Long-term patency was achieved, but paralysis of the peroneal nerve and chronic swelling persisted.

Both Miller et al. [16] and Critchley et al. [17] reported cases in which the CVF had been torn. In the first report, primary repair was successful. In the latter, the vein was repaired with a vein patch but chronic swelling persisted. More recently, Frings et al. [18] communicated a case in which the patient's CFV had inadvertently been excised. It was replaced after three days with a PTFE graft. The patient recovered without symptoms. Aleksic et al. [19] reported a patient whose superficial femoral and popliteal veins had been stripped and reimplanted thereafter. The *graft* remained patent but swelling persisted.

Compartment Syndromes

Compartment syndromes are a rare complication of varicose vein surgery. From the literature, we are aware of three cases published by Widmer et al. [20]. If early symptoms have been missed and decompression of the compartments delayed, disturbances of the sensomotory function are inevitable.

Observational studies

Vascular Injury

The largest observational study on complications of varicose vein surgery was published by Frings et al. in 2001 [18]. It covers a total of 40 636 treated limbs. Seven major vascular complications were observed (0.02%). These complications invariably affected veins and no arterial injury was observed in this series. The authors make a distinction between complications of crossectomy of great saphenous veins vs. small saphenous veins. A number of 31 838 crossectomies in the groin led to 4 major vein injuries (0.01%), none of which entailed a chronic post-thrombotic syndrome. In contrast, 3 major vein injuries occurred in 6 152 crossectomies in the popliteal fossa (0.05%). Thus, the risk of vein injury in small saphenous vein crossectomy was more than three times higher. Furthermore, all of them entailed post-thrombotic syndromes.

The second largest series was published by Balzer [21] in the same year. This series covers a total of 25 457 treated limbs. Five major vascular injuries were observed. Of these, 3 were transsection of femoral arteries (0.01%) and 2 were divisions of femoral veins (0.01%).

In 1992, Hagmüller [5] reported a series of 3 300 limbs. One occurrence of femoral vein ligature was observed (0.03%). In 1997, Critchley et al. [17] reported a total of 973 treated limbs with one vein injury (0.1%).

My own single surgeon experience from 1997 to August 2004 comprises 1923 limbs. Within this series, two minor tears in the CFV resulted from traction on vein branches. These were repaired by simple sutures and had no sequelae. Major vascular injuries did not occur during this period.

Deep Vein Thrombosis and Pulmonary Embolism

The large study by Frings et al. [18] is focused on vascular injuries and does not itemize thromboembolic events. Balzer [21], in contrast, reports 7 occurrences of deep vein thrombosis (DVT) and 5 cases of pulmonary embolism (PE) out of a total of 25 457 treated limbs. This corresponds to 0.03% of DVT and 0.02% PE. One PE was fatal.

After treating 3 300 limbs, Hagmüller [5] observed 8 occurrences of DVT (0.24%) and 2 cases of PE (0.06%). Out of 973 treated limbs, Critchley et al. [17] mention 2 cases of DVT (0.21%) and 1 PE (0.1%). Miller et al. [16] found in a series of varicose vein surgery totaling 1 322 limbs (997 patients), 4 occurrences of DVT (0.3%) and one non-fatal PE.

In my personal experience, one case of DVT was observed (0.05%). This resulted in moderate chronic swelling which was managed by the use of compression stockings. Another patient sustained non-fatal PE (0.05%). The source remained unknown.

Nerve Injury

Nerve injuries in varicose vein surgery almost never have disastrous consequences. Therefore, they are not the primary focus of this meta-analysis. Nevertheless, some mention of such occurrences will complete the picture of complications of varicose vein surgery.

Critchley et al. [17] reported one case of major nerve damage in 973 treated limbs (0.1%). Pressure of a retractor on the common peroneal nerve in the popliteal fossa led to a drop foot, which had almost completely disappeared after two years. In the same series, minor nerve injuries occurred in 6.6% of the limbs operated upon. Typically, a branch or the trunk of the saphenous or the sural nerve were affected with the consequence of transient or permanent numbness of restricted skin areas. In the study of Frings et al. [18], no major nerve lesion occurred during crossectomy in the groin, whereas 3 major injuries occurred in the popliteal fossa (0.05%). Of these, two were reversible and one irreversible. In a series of 20 000 treated limbs, Mildner and Hilbe [22] found no major nerve injuries, but minor injuries were frequent. Lesions of the saphenous nerve occurred in 14% of treated limbs. Of these, about half recovered within one year. Damage to the sural nerve occurred in less than 1% and more severe nerve injuries were not observed.

In our own series, no motor nerve injury occurred. In contrast, two patients suffered from chronic pain following injury to the sural nerve after SSV *stripping.*

WOUND COMPLICATIONS

According to Critchley et al. [17], the incidence of wound complications was 2.8% of all limbs (4% of patients). In the same series, leakage of lymph from the groin only occurred in re-explorations, with an incidence of 5/111 limbs.

MAJOR BLEEDING

Intra- or postoperative bleeding classified as "threatening" occurred 5 times out of 3 300 in the series of Hagmüller [5] (0.15%) and 15 times out of 25 457 in the series of Balzer [21] (0.06%). In our own series, one groin needed revision due to bleeding from the great saphenous vein stump (0.05%).

MORTALITY

One fatal PE is reported in the series published by Balzer [21]. Apart from this, no fatal complications appear from the papers quoted in this chapter.

Discussion

As early as 1948, Luke and Miller [2] reported two patients who had sustained inadvertent injection of sclerosing agents into the superficial femoral vein. Vollmar reported a similar case in 1968. All three cases resulted in major limb amputations. At present *PubMed* (the website of the *National Library of Medicine and National Institutes of Health*) lists papers published since 1950. However, the earliest reports focusing on complications of varicose vein surgery appear much later. In 1967, Stern published an article entitled *Dealing with difficulties and complications of varicose vein operations* [23].

A large body of literature on complications of varicose veins surgery, including many papers in German, was published in the 1970's.

Arterial injuries were reported in a surprisingly high number of case reports. Table I lists such reports in the order of severity of the lesion (as far as can be judged from the report). Of 24 limbs having sustained arterial lesions, 12 underwent one or more arterial reconstructions. Three of the affected limbs ultimately underwent major amputations.

In contrast, only 13 case reports on venous injuries have been retrieved via PubMed (Table II).

Apart from minor measures including removal of ligations or reanastomosis, venous reconstructions were carried out in four limbs. No amputations were reported.

Five observational studies have been identified. They are listed in Table III [5,17,18,21] and encompass a total of 72 289 limbs operated upon for varicose veins. Among these, only 3 arterial injuries were observed (0.01%). Venous injuries occurred in 12 cases (0.02%). Thus, venous injuries were four times more frequent than arterial injuries. This is no surprise as the great and small saphenous veins are connected immediately to the great veins while the arteries are separate. Furthermore, deep veins are more easily mistaken for varicose veins due to the quality of the wall and lack of pulse. Nevertheless, more case reports address arterial than venous injuries (24 vs. 13, Tables I and II). Thus, the chance of an arterial injury being published is manifold compared to a venous lesion. This may be due to the more dramatic consequences of arterial injuries. Indeed, 12 of 24 reported arterial injuries were followed by arterial reconstructions and 3 resulted in major amputations. In contrast, only 4 of 13 reported cases of vein injury prompted major reconstructive measures. Only a minority of the reported venous injuries entailed chronic post-thrombotic syndromes and, perhaps more importantly, no major amputations ensued.

The disproportionate numbers in case reports suggest that venous injury is underreported and probably underdiagnosed. We may hypothesize that in an unknown number of cases *postoperative DVT* and *post-thrombotic syndrome* are due to inadvertent and perhaps unadmitted severance of deep veins.

DVT was reported in 18 instances and PE in 9 from the observational studies listed in Table III. However, thrombo-embolic events are not itemized in the largest study [18]. Therefore, their incidence was calculated on the basis of four studies encompassing 31 653 treated limbs. The incidence of DVT ranges from 0.03% [21] to 0.24% [5], and was, on average, 0.06%. The incidence of PE was half as much (0.03%). PE was fatal in one patient and PE was the only cause of death.

Pharmacological prophylaxis against thromboembolic complications is not clearly defined in these studies and was probably not routinely administered. Today, low molecular weight heparin is widely used although the evidence of its efficacy is not strong and its controversy continues. The potential benefits of low molecular weight heparin

(LMWH) may be offset, in part, by an increased incidence of hematoma that may cause pain and compromise early mobilization [21]. Therefore, some authors believe in early mobilization rather than drug treatment [21]. Nevertheless, in our practice we routinely use LMWH, in part due to forensic considerations. The duration of treatment ranges between one and eight days and sometimes longer, depending on the individual risk profiles.

Medico-legal consequences of complications of varicose vein surgery were studied by Tennant and Ruckley [24] on the basis of the medico-legal literature. According to their report, in the United Kingdom an average of 34 patients per annum - against a background of an estimated 100 000 procedures performed - begin legal action against their medical attendants in connection with the treatment of varicose veins. The distribution of injury types is fairly constant as outlined below.

Injury of the femoral veins in the groin is responsible for 11% of cases proceeding to legal action. The commonest mechanism of injury is ligation or division of a femoral vein which had been mistaken for the long saphenous vein. Injury to the popliteal vein is much rarer and reflects the comparably low frequency of procedures performed at this site.

Arterial trauma leads to only 2% of actionable injuries. In order of decreasing frequency, the superficial femoral, the common femoral and the popliteal arteries are involved, and repair is often successful if the injury is recognized at the time of the venous procedure.

The most frequent complications resulting in legal action are nerve injuries, which account for

Table I ARTERIAL COMPLICATIONS IN CASE REPORTS (LISTED IN A PRESUMED ORDER OF SEVERITY)

First author [ref.]	Year	Cases	Lesion	Delay	Repair	Outcome
Natali [3]	1964	5	Ligation SFA	< 12 hours	Removal	All good
Buri [4]	1973	1	Ligation SFA	44 days	Removal	Good
Hagmüller [5]	1992	2	Ligation SFA		Suture	Good
Liddicoat [3]	1975	2	*Interruption*		Reconstruction	No amputation
Ramsheyi [7]	1998	3	*Arterial injuries*		2 *revascularizations*	Salvaged
Largiadèr [8]	1979	2	Tears SFA		Vein p/graft	Good
Morton [9]	1966	1	Excision SFA		Futile	Amputation
Eger [10]	1973	1	Excision SFA		Composite graft	Good
Leitz [11]	1974	1	Excision SFA+DFA	28 hours	Vein graft	Amputation
Hagmüller [5]	1992	1	*Stripping* SFA		Graft	Good
Becker [12]	1975	1	*Stripping* SFA-CA	7 hours	Vein graft	Good
Denck [13]	1979	1	*Stripping* SFA-CA	24 hours	Composite graft	Equinus
Denck [13]	1979	1	*Stripping* SFA-CA	48 hours	None	Amputation a-k
Pegoraro [14]	1987	1	*Stripping* SFA-CA	10 hours	Composite graft	Viable, occlusion
Hagmüller [5]	1992	1	*Stripping* SFA-CA		Vein graft	Equinus
Total		**24**			**~ 12 grafts**	**3 amputations**

CA : crural artery
DFA: deep femoral artery
SFA : superficial femoral artery

Table II   Venous complications in case reports (listed in a presumed order of severity)

First author [ref.]	Year	Cases	Lesion	Delay	Repair	Outcome
Denck [13]	1979	2	Stenose CFV	Long	None	Swelling
Largiadèr [8]	1979	1	Tear CFV	None	Suture	Good
Miller [16]	1996	1	Tear CFV	-	-	-
Critchley [17]	1997	1	Tear CFV	None	Vein patch	Patent, swelling
Largiadèr [8]	1979	1	Ligation CFV	4 weeks	None	Lost to follow-up
Largiadèr [8]	1979	1	Division CFV	5 hours	Thrombectomy, anastomosis	Rethrombosis, recanalization
Largiadèr [8]	1979	1	Division CFV	None	Anastomosis	Good
Denck [13]	1979	1	Division CFV	Short	Anastomosis	Good
Frings [18]	2001	1	Excision CFV	3 days	PTFE graft	Good
Denck [13]	1979	1	*Stripping* CFV	None	Vein graft	Good
Flis [15]	1995	1	*Stripping* "FV"	-	*Reconstrution*	
Aleksic [19]	2001	1	*Stripping* SFV-DFV	-	*Replantation*	Patent
Total		**13**			**~ 4 grafts**	**No amputation**

CFV: common femoral vein
DFV: deep femoral vein
FV : femoral vein
SFV : superficial femoral vein

15% of all cases [24]. Of these, the commonest injury is to the common peroneal nerve by blind avulsion of varices through stab incisions, with resultant drop foot. Almost equally frequent is injury to the saphenous nerve through *stripping* of the long saphenous vein in the lower leg. However, the sensory loss is less likely to lead to legal action.

Considering the grade of medical staff involved in litigation, there is a fairly even distribution across all grades. Tennant [24] states, in agreement with most other authors [17,21], that senior staff are by no means immune to effecting complications, both major and minor.

Conclusion

In summary, true disasters after varicose vein surgery are rare. Nevertheless, they keep occurring at a fairly constant rate and the risk of legal action,

although constant in the United Kingdom, may increase in other countries. Therefore, the treatment of varicose veins should be carried out by properly trained surgeons [5] who are also familiar with the preoperative investigation of the condition and who can communicate to the patient a realistic expectation of outcome in the light of previous results.

The most disastrous complications invariably result from misidentification of large vessels. At least in theory, they may be reduced by improved knowledge of the anatomy, especially of the groin and of the popliteal fossa. A high level of suspicion and a defensive attitude may further reduce such risks.

After surgery, any sign of venous or arterial interruption should lead to an immediate exploration of the temperature, the color, of peripheral pulses and leg circumferences, followed by duplex sonography, arteriography or venography, if indicated. Reconstruction of interrupted great vessels should

Table III SEVERE COMPLICATIONS

First author [ref.]	Year	Limbs	Arterial injury lig/div/tear	excis/strip	Venous injury lig/div/tear	excis/strip	DVT	PE	Major bleeding
Severe complications in five observational studies									
Hagmüller [5]	1992	3 300	-	-	1	-	8	2	5
Critchley [17]	1997	973	-	-	1	-	2	1	NA
Frings [18]	2001	40 636	-	-	6	1	NA	NA	NA
Balzer [21]	2001	25 457	3	-	2	-	7	5	15
Personal experience	2004	1 923	-	-	0	-	1	1	1
Total		**72 289**	**3**	**0**	**10**	**1**	**18**	**9**	**21**
Incidence of severe complications									
Hagmüller [5]	1992	3 300	-	-	0.030	-	0.242	0.061	0.152
Critchley [17]	1997	973	-	-	0.103	-	0.206	0.103	NA
Frings [18]	2001	40 636	-	-	0.015	0.002	NA	NA	NA
Balzer [21]	2001	25 457	0.012	-	0.008	-	0.027	0.020	0.059
Personal experience	2004	1 923	-	-	-	-	0.052	0.052	0.052
Total		**72 289**	**0.004**	**0**	**0.014**	**0.001**	**0.057**	**0.028**	**0.029**

DVT: deep venous thrombosis
PE : pulmonary embolism
NA : not available

be attempted in most instances. If necessary, the patient should be referred to a vascular surgeon with minimal delay. Furthermore, the unfortunate patient deserves and needs to be told the truth, not only from an ethical but also from a medico-legal viewpoint. Unrestricted information may facilitate greater cooperation from the patient than secretiveness. Prior to surgery, obtaining fully informed consent from the patient is mandatory. Some authors claim that this should include even the most serious potential risks of varicose vein surgery, such as loss of limb and loss of life [17].

REFERENCES

1 Keller WL. A new method of extirpating the internal saphenous and other veins in varicose conditions. A preliminary report. *NY Med J* 1905; 82: 385.
2 Luke JC, Miller GG. Disasters following the operation of ligation and retrograde injection of varicose veins. *Ann Surg* 1948; 127: 426.
3 Natali J. Surgical treatment of varices: enquiry into 87,000 cases. *J Cardiovasc Surg* 1964; 15: 713-721.
4 Buri P. Iatrogene Schaedigung von Glutgefaessen (Iatrogenic blood vessel injuries). *Helv Chir Acta* 1971; 38: 151-152.
5 Hagmüller GW. Komplikationen bei der Chirurgie der Varikose. *Langenbecks Arch Chir* Suppl (Kongressbericht). 1992; 470-474.

6 Liddicoat JE, Bekassy SM, Daniell MB, DeBakey ME. Inadvertent femoral artery "stripping": surgical management. *Surgery* 1975; 77: 318-320.

7 Ramsheyi A, Soury P, Saliou C et al. Inadvertent arterial injury during saphenous vein stripping: three cases and therapeutic strategies. *Arch Surg* 1998; 133: 1120-1123.

8 Largiadèr J, Brunner U. Grossvaskuläre Komplikationen der Krossektomie. *Die Leiste* 1979; 160-166.

9 Morton JH, Southgate WA, DeWeese JA. Arterial injuries of the extremities. *Surg Gynecol Obstet* 1966; 123: 611-627.

10 Eger M, Golcman L, Torok G, Hirsch M. Inadvertent arterial stripping in the lower limb: problems of management. *Surgery* 1973; 73: 23-27.

11 Leitz KH, Schmidt FC. Iatrogene Arterienverletzung bei Babcockscher Venenexhairese. *VASA* 1974; 3: 45-49.

12 Becker H-M. Ueber eine erfolgreiche Gefässrekonstruktion nach versehentlicher Arterienexhairese bei Varicenoperation. *Chirurg* 1975; 46: 367-370.

13 Denck H, Hugeneck J, Garaguly G. Folgenschwere Fehler bei Varizenoperationen speziell in der Leiste. *Die Leiste* 1979; 148-159.

14 Pegoraro M, Baracco C, Ferrero F, Palladino F. Successful vascular reconstruction after inadvertent femoral artery "stripping". *J Cardiovasc Surg* 1987; 4: 440-444.

15 Flis V. Reconstruction of venous outflow after inadvertent stripping of the femoral vein. *Eur J Vasc Endovasc Surg* 1995; 10: 253-255.

16 Miller GV, Lewis WG, Sainsbury JR, Macdonald RC. Morbidity of varicose vein surgery auditing the benefit of changing clinical practice. *Ann R Coll Surg Engl* 1996; 78: 345-349.

17 Critchley G, Handa A, Maw A et al. Complications of varicose vein surgery. *Ann R Coll Surg Engl* 1997; 79: 105-110.

18 Frings N, Glowacki P, Kohajda J. Prospective documentation of complication rate in surgery of the V. saphena magna and V. saphena parva. *Chirurg* 2001; 72: 1032-1035.

19 Aleksic I, Busch T, Sirbu H et al. Successful reconstruction of stripped superficial femoral vein. *J Vasc Surg* 2001; 33: 1111-1113.

20 Widmer MK, Hakki H, Reber PU, Kniemeyer HW. A rare, but severe complication of varicose vein surgery: Compartment syndrome. *Zentralbl Chir* 2000; 125: 543-546.

21 Balzer K. Complications in varicose vein operations. *Zentralbl Chir* 2001; 126: 537-542.

22 Mildner A, Hilbe G. Complications in surgery of varicose veins. *Zentralbl Chir* 2001; 126: 543-545.

23 Stern W. Dealing with difficulties and complications of varicose vein operations. *Med J Aust* 1967; 1: 554-556.

24 Tennant WG, Ruckley CV. Medicolegal action following treatment for varicose veins. *Br J Surg* 1996; 83: 291-292.

Conception et réalisation
ODIM, z.a. La Carretière
04130 VOLX

Achevé d'imprimer sur ses presses
en février 2005
N° d'imprimeur: 04.471
Dépôt légal: 1er trimestre 2005

Imprimé en FRANCE